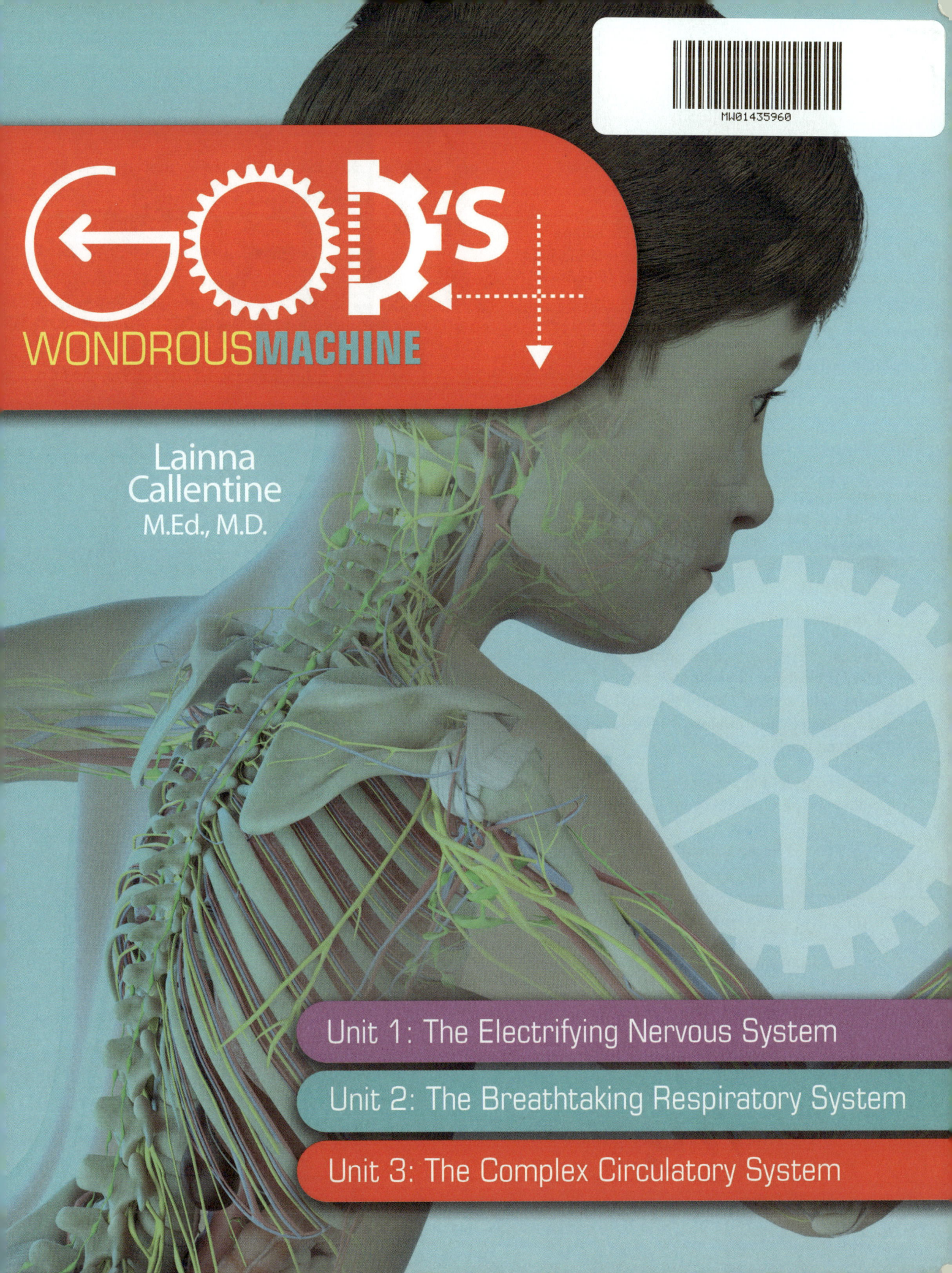

First printing: November 2014
First revised printing: September 2022

Copyright © 2014, 2015, 2016 by Dr. Lainna Callentine and Master Books®. No part of this book may be reproduced, copied, broadcast, stored, or shared in any form whatsoever without written permission from the publisher, except in the case of brief quotations in articles and reviews. For information write:

Master Books, P.O. Box 726,
Green Forest, AR 72638

Master Books® is a division of the
New Leaf Publishing Group, Inc.

ISBN: 978-1-68344-318-6
ISBN: 978-1-61458-822-1 (digital)
Library of Congress Numbers: 2014950463, 2015932194, 2015960972

Cover and Interior Design by Diana Bogardus

Unless otherwise noted, Scriptures taken from the Holy Bible, New International Version®, NIV®. Copyright © 1973, 1978, 1984, 2011 by Biblica, Inc.™ Used by permission of Zondervan. All rights reserved worldwide.

Please consider requesting that a copy of this volume be purchased by your local library system.

Printed in the United States of America.

Please visit our website for other great titles:
www.masterbooks.com

For information regarding promotional opportunities, please contact the publicity department at pr@nlpg.com.

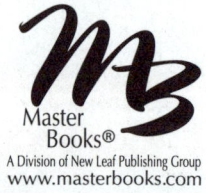

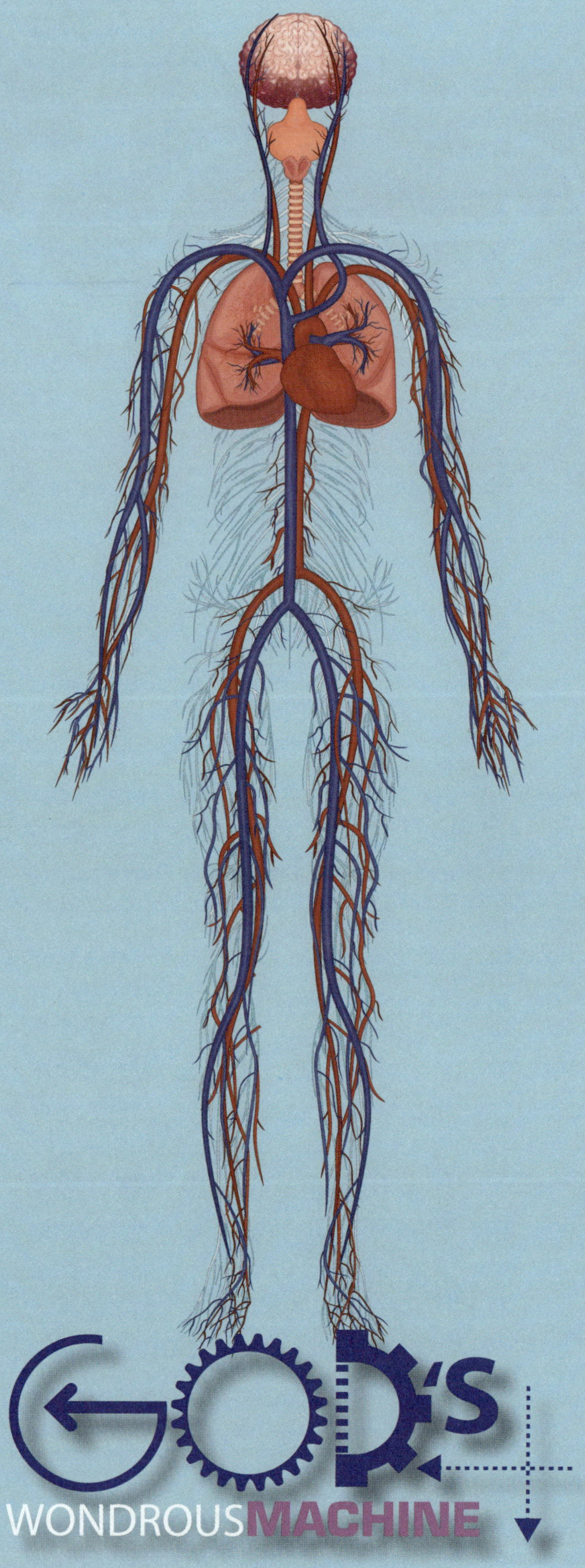

TABLE OF CONTENTS

How to Use This Book (All about us!) 5
About the Author 6
A Note from the Author 7
Using the Curriculum guide 8

THE ELECTRIFYING NERVOUS SYSTEM 9

Vocabulary Levels 10
See It, Say It, Know It! 11

1. Let's Start at the Beginning: Historical Points of Interest 14
2. Seeing is Believing: Looking inside the Brain 22
3. The Basics of the Nervous System 24
4. Anatomy & Physiology: The Brick & Mortar of the Nervous System 28
5. The Developing Brain 40
6. A Case for the Brain 44
7. The Gate Keeper: The Blood Brain Barrier 46
8. The Great Stabilizer: The Backbone 48
9. It's Simply Automatic 50
10. Take Good Care: Health Facts 54
11. Facts: The Wacky, the Weird, and Wow 66

THE BREATHTAKING RESPIRATORY SYSTEM 75

Vocabulary Levels 76
See It, Say It, Know It! 77

1. Introduction: Why Do We Breath 82
2. Respiratory History Timeline: A Walk Back in Time 84
3. The Structure of the Respiratory Tract 90
4. The Structure of the Lower Respiratory Tract 98
5. Respiration — Ventilation Getting Into the Act 104
6. The Development of the Lungs 108

7	Technology	112
8	Health and Illness	116
9	The Story of Polio	130
10	Ponder This	136
11	Fun Stuff	140

THE COMPLEX CIRCULATORY SYSTEM ... 145

	Vocabulary Levels	146
	See It, Say It, Know It!	147
	Introduction	150
	Biblical References to the Heart	151
1	Historical Timeline of Circulatory System	152
2	Blood	162
3	Highways of Blood	174
4	Blood-Sucking Critters	176
5	Take Heart: Getting to the Heart of the Matter	180
6	In the Beginning: The Development of the Heart	188
7	Technology	192
8	An Apple a Day Keeps the Doctor Away: Good Health	196
9	Ponder This	198
10	Facts: Bizarre and Gross	202
11	Fun Stuff	204

Bibliography	212
Index	216

How to Use This Book (All about Us!)

About this *God's Wondrous Machine* series:

Developed by a master's-trained teacher and homeschooling mother who happens to be a pediatrician, this book focuses on the human body's nervous system, respiratory system, and circulatory system. It will create engaging opportunities for children to discover the wonders and workings of the human body.

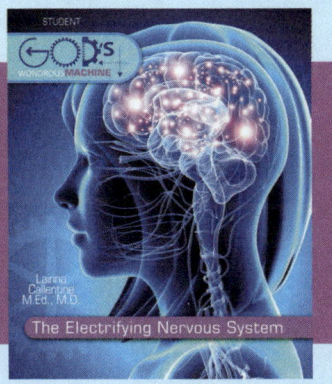 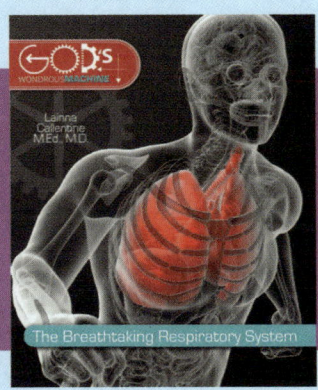 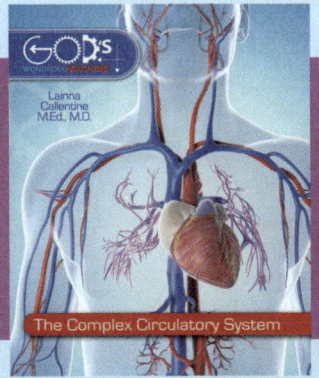

Three units — One book!

This book is bursting with vibrantly colorful images, interesting historical and weird facts, anatomy, physiology, and modern innovations. You will engage your senses and have a multitude of choices for hands-on exploration. You will discover aspects of the human body from a doctor's perspective. Each unit focuses on a particular system of the body, discussing how it works and how it doesn't at times. Common questions kids ask are answered to stimulate curiosity, and your senses will be engaged as the world of medicine is demystified.

This book gives many perspectives in science education by connecting to other fields of study (i.e., history, sociology, psychology, and theology), and it encourages the reader to appreciate God's magnificent handiwork: your body.

God's Wondrous Machine recognizes that every learner is not the same. Whether used in a homeschool or classroom setting, the hands-on activities are based on the educational theory of Multiple Intelligence by Howard Gardner (which states there are many types of intelligences and recognizes different learning styles: musical–rhythmic, visual–spatial, verbal–linguistic, logical–mathematical, bodily–kinesthetic, interpersonal, intrapersonal, and naturalistic). It is flexible enough for endless customization for the skills, interests, and abilities of each student.

Dedication
To my dear family, thanks for standing by my side.
D.R., my best friend, thanks for your steadfast love and unending encouragement.
You have been there in sickness and health.
My children: Michael, Jay, and Hannah, where does time go? Thank you for your support and love.

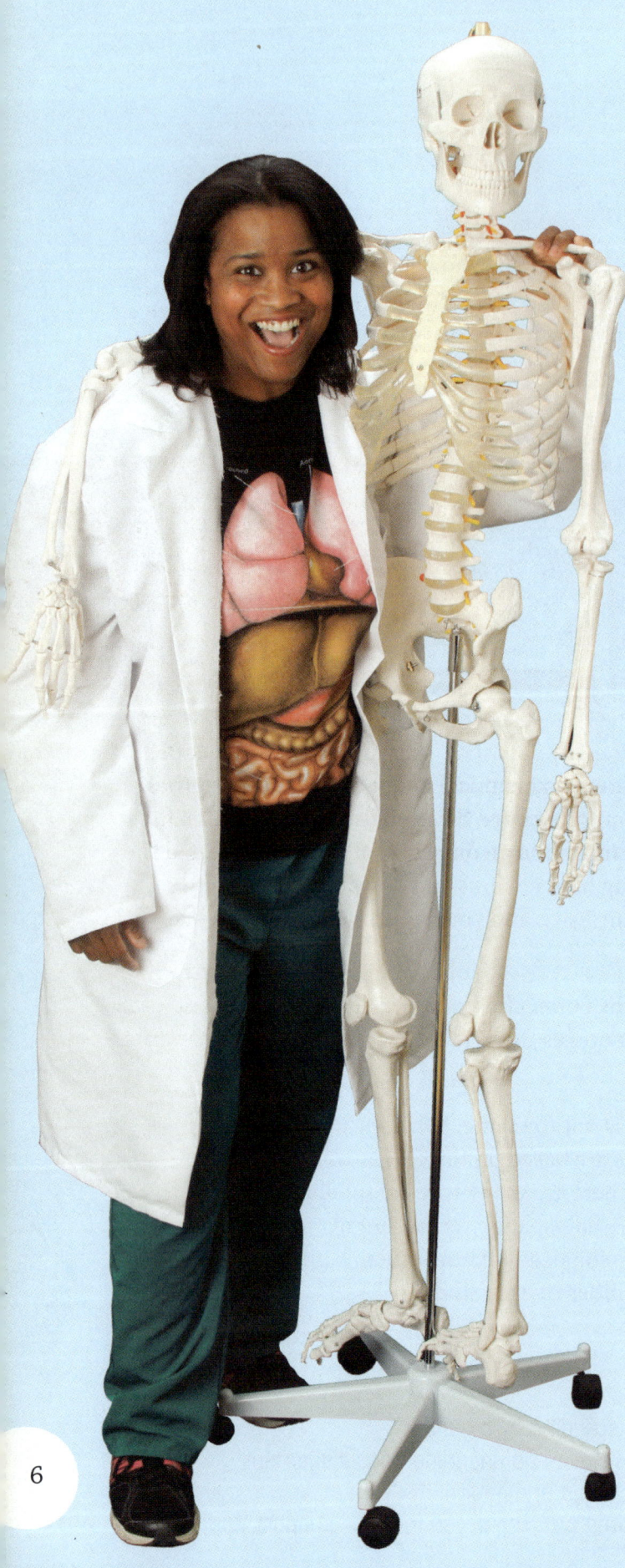

About the Author

Dr. Lainna Callentine has a passion for science. She spent many hours as a child turning over rocks and wading through streams chasing tadpoles. She is from a family of six children. Her parents grew up in the inner city housing projects of Chicago, and her parents felt that education was a powerful tool. They instilled in her and her siblings a great love for learning.

Dr. Callentine wears many hats. She is a coach, teacher, pediatrician, and homeschool mother. She obtained her bachelor's degree in human development and social policy from Northwestern University in the school of education while competing as a full–scholarship athlete. She began her professional career as an elementary school teacher. She obtained her master's degree in education from Widener University. Then she went on to pursue her lifelong dream of becoming a doctor. Dr. Callentine obtained her medical degree from University of Illinois College of Medicine. She worked in one of the busiest emergency rooms in Illinois before answering the call to go home and homeschool her three children.

She founded Sciexperience and travels nationally as a speaker doing inspiring hands-on science workshops for all ages. She continues to utilize her medical training as a missionary doctor in a clinic for the uninsured in the suburbs of Chicago. She is a member of the Christian Medical and Dental Society and The Author's Guild. She enjoys basketball, time with her husband and three kids, and the outdoors.

A Note from the Author

I have always been fascinated by the complexity and intricacy of the human body — how it works and why it doesn't. To be sure, there is more to us than just a physical body. But this wondrous machine that God has fashioned for us is something to marvel. It reveals His very handiwork. There are two fundamental ways God has chosen to reveal Himself to us through His Word and through His creation. We are part of that creation. This book guides and teaches the student to see the evidence of God's design. We truly are "fearfully and wonderfully made."

This book was a culmination of two reinforcing factors in my life: my passion for the life sciences and my desire to see those same sciences presented in a technical but biblically accurate way. Some may feel that the Bible has no bearing on science and only serves to dilute or confuse our understanding of it. This book does not present science apart from the Bible but in light of it. Others may feel that science, especially anatomy and biology, have much more to say about God and the Bible than this book offers. I believe indeed it does. This would require a much broader investigation across multiple disciplines to fully develop.

One issue challenged in Christian books is the controversy between "evolutionary theory" and the Genesis creation account. The immune system, DNA, the complexity of the brain, and virtually every aspect of the human body demonstrates design. This is readily apparent. And this book looks at the parts and systems of the body, how they work, and why they don't, giving credit to God as the author. My hope is that by developing an understanding and appreciation for the miracle that is the human body, one more stumbling block will be removed from trusting in an omnipotent God who created the world as described in Genesis.

To be sure, all science flows from the Creator of the universe, the Designer of its laws, and the One who fashioned our bodies from the dust of the earth and breathed life into them. My hope is that you will see the human body as an amazing example of God's love for us and want to dig deeper into the science that attempts to understand this amazing machine, seeking to know more about the One who designed it. May God bless you as you begin this journey.

In His Service,

Dr. Lainna Callentine

Using the teacher guide

This student book and the available teacher guide were developed to challenge children in all facets of multiple intelligence. The parent/instructor is able to choose and customize hands-on activities that engage a multitude of learning styles and challenge the student to explore life's big issues. The program is specially designed for lower and upper elementary level students, including advanced learners with middle school proficiency!

You can use this book as an interesting:

▸ Unit Study

▸ Curriculum

▸ Supplemental Resource

The teacher guide contains perforated sheets for worksheets, and tests, in addition to a flexible educational calendar. This additional material allows for a multiple array of assessment for the instructor (i.e. project based, traditional testing, or portfolio assessment). It is designed to maximize the learning opportunities and retention of information from the book, as kids have fun learning about the mechanics and mysteries of themselves!

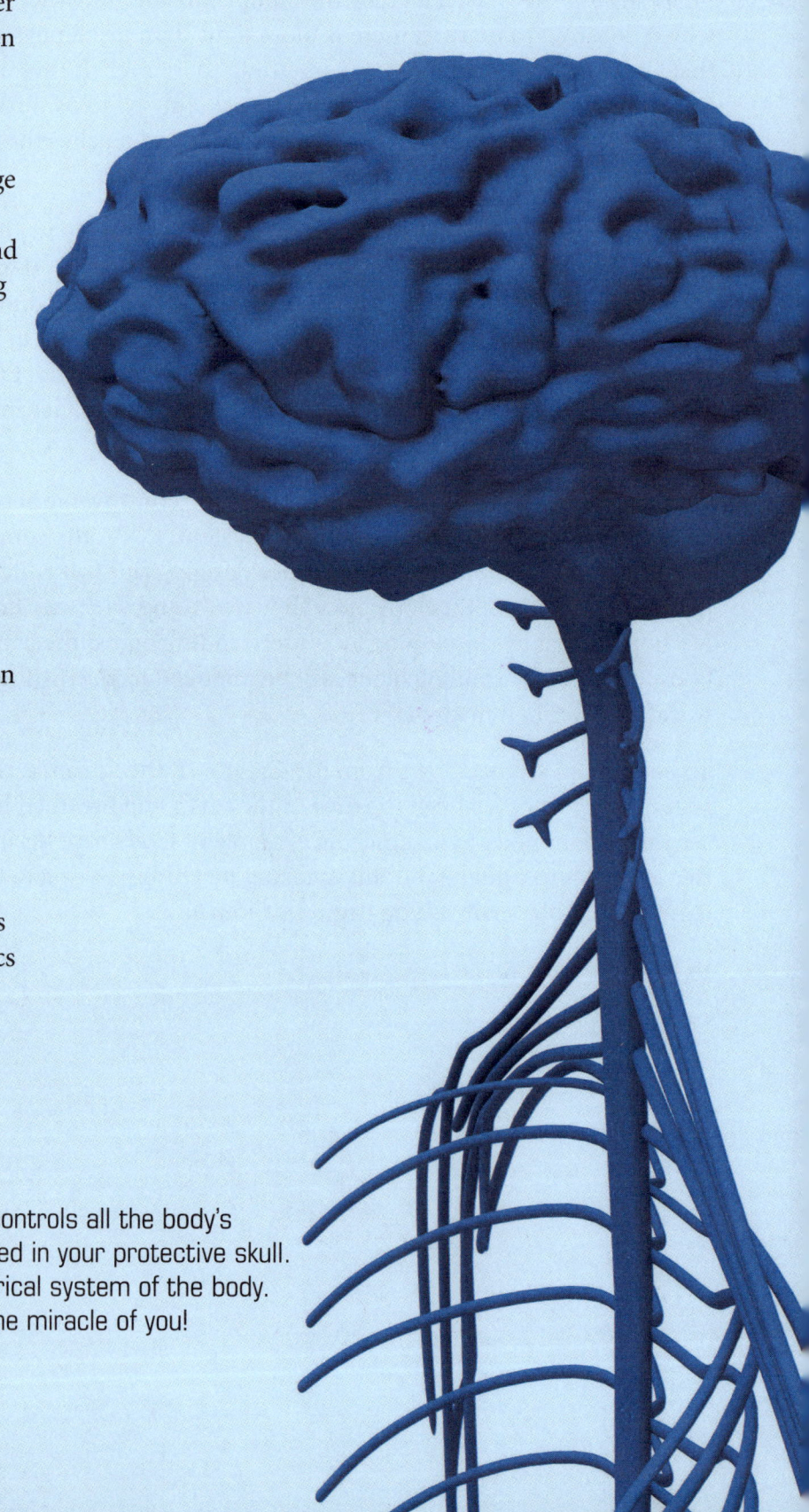

From laughing to crying, your brain controls all the body's functions. Your brain lays safely tucked in your protective skull. You will take a trip through the electrical system of the body. Come learn how God has designed the miracle of you!

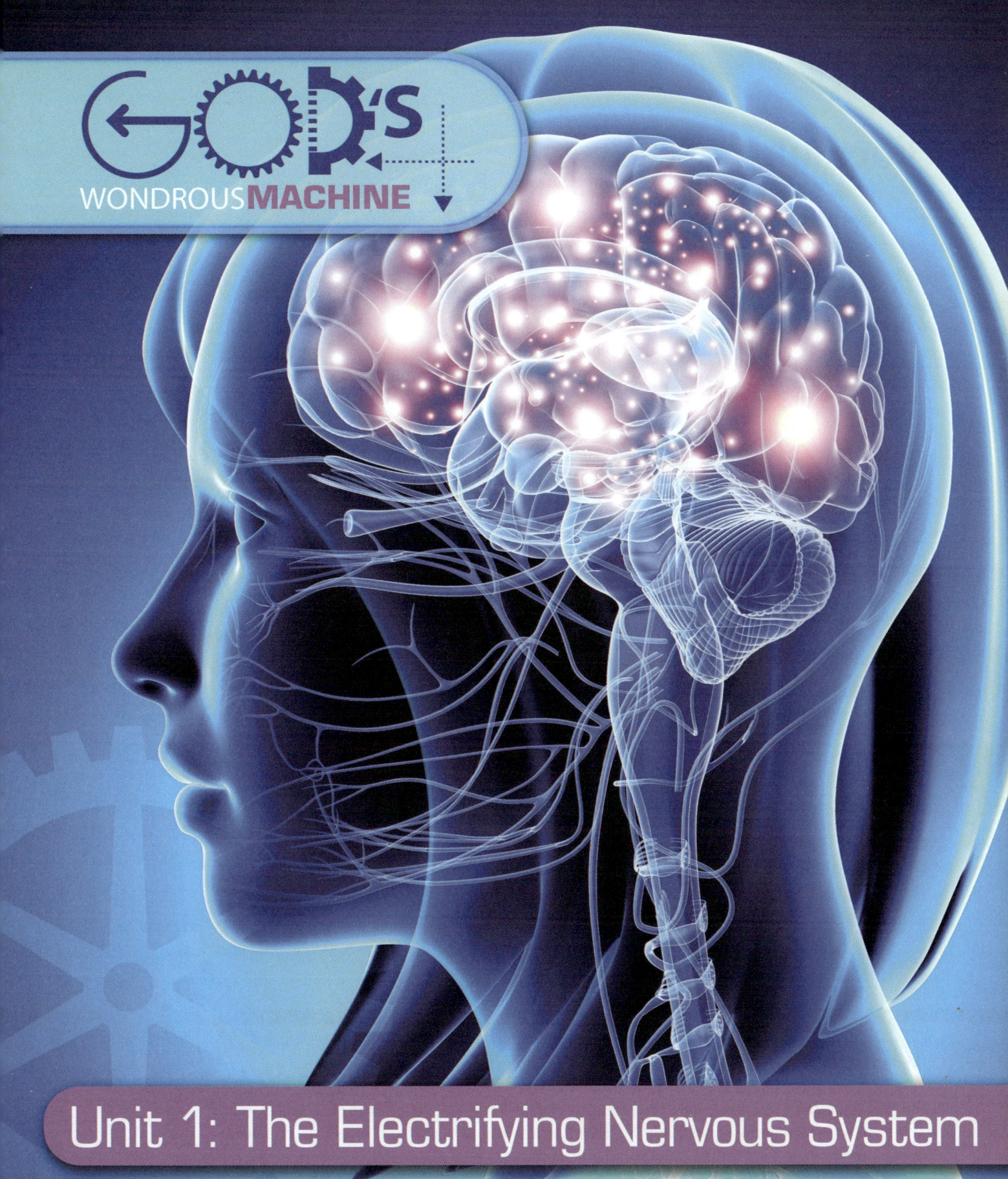

VOCABULARY LEVELS

Choose the word list based on your skill level. Every student should be able to master Level 1 words. Add words from Levels 2 and 3 as needed. More proficient students should be able to learn all three levels.

Level 1 Vocabulary

- Arbor Vitae
- Central Nervous System
- Cerebral Hemispheres
- Cerebellum
- Cerebrum
- Frontal Lobe
- Gray Matter
- Neurons
- Occipital Lobe
- Parietal Lobe
- Temporal Lobe
- White Matter

Level 2 Vocabulary

Review and Know Level 1 Vocabulary

- Autonomic Nervous System
- Blood-Brain Barrier
- Cerebral Spinal Fluid
- Corpus Callosum
- Dermatomes
- Homunculus
- Meninges
- Pituitary Gland

Level 3 Vocabulary

Review and Know Level 1 and 2 Vocabulary

- Astroglia
- Axon
- Broca's and Wernicke's Areas
- Cerebral Palsy
- Dendrites
- Diencephalon
- Ependymal Cells
- Gyrus
- Hypothalamus
- Medulla Oblongata
- Mesencephalon
- Microglia
- Myelin Sheath
- Neuroglia
- Oligodendroglia
- Pons
- Pyrogens
- Shingles
- Synapse
- Thalamus
- Ventricles

God created you with much care, love, and incredible design! The human brain has 1 quadrillion synapses (that is a 1 followed by 15 zeroes or 1,000,000,000,000,000). All those synapses fit into the tiny compartment of your brain. In comparison to man's design, a typical computer has approximately 16,000,000,000 bytes of memory. It would take a million computers to have the equivalent amount of connections to rival the brain!

See it, Say it, Know it!

Word [Pronunciation]	Definition
Arbor Vitae [Arbor ˈvaɪtiː/]	"Tree of life" located in the middle section of the cerebellum; helps to coordinate movement.
Astroglia [ăs-trŏg′lē-ə]	A type of brain cell that supplies nutrients to the neuron.
Autonomic Nervous System [ô′tə-nŏm′ĭk]	Self-controlling part of the nervous system that does not require conscious thought to operate.
Axon [ăk′sŏn′]	The part of the neuron through which electrical impulses travel down the body of the nerve cell to other nerve cells; many are wrapped in a white fatty substance called the myelin sheath.
Blood-Brain Barrier	A special barrier that surrounds the brain and acts like the gate keeper from the rest of the body. It is composed of small blood vessels and cells packed close together that act as a filter that blocks unwanted materials from entering the brain.
Broca's Area [Brō′kəz]	Located on the left hemisphere; the area that houses the motor speech region, which provides the ability to form spoken words.
Central Nervous System	The central nervous system consists of the brain and the spinal cord.
Cerebral Hemispheres [Sĕr′ə-brəl]	The two halves of the brain, right and left.
Cerebral Palsy [Sĕr′ə-brəl pôl′zē]	A group of disorders that affects the brain and nervous system functions that can affect movement, learning, hearing, vision, and speech. There are different types of cerebral palsy; in one type, an individual may experience spasticity, which means his or her movements are jerky and difficult to coordinate.
Cerebral Spinal Fluid [Sĕr′ə-brəl]	A clear fluid that bathes the brain and spinal cord and transports nutrients, chemical messengers, and waste products.
Cerebellum [sĕr′ə-bĕl′əm]	The region of the brain located behind the brain stem. The arbor vitae resides here.
Cerebrum [sĕr′ə-brəm]	The main part of the brain composed of the two hemispheres.
Corpus Callosum [kôr′pəs kə-lō′səm]	The arched white matter found in the center of the cerebrum that connects the two hemispheres of the brain.
Dendrites [dĕn′drīt′]	Tentacle-like structures that extend from the cell body of the neuron and reach out to other neurons.

Unit 1: The Electrifying Nervous System

Word [Pronunciation]	Definition
Dermatomes [dûr′mə-tōm′]	Areas or zones of the skin where sensation arises from a particular spinal nerve root.
Diencephalon [dī′ĕn-sĕf′ə-lŏn′, -lən]	A structure in the middle of the brain that connects to the brainstem; also the location of the thalamus and the hypothalamus.
Ependymal Cells [ĕ-pen′di-măl]	The cells that make up the lining of the ventricles of the brain and of the spinal cord that help in producing spinal fluid.
Fissures [fis·sure]	A groove or deep fold in the cerebral cortex.
Frontal Lobe	The front (anterior) part of the brain involved in reasoning and personality.
Gray Matter	The thin outer rim on the surface of the brain where memory storage, processing, and conscious and subconscious regulation of skeletal movement occur.
Gyrus [Ji´rus]	A rounded convolution (folded or ridged part) on the surface of the brain.
Homunculus [Hō-mŭng′kyə-ləs]	"Very small man," a visual representation of the connection between different body parts and the areas in the brain hemisphere that control them.
Hypothalamus [Hī′pō-thăl′ə-məs]	The part of the brain that regulates body temperature, sleep, and puberty.
Medulla Oblongata [Me·dul·la ŏb′lŏng-gā′tə]	Located in the lower half of the brainstem, connecting to the pons, it regulates the vital functions of breathing, swallowing, and heart rate.
Meninges [Mĕn-in´jēz]	The tough fibrous membranes that cover the brain and spinal cord.
Mesencephalon [Mez″-en-sef´ah-lon]	The midbrain located below the cerebral cortex near the center of the brain. The key in sorting through the visual and auditory data received by the brain.
Microglia [Mi-krog´le-ah]	The "garbage collector" cells of the brain that kill unwanted organisms and remove waste products produced by the neurons.
Myelin Sheath [Mī′ĕ-lin shēth]	A substance that coils around and insulates (coats) the nerve cell; made from a lipid (fat).
Neuroglia [Noo-rog-lee-a]	General term for the glia cells of the brain that support nerves. Glia comes from the Greek word meaning "glue."

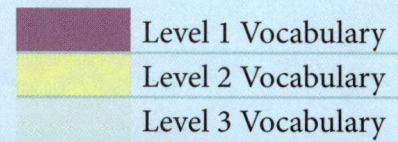

Word [Pronunciation]	Definition
Neurons [Noŏr′ŏn′]	An electrical conducting cell of the nervous system.
Occipital Lobe [ŏk-sĭp′ĭ-tl]	The back or posterior part of the brain that houses the visual processing center.
Oligodendroglia [ŏl′ĭ-gō-děn-drŏg′lē-ə]	The "protector" cells of the nervous system that support, protect, and insulate the axons by helping to form the myelin sheaths.
Parietal Lobe [pa·ri·e·tal]	Located between the frontal and occipital lobes of the brain; serves as the primary sensory cortex. Enables conscious perception of touch, pressure, vibration, pain, taste, and temperature. Memory storage, processing, and conscious and subconscious regulation of skeletal movement also originate in this area.
Pituitary Gland [pi·tu·i·tary]	A pea-sized structure at the base of the skull that secretes hormones. It is the "master gland" of the body by overseeing key functions, such as growth during childhood and the onset of puberty, by controlling male and female hormones.
Pons	Latin for "bridge." Located anterior to (in front of) the cerebellum, it serves as a bridge between the cerebellum and the thalamus, acts as a relay station for sensory information between the structures.
Pyrogens [pī′rə-jən]	A substance released from the brain that tells the hypothalamus to increase the body's temperature, causing a fever.
Shingles	A painful, blistering skin rash caused by the chicken pox virus. Pain, tingling, or burning occurs along a dermatome.
Synapse [sĭn′ăps′]	A small gap between neurons across which electrical information travels from one neuron to the next.
Temporal Lobe [těm′pər-əl]	The side (lateral) region of the brain in which the auditory perception, and language comprehension are located.
Thalamus [thăl′ə-məs]	Buried under the cerebral cortex, it serves like a communications center; relays and processes sensory information to various destinations in the brain.
Ventricles [věn′trĭ-kəl]	Spaces in the middle part of the brain that produce and are filled with cerebrospinal fluid.
Wernicke's Area [věr′nĭ-kēz]	The region of the brain that interprets what one hears and makes sense of spoken communication.
White Matter	Regions of the brain that lie at a deeper depth in brain; the area where neurological nerve tracts are housed.

*Pronunciation Keys from: http://medical-dictionary.thefreedictionary.com

Unit 1: The Electrifying Nervous System

1 Let's Start at the Beginning: Historical Points of Interest

Thinking, crying, breathing, running, skipping, singing, smiling, itching, sneezing, and your beating heart — all of these activities have one thing in common: your brain. Tipping the scales at a mere 3 pounds, it is the integral organ of your body. Your brain operates 24 hours a day, 7 days a week, 365 days a year. It works tirelessly, day in and day out. Serving as the central control center of your body, this marvelous machine is composed of billions of cells that make hundreds of billions of connections without any traffic jams. Through this super highway of connections, we perceive and process impulses that originate inside and outside our bodies.

In this unit, we will explore the mysteries of the brain through investigation of its anatomy (name and location of parts of the body), physiology (how the body functions), histology (microscopic cell structure), and pathology (abnormal health consequences of disease). Let's pick our brains and peer into the ultimate multi-tasker.

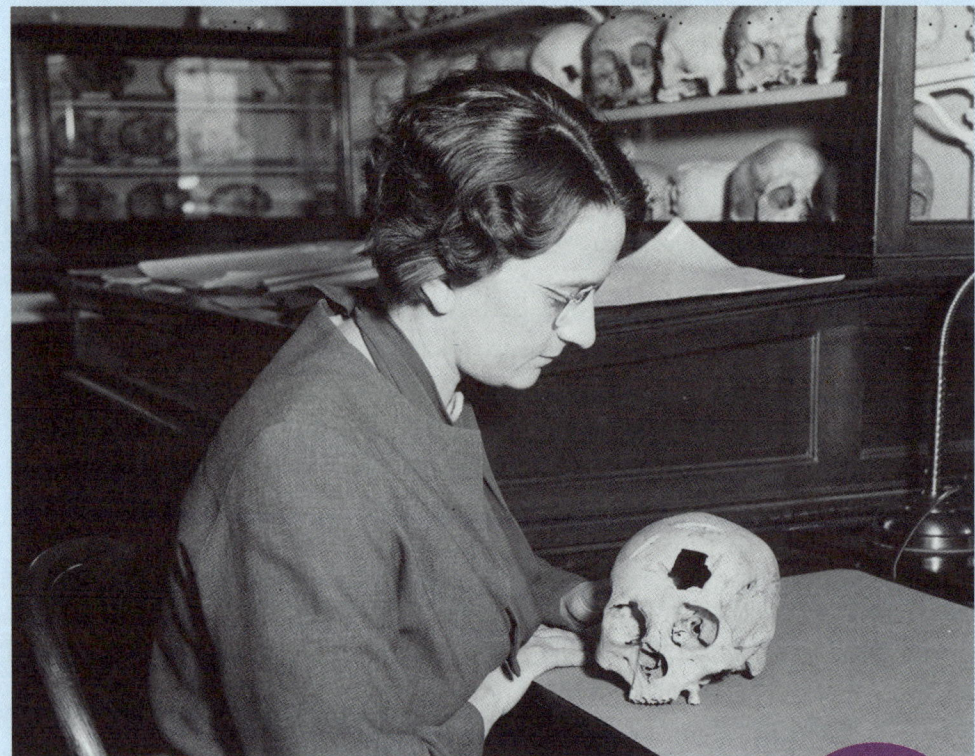

A curator for the Smithsonian Institution in 1935 looking at a skull that possibly shows signs of brain surgery from thousands of years ago. Other skulls have been found that also detail new bone growth, indicating that patients survived the initial procedure.

KNOW IT ALL

The brain and nervous system are an important control center for your body. It can send signals throughout the body at over 320 feet per second. That is nearly the distance of a football field!

14

God's Wondrous Machine

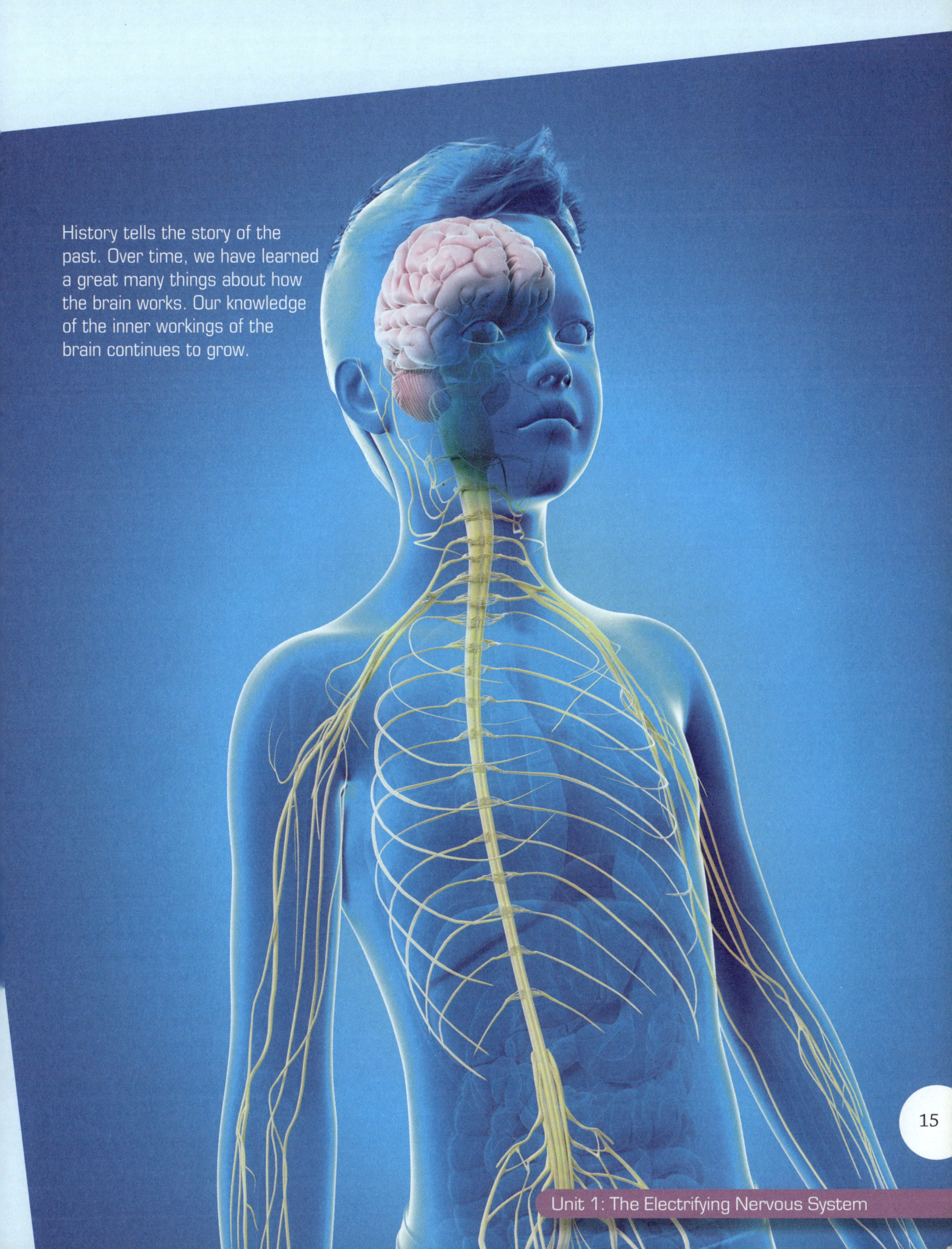

History tells the story of the past. Over time, we have learned a great many things about how the brain works. Our knowledge of the inner workings of the brain continues to grow.

Unit 1: The Electrifying Nervous System

But we have this treasure in jars of clay to show that this all-surpassing power is from God and not from us. We are hard pressed on every side, but not crushed; perplexed, but not in despair; persecuted, but not abandoned; struck down, but not destroyed. We always carry around in our body the death of Jesus, so that the life of Jesus may also be revealed in our body (2 Corinthians 4:7-10; NIV).

Mankind has been on a quest since the beginning of time to understand our external and internal environments. Understanding the brain has been one of those perplexing pursuits. The Bible reminds us that God's power is "all surpassing" and that the life of Jesus is revealed in our bodies. Throughout time, man has continued to gain insight and understanding about the brain and its functions. Yet, even with the achievements of modern neuroscience, the inner workings of the mind are still great mysteries.

Without a doubt, the quality of life for men has improved dramatically through the centuries because of the advances and discoveries that men have made in medicine. The time-line below depicts some of the discoveries made in neuroscience. It provides an idea of how we have acquired knowledge through time.

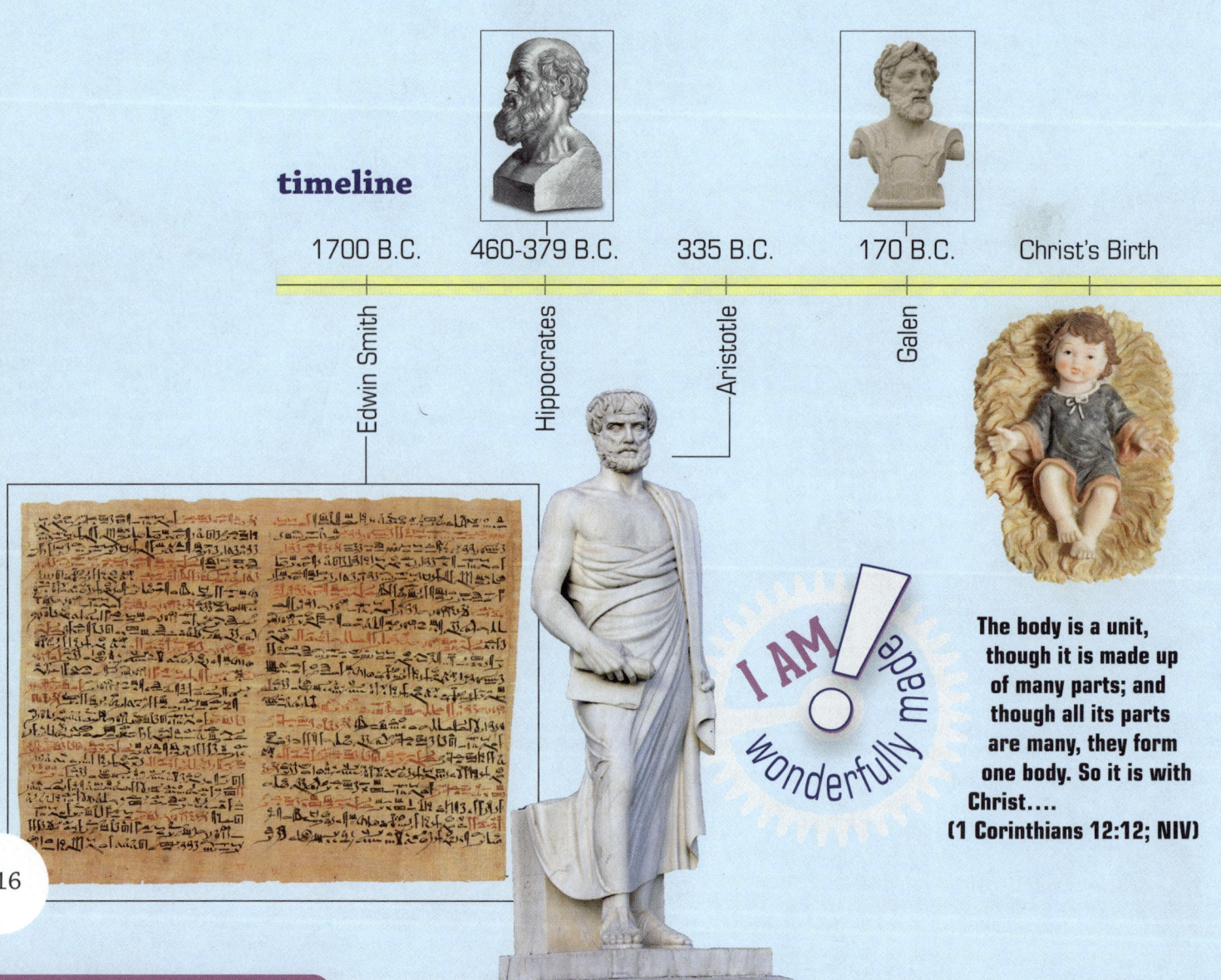

timeline

1700 B.C.	460-379 B.C.	335 B.C.	170 B.C.	Christ's Birth
Edwin Smith	Hippocrates	Aristotle	Galen	

The body is a unit, though it is made up of many parts; and though all its parts are many, they form one body. So it is with Christ....
(1 Corinthians 12:12; NIV)

I AM wonderfully made!

God's Wondrous Machine

Traveling through the course of time, in 1700 B.C. the Edwin Smith Surgical Papyrus was written. It is the first written record of the nervous system to appear in Egyptian documents that describe cases of brain injury.

Hippocrates (460–379 B.C.) was born 460 years prior to Jesus' birth and was an early doctor known as the "Father of Medicine." Hippocrates felt that it was important that all doctors take an oath, or special promise before they began practicing medicine. He developed the Hippocratic Oath, in which all doctors promise never to use their knowledge to cause harm to anyone under their medical care.

In addition, Hippocrates discussed epilepsy as a problem in the brain. He also believed that the ability to feel sensations and intelligence originated in the brain. This was a very revolutionary idea, because prior to this the consciousness of the mind was believed to reside in the heart.

In 335 B.C., Aristotle wrote about sleep, but believed that mental processes originated in the heart, and that the brain was merely a place to cool hot blood pumped from the heart.

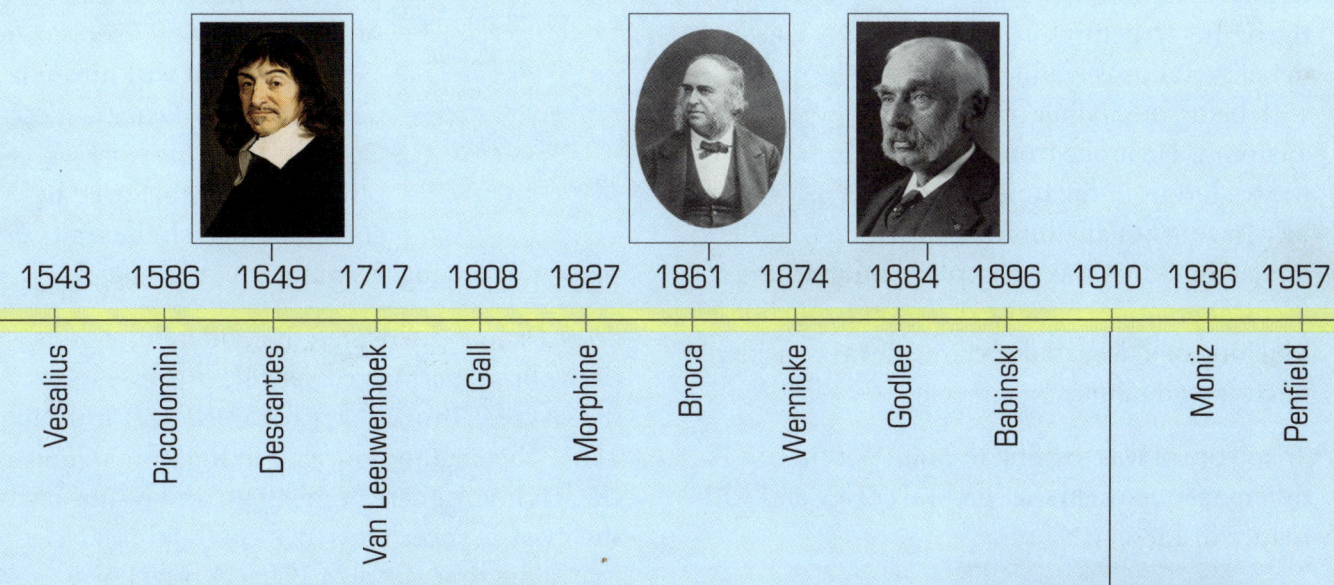

1543　1586　1649　1717　1808　1827　1861　1874　1884　1896　1910　1936　1957

Vesalius　Piccolomini　Descartes　Van Leeuwenhoek　Gall　Morphine　Broca　Wernicke　Godlee　Babinski　　Moniz　Penfield

Lead Poisoning

Alice Hamilton (1869-1970), a physician who was the world's leading authority on industrial medicine. In 1910, she discovered the cause of a common illness that produced deadly outcomes in factory workers. The workers would suffer from shakiness, headaches, and loss of muscle control that sometimes lead to paralysis and death. She discovered "plumbism" or lead poisoning. *Plumbum* is the Latin word for lead.

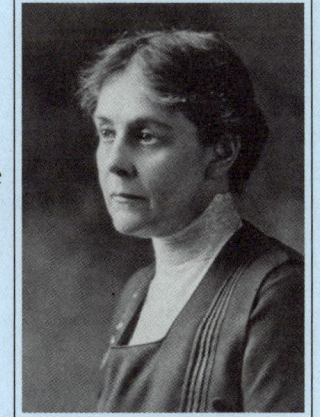

Unit 1: The Electrifying Nervous System

A Roman physician to the gladiators named Galen dissected the brains of animals in 170 B.C. From his studies, he believed the cerebellum controlled the muscles and the cerebrum, which allows us to sense our environment.

In 1543, Andreas Vesalius published his book, *On the Workings of the Human Body,* which discussed human anatomy, including the brain's structures in detail. Vesalius is credited with being the "father of anatomy." He broke from the traditions of the time by carrying out anatomical dissections. This was a sharp deviation from medical practices because dissection, much less touching of a deceased specimen, was considered unclean and taboo.

Piccolomini was the first to point out the differences between the cerebral cortex and white matter in 1586.

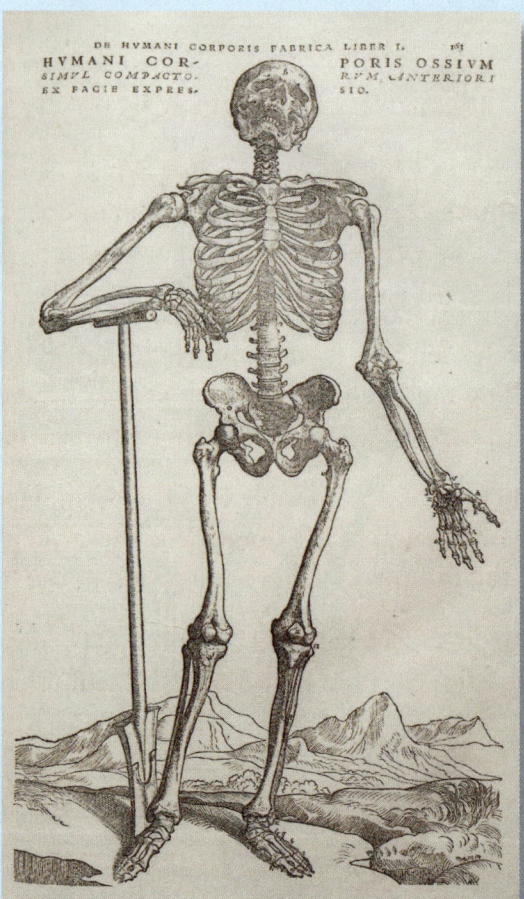

Image from Andreas Vesalius' De humani corporis fabrica (1543), page 163

Rene Descartes, in 1649, described the Pineal gland as the control center of the body and mind. The Pineal gland, located in the brain, produces Melatonin, which regulates the sleep cycle (circadian rhythm). A cross-section of a nerve cell was seen in one of the first microscopes by Antonie Van Leeuwenhoek in 1717. Although we know it is now incorrect, Franz Joseph Gall published his work on phrenology. He believed he could distinguish the traits of a person by feeling the bumps on their head.

Paul Broca discovered that different regions of the brain performed specific processes. He discovered "Broca's" Area (named after him) in 1861. This region is located in the frontal lobe of the left hemisphere of the brain and is intimately involved in speech articulation (talking). Near that same time, in 1874, Carl Wernicke published *Der Aphasische Symptomencomplex,* a book on aphasias. Aphasia is the term used to identify a difficulty in forming and understanding language. Wernicke's Area is located close to Broca's Area.

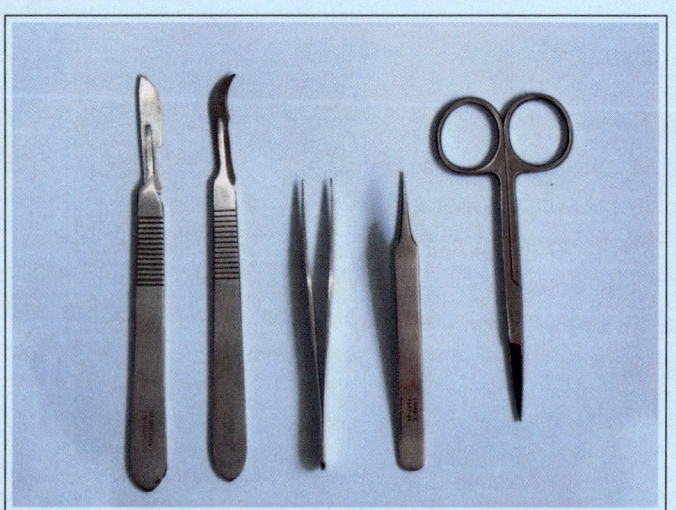

18

God's Wondrous Machine

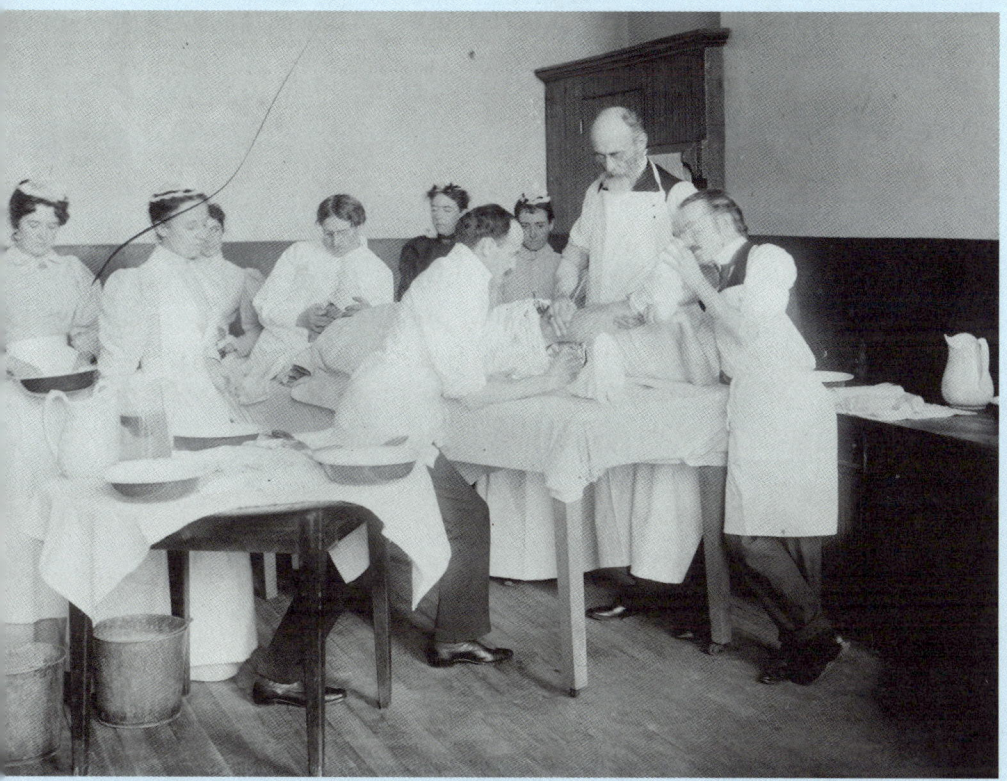
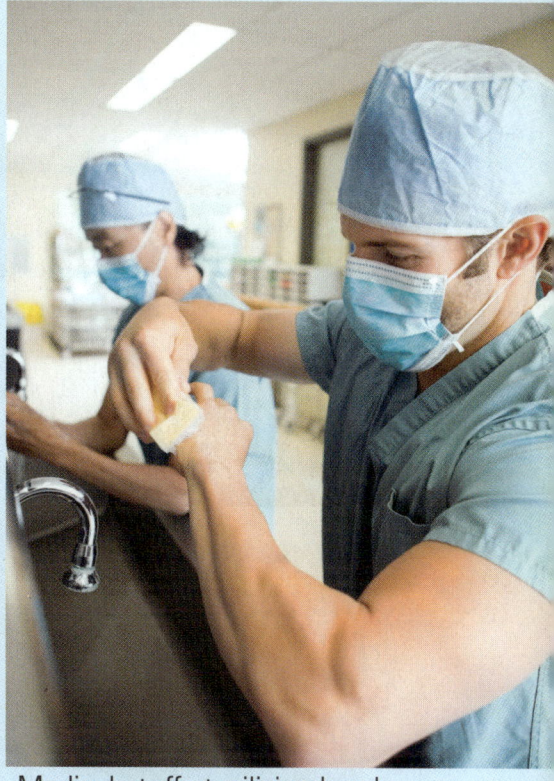

Observe the picture above. Do you see anything missing (a lack of masks, gloves, substances….)? Unlike very advanced and sterile (germ-free) environments for modern surgery, proper sanitary procedures were not practiced.

Medical staff sterilizing hands and arms before surgery

Your brain is a very complex and delicate organ. Unlike other parts of the body, disorders of the brain could not be treated or even diagnosed correctly. It wasn't until 1884 when the first successful surgical removal of a brain tumor was performed by Sir Rickman John Godlee. Joseph Babinski was the first to describe the Babinski Reflex. It is a normal reflex in infants but an abnormal reflex in older children and adults. We will learn more on this reflex later.

One of the most grotesque practices in neuroscience was developed in 1936 by Dr. Antonio Egas Moniz, who invented the procedure of frontal lobotomies for the treatment of mental illnesses. This caused changes in the person's personality and sometimes death. Fortunately, this is not practiced today.

Dr. Wilder Penfield developed a visual representation of the brain — called the homunculus — that identifies the sensory regions. We will visit with Dr. Penfield in an upcoming section.

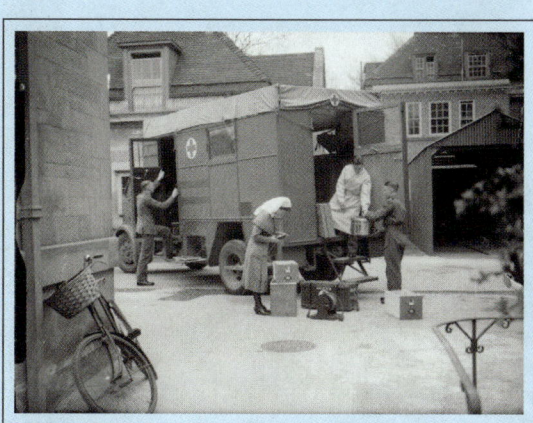

The British Army's first mobile brain surgery unit shown being stocked in 1940. It was staffed with five specialist doctors and two nurses.

Unit 1: The Electrifying Nervous System

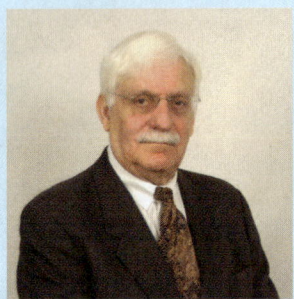
And last on our timeline is Dr. Raymond Damadian, who became a pioneer in the field of magnetic resonance imaging (MRI) through his development of several patents and a working machine named Indomitable that could be used for non-invasive detection of cancer in the human body. The first commercial MRI scanner was produced in 1980. This important technology can show disease or any damage in the brain in several ways without using surgery.

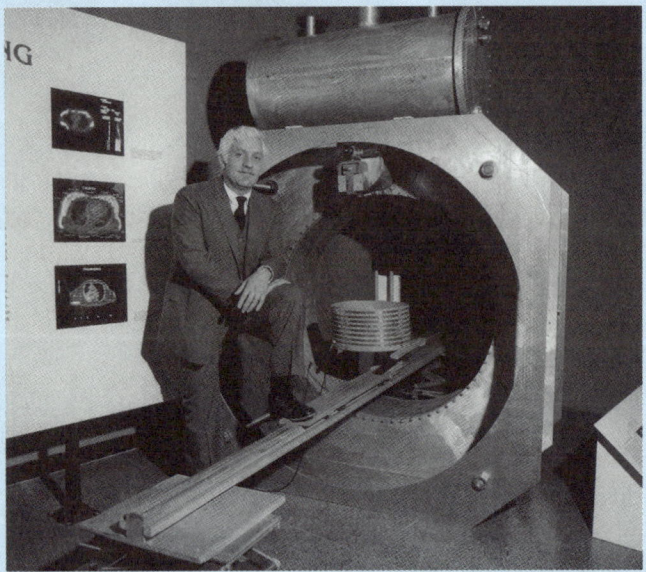
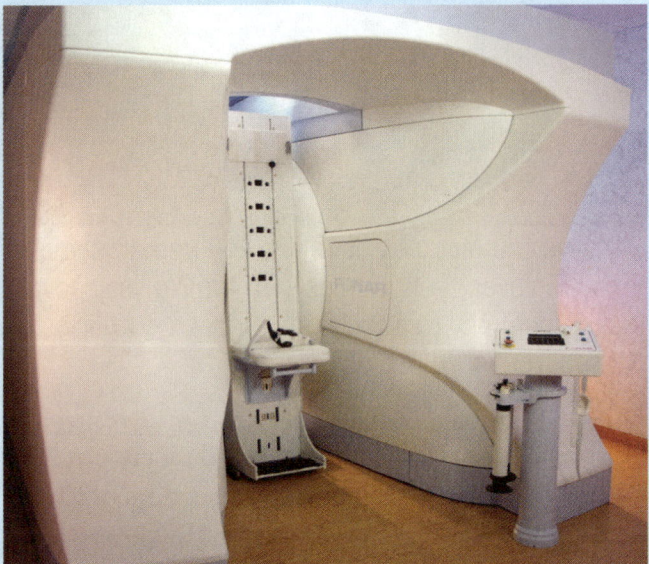

Continuing improvements to MRI technology are helping to discover new details of how our bodies function and ways to discover when there are problems. At left, Dr. Damadian with his pioneering machine, Indomitable.

Word Wise!

ANATOMY refers to the study of the body structure, systems, and organs of living things. The word developed from the Greek words "ana" meaning "up," and "tomia" for cutting.

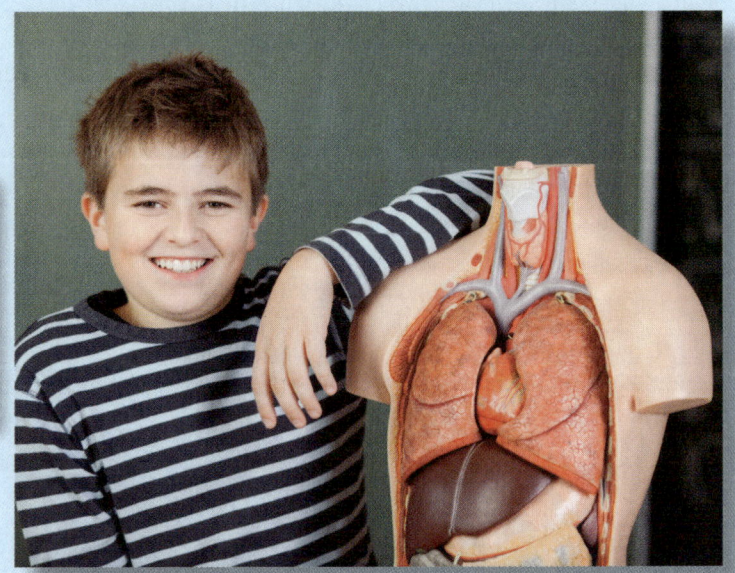

God's Wondrous Machine

MODERN MARVELS

You may have seen a mortar and pestle in the drug store – either as a symbol or as a decorative object. While also used for some cooking techniques, these were traditionally used in many cultures to mix up the ingredients in medicine.

Good or Bad Medicine?

When a doctor gives you a prescription for medicine, you go to a pharmacy. Pharmacists are a type of doctor who have special training in drugs and their effects on the body. Before there were pharmacists, there were apothecaries. If you lived in the 15th century, in the times of Christopher Columbus, and became ill, you may have gone to an apothecary. They mixed their own medicines and gave advice on healthcare. Many doctors were able to formulate their own medicines as well. Evidence of prescriptions and instructions for how they were made have even been found on clay tablets as early as ancient Babylon.

There were no rules in how this had to be done. This meant that while a doctor in one place might have created a specific type of medicine, a doctor in a nearby town might make the same medicine only it would be slightly different in its formula of ingredients. Both might have prescribed a different amount of the medicine for the same type of injury. Now there are strict regulations and professional standards that help to insure uniformity in the formulas and prescriptions for medicine. Drugs for mental health, or psychotropic drugs, are a relatively new invention. Drugs developed for the specific treatment of mental health problems only came into existence after World War II.

Today many medicines are developed by huge corporations who spend billions of dollars in formulating these new drugs. They then have to go through a strict testing and approval process. The Food and Drug Administration is the government agency tasked with approving new medicines in the United States.

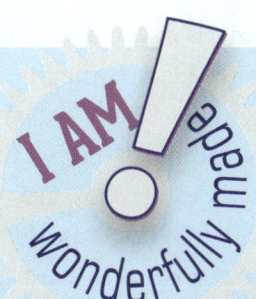

BIBLICAL REFERENCES: The Bible has a multitude of references to the body's organs and systems. However, it does not directly mention the brain.

Mind	Think	Meditate
Psalm 26:2	Romans 12:3	Psalm 48:9
Matthew 22:37	Philippians 4:8	Psalm 143:5
Luke 10:27	Proverbs 23:7	Psalm 119:15, 23, 27, 48, 78, 97, 99, 148
1 Peter 4:7	2 Peter 3:1	
Psalm 7:9	1 Corinthians 14:20	Colossians 3:2

Unit 1: The Electrifying Nervous System

2 Seeing Is Believing: Looking inside the Brain

We have just learned about how medical and scientific discoveries were made in the past. What are some of the kinds of technology used today in studying the brain?

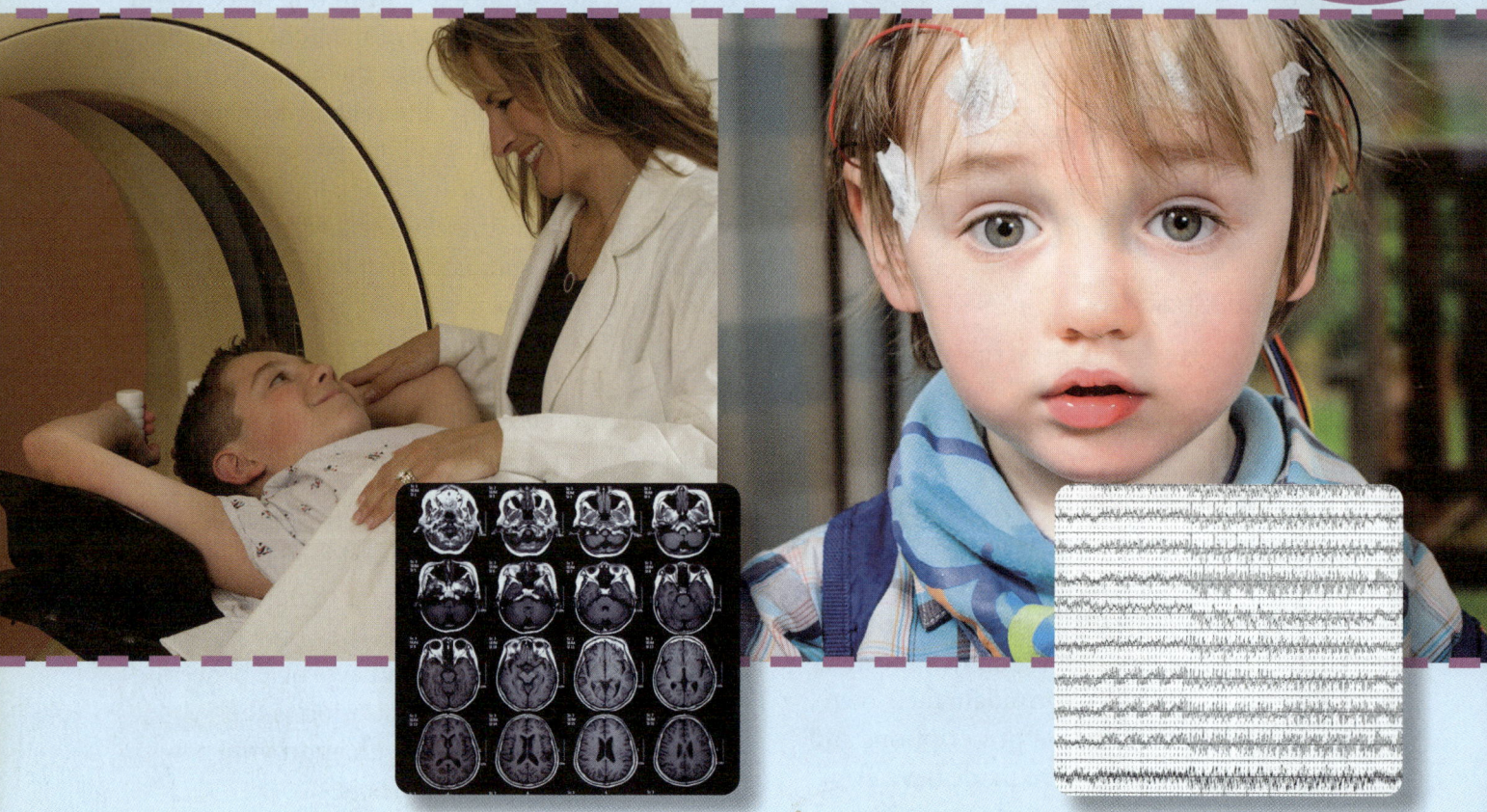

CT Scans

CT Scans, Computerized Tomography, is a painless way to take images inside the body and provides far more detail than an x-ray. These are images that are computer processed and combined to show images of the brain and other parts of the body. This type of study is best used for diagnosing bone injuries, lung/chest problems, and cancers. It takes less than 5 minutes to perform. To the CT scanner, the body is like a loaf of bread. Images are taken of the body and stacked like slices of bread without causing any harm to the patient.

EEG

EEG, Electroencephalogram, is a way of recording electrical activity of the brain. Electro-means electric. Encephalo-means brain. Gram is derived from the Greek meaning something that is recorded. The special sensors, electrodes, are placed on various areas on the scalp in a sticky paste. These electrodes are hooked to wires to a computer that records the brain's electrical activity. It can record abnormal electrical waves that are seen in seizure disorders. Just like throwing a pebble into a pond when it hits a spot on the water, ripples are made across the surface. The brain's neurons send electrical waves that are conducted through adjacent neurons across the brain like ripples across a lake. The EEG measures these waves.

God's Wondrous Machine

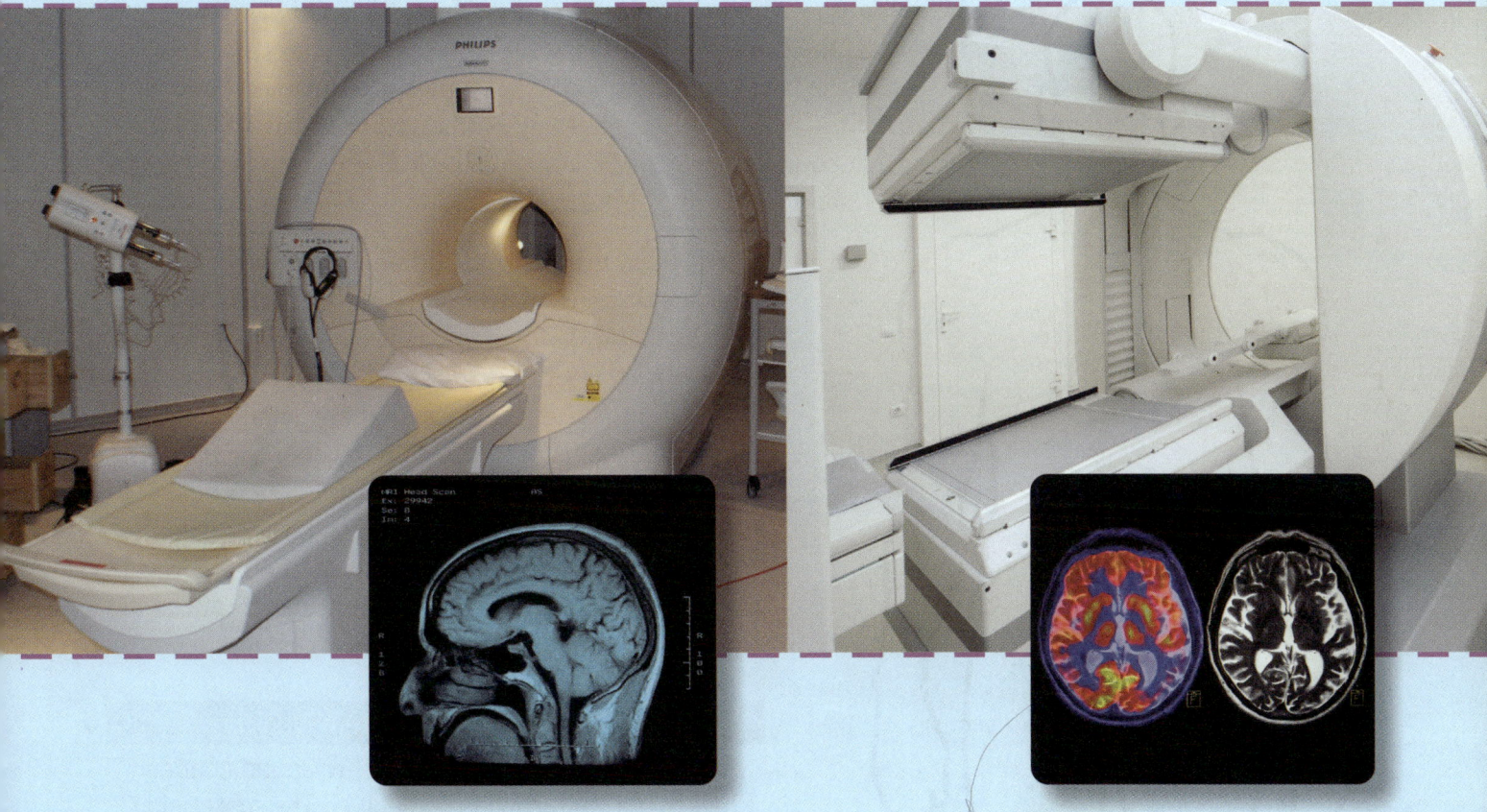

MRI

MRI, Magnetic Resonance Imaging, are scanners that use powerful magnetic fields and radio waves to form images of the body. It is often more sensitive than a CT scan and is best used to diagnose injuries to soft tissues of the body, brain tumors, and problems with the spinal cord. It takes at least 30 minutes or more to perform.

PET scan

The PET scan (Positron Emission Tomography) is a type of scanner that uses radioactive tracers. The body breaks down these tracers, causing them to emit energy. This energy is detected and used to create images that reveal which areas of the brain are active.

MEDI+MOMENT

Doctors can look at your outsides and your insides. Special medical inventions allow doctors to peer inside the body without surgery. The CT Scan allows the doctor to see small sections of the body.

Unit 1: The Electrifying Nervous System

3   The Basics of the Nervous System

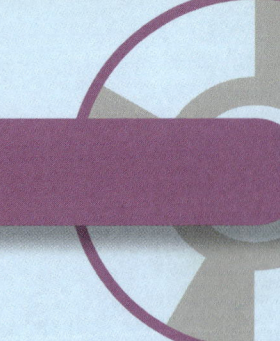

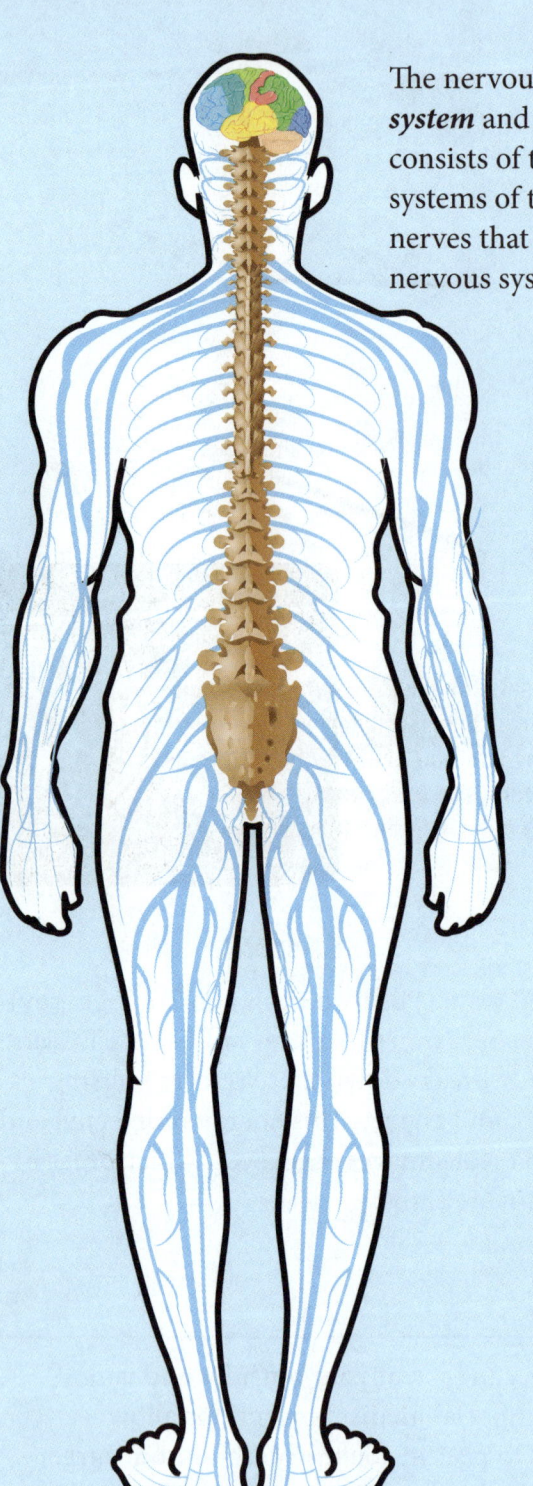

The nervous system has two major parts: *the peripheral nervous system* and the *central nervous system.* The central nervous system consists of the brain and the spinal cord, which are the main control systems of the body. The peripheral nervous system consists of all the nerves that connect to the brain and spinal cord, which link the central nervous system to the rest of the body.

The neuron is the most fundamental unit of the nervous system. In order to read this sentence, you can see that individual letters are placed together to form words. A letter is the smallest part of a word. The nervous system is made of many small parts. The smallest part of the nervous system is a *neuron.* Billions of neurons link together in the nervous system. The neurons connect to send information to and from the brain and body. These impulses travel very fast along the neurons; the quickest impulses go as fast as 250 miles an hour!

A Central Nervous System Neuron	
Myelin Sheath	Protective spiral-wrapped coating around the neuron. The materials to make myelin begin from the Oligodendroglia.
Mitochondrion	Place where energy for the neuron is generated.
Node of Ranvier	Intermediate gaps in the myelin that occur along the axon that allow the nerve impulse to travel at a greater velocity, jumping from one gap to the next.
Axon Terminal	The end of the neuron that forms a synapse (connection) with another neuron.

God's Wondrous Machine

The central cell body

DENDRITES: tentacle-like structures that extend from the cell body of the neuron and reach out to the other cells

AXON: the long, tail-like extension of the cell body that is covered with a white, fatty, segmented substance called the myelin sheath. This allows electrical signals to be sent quickly along nerve cells.

Neurons communicate with neighboring neurons and form the electrochemical highway system through which electrical impulses are transmitted through the brain.

However, the neuron is not the only cell housed in the central nervous system. Another cell of the central nervous system is the neuroglial cell. The word "glia" derives from the Greek meaning "glue." These cells "glue" the neurons together.

There are four types of neuroglial cells

ASTROGLIA: are like the brain's "store grocer" who supplies nutrients to the neuron.

EPENDYMAL CELLS: which serve as "the lining." These cells line the small cavities in the brain and produce cerebral spinal fluid (CSF).

MICROGLIA: which serve as "the garbage collectors." These cells are phagocytic (phago means to eat), which means that they digest microorganism invaders and waste products made by the neurons.

OLIGODENDROGLIA: which serve as "the protectors." These cells support and insulate the axons and assist in forming the myelin sheaths that protect neurons.

The vessels for the hard-working brain transport the vital oxygen and nutrients that are vital to its function. The brain has 100,000 miles (160,934.4km) of blood vessels. That is the distance four times around the Earth at the equator! This is all a part of God's amazing design.

I AM wonderfully made

The main parts of a neuron are:

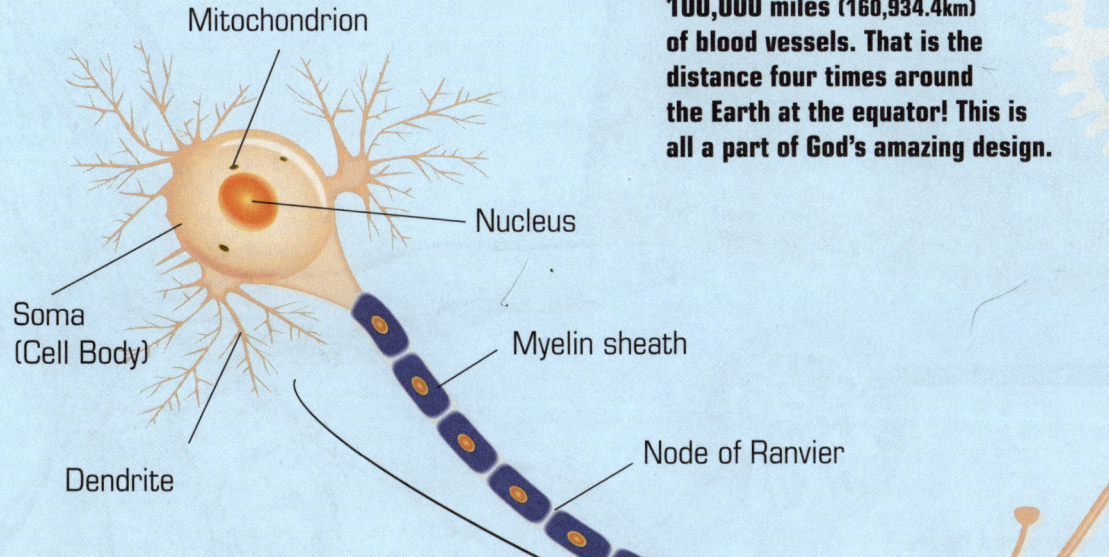

- Mitochondrion
- Nucleus
- Soma (Cell Body)
- Myelin sheath
- Dendrite
- Node of Ranvier
- Axon
- Axon terminal

Unit 1: The Electrifying Nervous System

MODERN MARVELS

Many researchers are focused on thought-controlled technologies. From planes controlled by thoughts to prosthetic limbs or even robotic suits, attempts to harness the power of the human mind are starting to show some amazing results. In May 2014 a breakthrough came with the efforts of Battelle, a nonprofit research group whose invention was being tested by Ian Burkhart, a young man who lost most of his mobility after breaking his neck in a swimming accident. Now requiring assistance with caring for himself, Burkhart hoped for a medical advance that would help to regain some of his independence. Surgeons implanted a tiny chip with electrodes in his brain. The chip is wired to an area on Burkhart's head, attached to a computer that "decodes" signals from the brain and even adds additional instructions that would ordinarily come from his spinal cord. The computer is connected to a group of electrodes attached to his wrist, designed to quickly activate in a sequence mirroring his brain thoughts about moving his hand. The experiment was successful, and while the process seems awkward, it represents a small, but important step in this research!

Science fiction come true: Moving a paralyzed hand with the power of thought," The Washington Post, June 24, 2014. http://www.washingtonpost.com/

Your Brain is in Charge!

The cerebrum is the largest part of your brain. It gives the wrinkled appearance of the brain. The Cerebrum makes up two-thirds of the brain's total weight. It is involved in hearing, vision, emotions, personality and muscle movements. In the next section, you will discover how the nervous system — including the cerebrum — is designed and functions!

Imagine how much brainpower goes into a thumb war! Reach out your hands, and curl your fingers together, keeping your thumbs up. To win the game you have to pin your challenger's thumb for a count of three — but that is easier said than done! Give it a try — put your brain to work and have fun!

KNOW IT ALL

Every minute enough blood flows through the brain to fill three soda cans.

26

God's Wondrous Machine

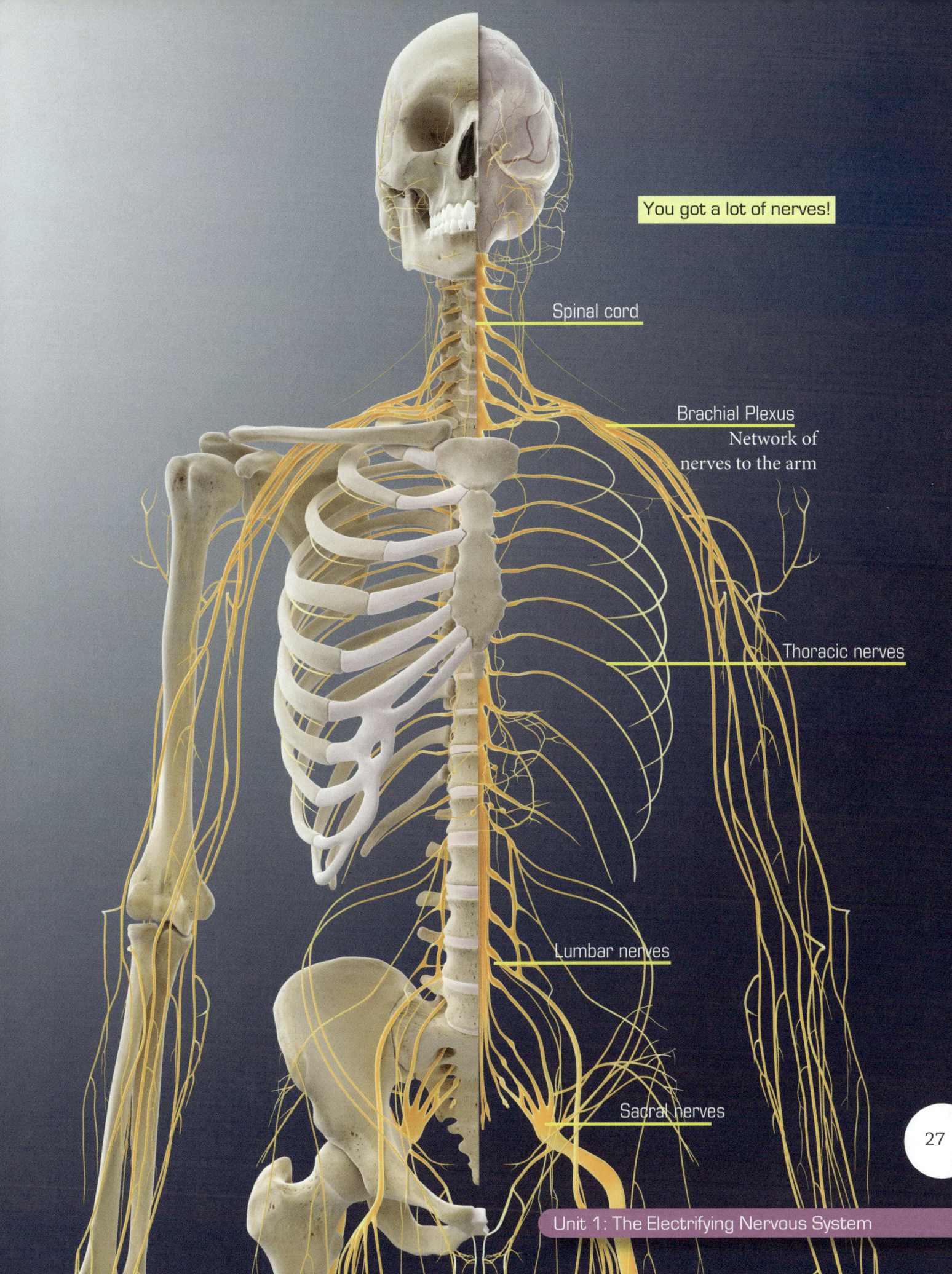

4 Anatomy & Physiology: The Brick & Mortar of the Nervous System

What is the difference in anatomy and physiology? It's simple! Anatomy is focused on the parts or structures of the system. Physiology is focused on the function or actions of the systems. Let's start with the brain — it is the main part or control center of the nervous system:

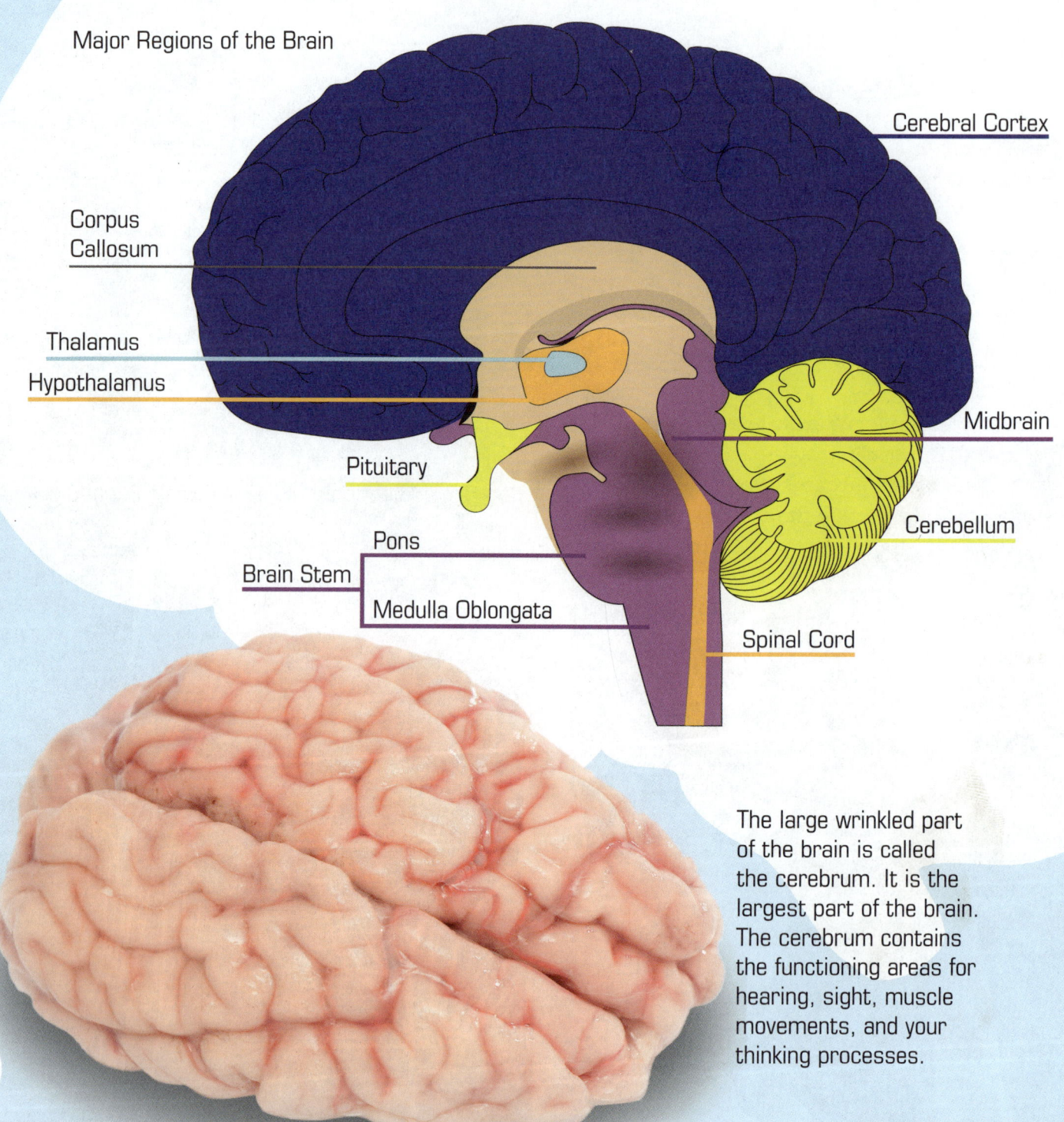

The large wrinkled part of the brain is called the cerebrum. It is the largest part of the brain. The cerebrum contains the functioning areas for hearing, sight, muscle movements, and your thinking processes.

God's Wondrous Machine

PARTS, BOLTS, AND COGS

The Cerebrum (sĕr′ə-brəm)

The *cerebrum* consists of two large, paired hemispheres (hemi- means half). The right and left *cerebral hemispheres* are where conscious thought processes occur. When someone refers to you using your "gray" matter, they are implying that you are using your intellect. The **gray matter** is the thin outer rim on the surface of the brain like the outer crust of a slice of bread. Memory storage, processing, and conscious and subconscious regulation of skeletal movement also originate in this area. **White matter** lies deeper in the brain and houses neurological nerve tracts. Neurological nerve tracts are pathways that contain bundles of myelin-coated neurons. They serve to connect to the gray matter and allow for communication with the rest of the body.

The cerebrum is the largest region of the brain. The two hemispheres connect only in the area of the *corpus callosum,* located in the center of the brain. The corpus callosum consists of arched neurofiber tracks that enable the two hemispheres of the brain to communicate with each other.

The right and left hemispheres of the brain have distinctly different functions. Have you ever heard the expression "Oh, she is totally a 'right-brained' person" or "He is really a 'left-brained' person"? Left brain functions deal with areas of logic and order. Right brain functions deal in the areas of imagination and feelings.

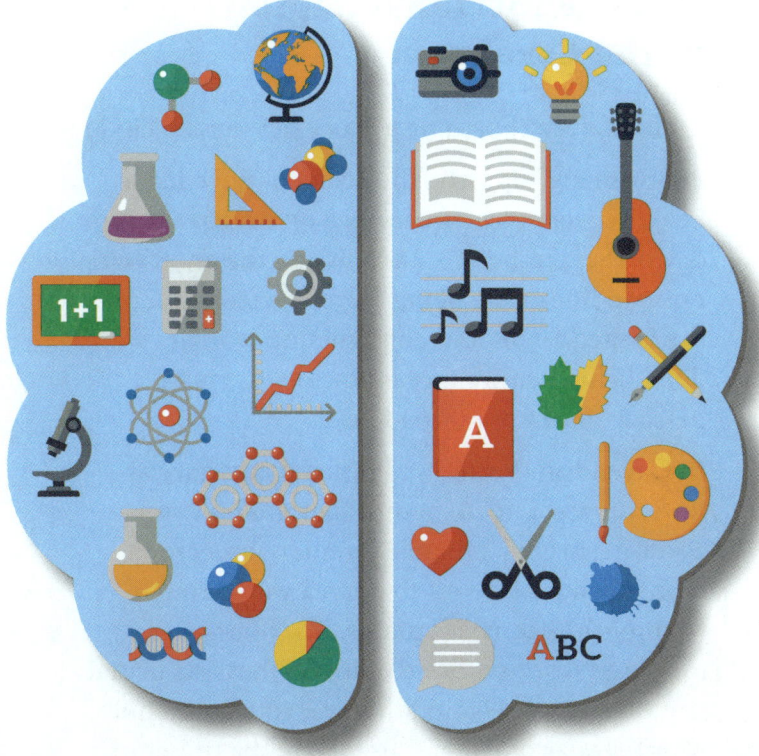

Left Brain Functions	Right Brain Functions
uses logic	uses feelings
detail oriented	"big picture"
facts rule	imagination rules
words and language	symbols and images
present and past	present and future
math and science	philosophy & religion
can comprehend	can "get it" (meaning)
knowing	believes
acknowledges	appreciates
order/pattern perception	spatial perception
knows object name	knows object function
reality based	fantasy based
forms strategies	presents possibilites
practical	impetuous
safe	risk taking

Major Functional Regions of the Cerebrum

Unfortunate/Fortunate Story of Phineas Gage

A "fortunate" unfortunate accident unveiled a key discovery in neuroscience on a crisp autumn day on September 13, 1848. It was the era when railroad lines were being forged westward across the United States and construction workers were demolishing entire mountainsides to create a passage for these railroad lines.

In Cavendish, Vermont, Phineas Gage gave an unfortunate "gift" to neuroscience. Phineas was a well-respected, amiable foreman for a crew of men whose job was to open a way through Vermont's Green Mountains. The hours were long, and work on these railroad lines was brutal and dangerous. During this era, you would not hear the roar of engines or take in the fumes of diesel fuel burning. No, the tools of the trade were shovels, pick axes, hand rock drills, and explosives. Phineas had a reputation for his great skill in blasting. During the blasting process, workers ignited gunpowder to break rocks apart.

On this particular day in September, Phineas used a tool of the blasting trade called a tamping iron. This iron bar was approximately 3½ feet long and it weighed 13 pounds. The process of blasting had several steps. First, Phineas drilled a hole in the rock by hand. He poured gunpowder into the hole and placed a piece of rope for a fuse. He then placed sand on top to fill the hole. With the flat end of the tamping iron, Phineas would tamp the sand tight in the hole. This was something he had done countless times before. However, on this particular day, he did not place the sand in the hole. With Phineas standing directly over the hole, a stray spark from the tamping iron descended into the hole and ignited the gunpowder. The

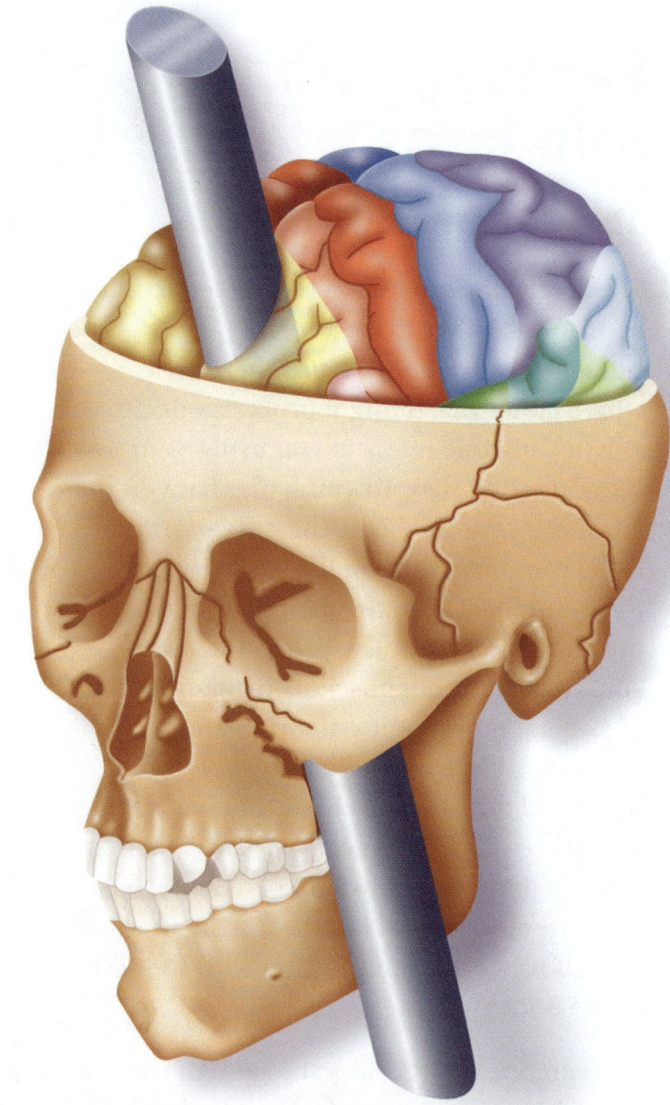

MODERN MARVELS

Scientists continue to study what areas of the brain's anatomy and functions were impacted when Phineas was injured over 165 years ago. With modern equipment that accurately detail the smallest structures and pathways within the brain, computers are now used to model the path of the damage to study what impact it may have had.

God's Wondrous Machine

resulting explosion turned the tamping iron into a ballistic missile traveling 30 feet up in the air.

The path of the projectile could be traced as it entered under Phineas' left cheekbone, passed behind his left eye, went through the front of his brain, and exited out the middle of his forehead. Phineas fell on his back and, remarkably, never lost consciousness. His men took him to the closest doctor in the nearby village. In the commotion, he insisted on retelling the doctor the details of his accident by himself. All were amazed.

It took many months for Phineas to "recover" from his injuries. Unfortunately, he was never the same. After the accident, Phineas' behavior became erratic. He was unable to hold a job or a meaningful relationship with another person. He was crude, rude, foul-mouthed, and impulsive. He made very unwise decisions.

The doctors at Harvard Medical School took an interest in Phineas and began to study him. They discovered, through Phineas' unfortunate accident, that the brain's frontal lobe (the part damaged by the tamping iron) is responsible for "executive functions." Executive functions oversee our social interactions and decision-making. Phineas provided a textbook case study on the frontal lobe of the brain. Some would argue that he "died" on the day of the accident, because he was never the same. However, he did not die physically from his injuries until 11 years, 6 months, and 19 days later, at the age of 37.

Phineas Gage never recovered from his injury. However, a remarkable trait children possess is something called brain plasticity. Certainly, this does not mean your brain is composed of plastic. What it does mean is that the brain of a child has the ability to reorganize neural connections. If one part of the brain is injured, then other areas of the brain may be retrained to take over the functions of the damaged area. There is so much yet to be discovered and understood about neuroscience.

Smithsonian Magazine shared an interesting article in 2010. A 19th-century picture of a man with one closed eye and a large metal bar led a couple who collect old photographic images to think it might be someone who had been injured hunting whales. After posting a scan of the photograph online, they quickly discovered the man was not a whaler, and after a suggestion that it might be Phineas Gage, contacted a librarian at Harvard who also felt it was probably Phineas Gage. The bar that is being held by the man in the image has an inscription that could only partially be read. The rod that injured Phineas had been engraved during his lifetime to read, "This is the bar that was shot through the head of Mr. Phinehas P. Gage." His name was mispelled.

LETS PICK OUR BRAIN

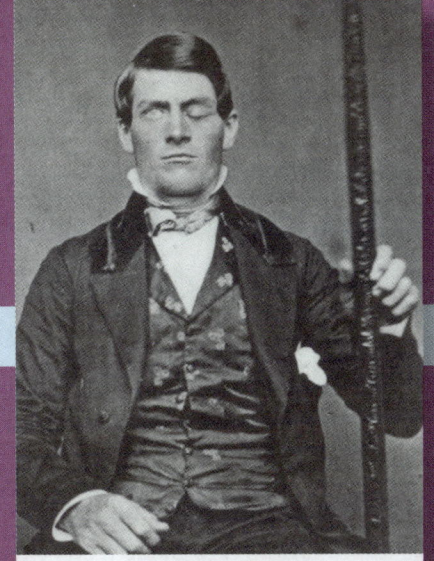
Phineas Gage

Unit 1: The Electrifying Nervous System

Let's take a closer look at the parts of the cerebrum!

Lobes	Location	Function
1. Frontal Lobe	The front (anterior) region of the brain	Personality, judgment, abstract reasoning, social behavior: location of the primary motor cortex, which controls movement
2. Parietal Lobe	Between the frontal and occipital lobes	Location of the primary sensory cortex — conscious perception of sensations, such as touch, pressure, vibration, pain, taste, and temperature; origination of memory storage and processing, as well as conscious and subconscious regulation of skeletal movement
3. Occipital Lobe	The back (posterior) region of the brain	Visual cortex
4. Temporal Lobe	The side (lateral) region of the brain	Auditory cortex, olfactory (smell) cortex, and language comprehension

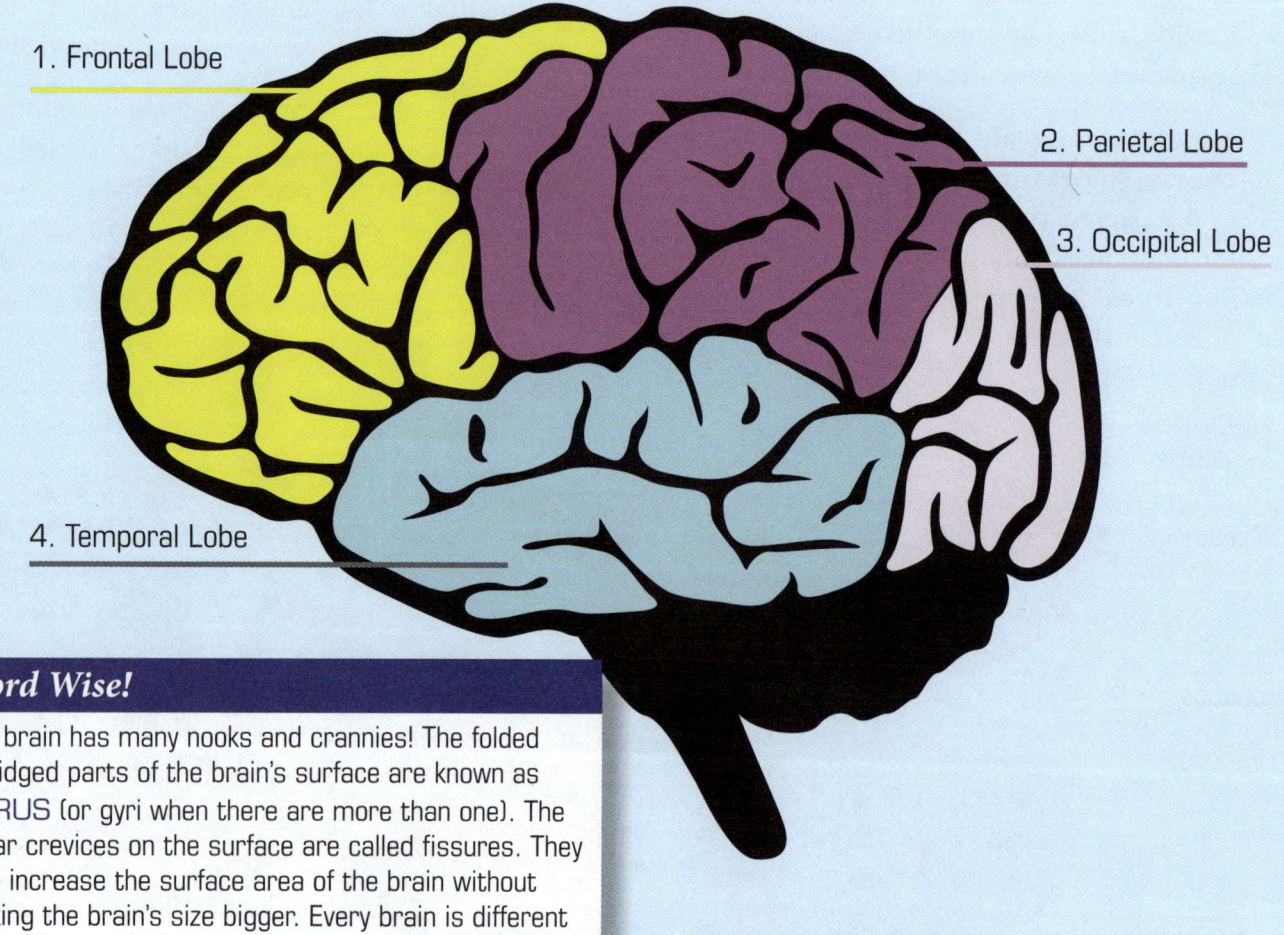

1. Frontal Lobe
2. Parietal Lobe
3. Occipital Lobe
4. Temporal Lobe

Word Wise!

The brain has many nooks and crannies! The folded or ridged parts of the brain's surface are known as GYRUS (or gyri when there are more than one). The linear crevices on the surface are called fissures. They help increase the surface area of the brain without making the brain's size bigger. Every brain is different so no one knows how many "wrinkles" every brain has!

God's Wondrous Machine

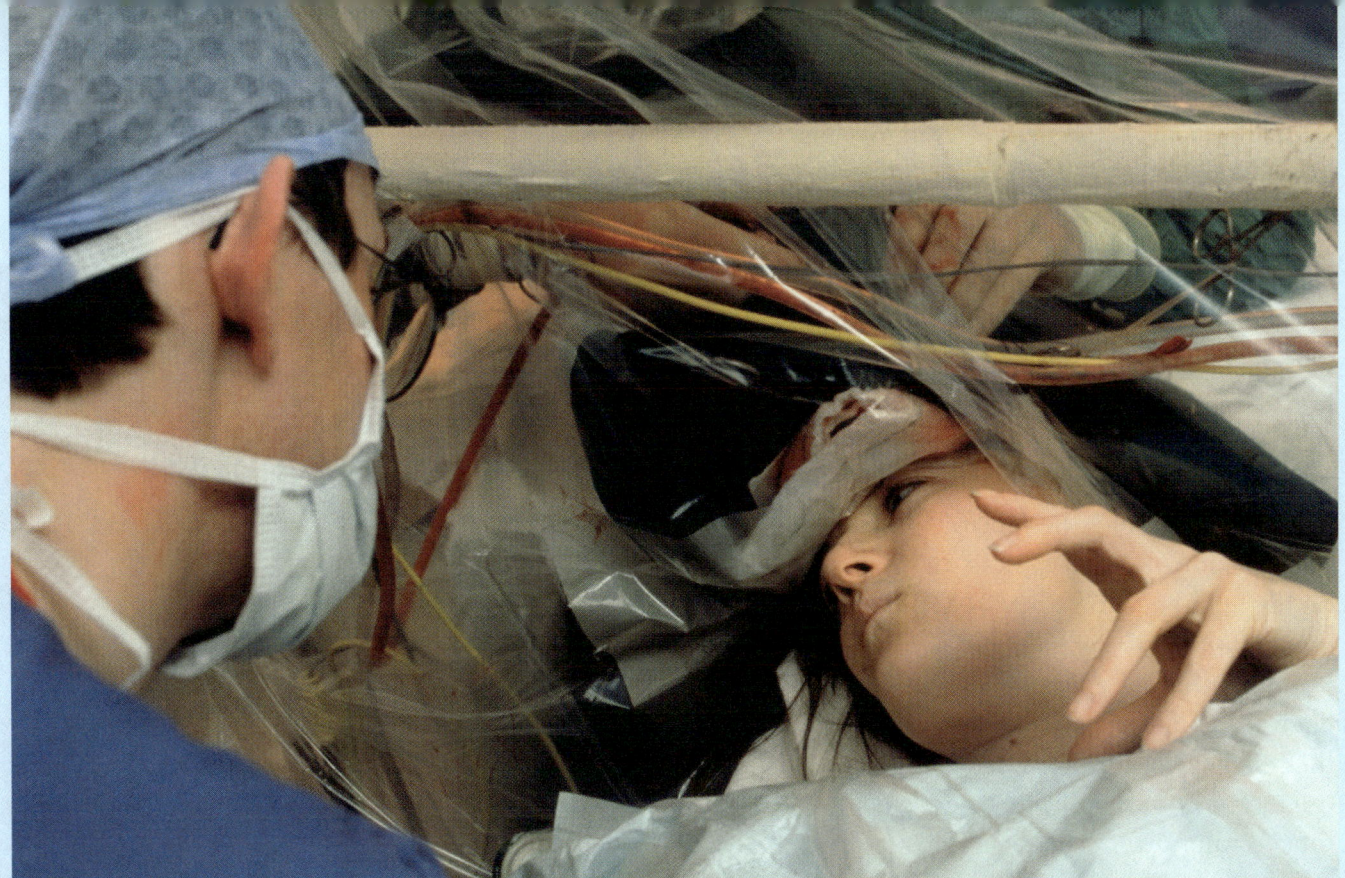

In some brain procedures or surgery, it is important for the patient to be alert and able to communicate with the doctors and support staff. While it may seem a little scary, the patient is not in pain.

Not only did Phineas Gage contribute to our understanding of the cerebrum, but Dr. Wilder Penfield made substantial contributions to the field of neuroscience. Dr. Penfield, an American-born Canadian neurosurgeon, is credited with the groundbreaking work on the *homunculus.* In the 1950s, Penfield attempted to treat patients with uncontrollable seizures, called epilepsy. A seizure occurs when abnormal electrical impulses travel through the brain.

A person who suffers from this condition can experience anything from a mild staring episode to a loss of consciousness and body-wide shaking. Epilepsy can be very debilitating. The types of patients in which Dr. Penfield dealt experienced cases of epilepsy that were so severe and debilitating that they could not live normal lives.

Dr. Penfield noted that many of his patients would experience an "aura" before the onset of a seizure. This "aura" served as a warning to the patient that a seizure was about to occur. Some saw flashing lights, heard a loud sound, or experienced unusual smells, like the smell of burnt toast. Penfield performed brain surgery on patients who were awake (the brain does not feel pain) and attempted to provoke an aura with a mild electric current to brain. He was able to localize the region in which the seizure activity began. Then he removed a small piece of brain tissue and the seizures improved. Through these surgeries, he was able to map the brain.

One of Dr. Penfield's most emotionally challenging brain operations was the one he performed on his own sister, Ruth. Ruth's life was in grave danger from a brain tumor that was causing life-threatening seizures. In a radical surgery, he removed most of her right frontal lobe. Ruth's only concern prior to the operation was embarrassing her talented younger brother in his distinguished work. Ruth's life was extended for a few more years.

Unit 1: The Electrifying Nervous System

What is that?

The *homunculus* is a visual representation of the connections between different body parts and the areas in the brain hemispheres that control them. The term "homunculus" is derived from Latin; it means "little man." The motor region (which controls muscle movement) is on the left hemisphere and is called the *motor homunculus.* The right hemisphere in the same area senses the external environment, which is appropriately called the *sensory homunculus.* It is similar to the motor homunculus, but it tells how much brainpower is dedicated to sensing different body parts.

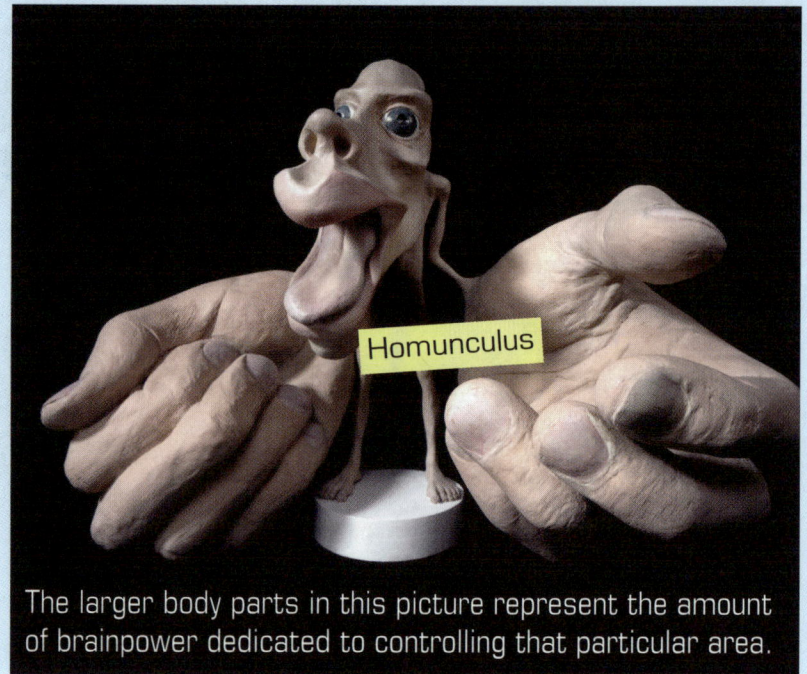

The larger body parts in this picture represent the amount of brainpower dedicated to controlling that particular area.

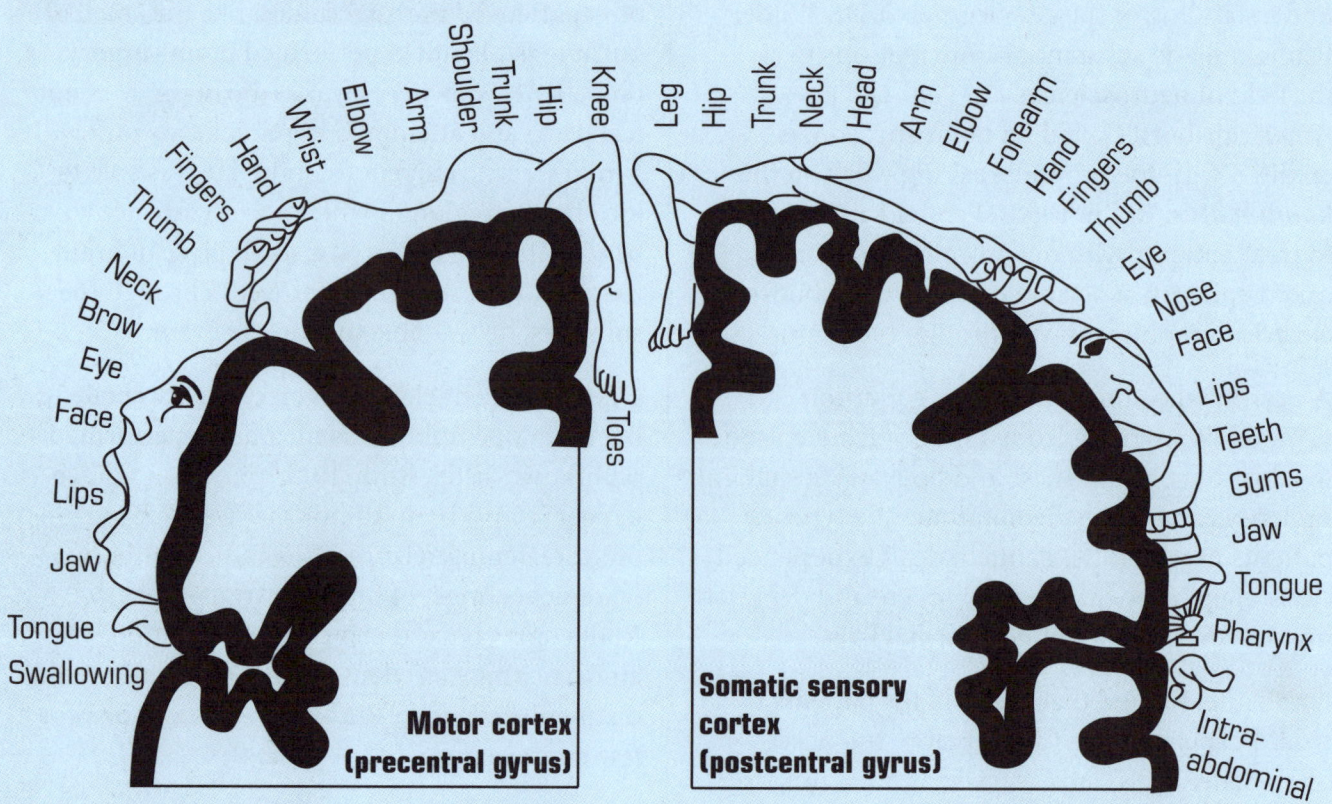

God's Wondrous Machine

Broca's Area and Wernicke's Area

Two unique areas of the brain are located in the left temporal region — *Broca's area* and *Wernicke's area.* These areas are very special areas. Broca's area controls the process of making intelligible sounds in speech. It transmits neurological impulses to the vocal cords and assists with articulating the exact words for communication. *Wernicke's area* interprets what the ear hears and makes sense of spoken communication. When someone experiences a stroke in one of these areas of the brain, problems arise in communication. (A stroke occurs when a blood vessel breaks in a particular part of the brain and causes an injury in that region.) People who experience damage to Broca's area can still make sounds, but their language is garbled. These people may completely understand what others say to them, but they are unable to articulate comprehensible dialogue.

Can you predict what would happen if the Wernicke's area was damaged? If damage occurs in Wernicke's area, the person loses the ability to interpret what others say to them. They can hear all the sounds, but what they hear sounds like nonsense. They can speak without difficulty, but are unable to make proper responses.

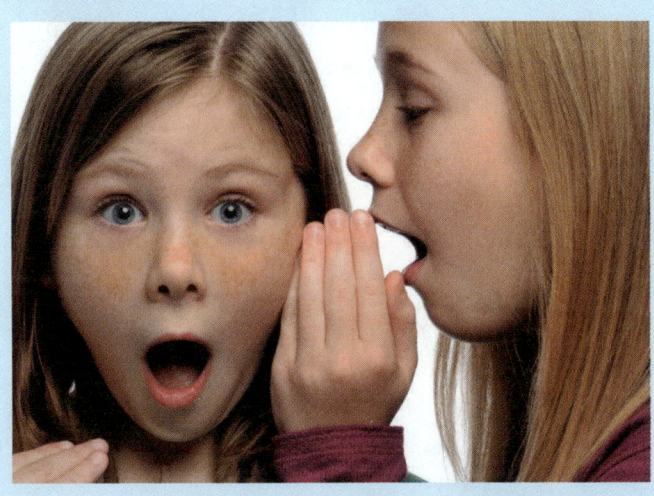

KNOW IT ALL

The adult human brain only composes 2% of the body's total weight. God has designed it to be amazingly efficient and occupy a small space.

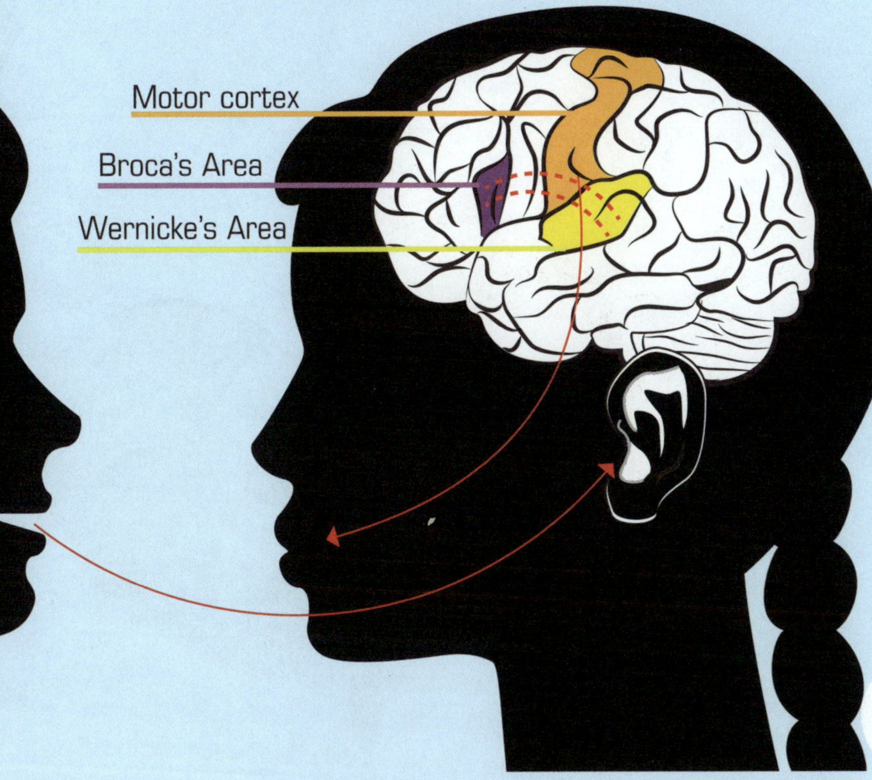

Motor cortex
Broca's Area
Wernicke's Area

Unit 1: The Electrifying Nervous System

Stay Balanced: The Cerebellum
(sĕr´ə-bĕl´əm)

The cerebellum is hidden below the depths of the cerebral hemispheres. This area coordinates movements and allows you to perform the same movements over and over. If one cuts the cerebellum in half, a visible white structure called the **arbor vitae** is present, which is Latin for the "tree of life." The name for this structure is quite appropriate. It is composed of white matter that is configured in a tree-like branch pattern resembling a fern. This structure brings both sensory and motor information to the cerebellum.

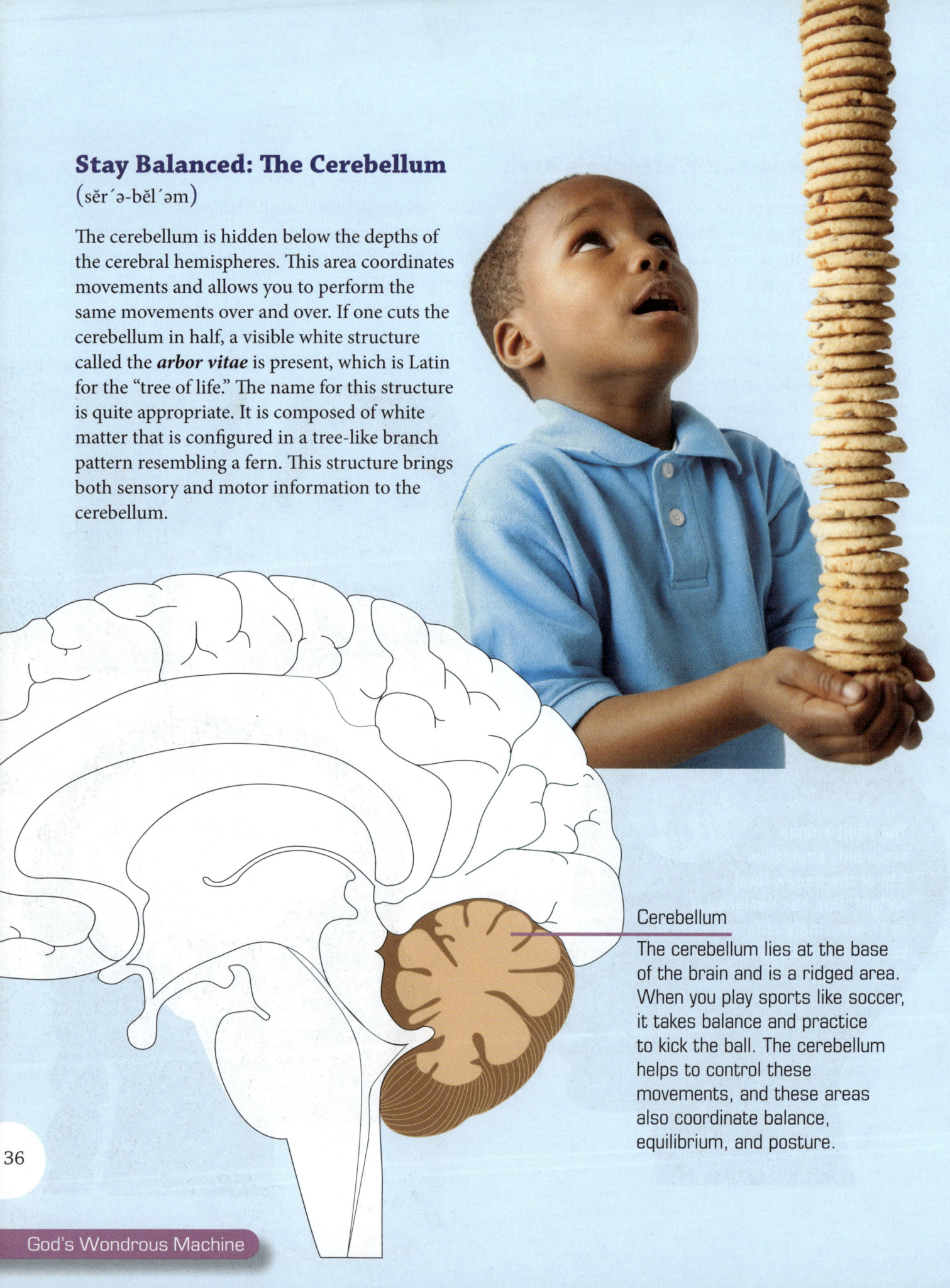

Cerebellum
The cerebellum lies at the base of the brain and is a ridged area. When you play sports like soccer, it takes balance and practice to kick the ball. The cerebellum helps to control these movements, and these areas also coordinate balance, equilibrium, and posture.

God's Wondrous Machine

Growing Like a Weed: The Diencephalon

The *diencephalon* lies deep in the middle of the brain, below the top ridge of the corpus callosum and connects the cerebrum to the brainstem. Two key structures in the diencephalon are the *thalamus* and the *hypothalamus.* The thalamus acts like a switchboard operator, relaying and sending sensory information to its various destinations. As a person senses his or her surroundings, this area helps to interpret the environment. The hypothalamus regulates body temperature and hormone production. It also controls reflexes associated with eating, such as swallowing. These unconscious operations are part of the *autonomic nervous system.* The autonomic nervous system is part of the body's control system and performs its vital functions without any conscious thought.

Another structure that lies within the diencephalon is the pituitary gland. The *pituitary gland* is a pea-sized structure that lies at the base of the brain and is cradled in a recess of the skull bone (see pg. 28). It secretes hormones that enable it to be the "master gland" of your body. It oversees key functions, such as growth during childhood and the onset of puberty, by controlling male and female hormones.

Gigantism is a disorder that sometimes occurs when a tumor forms in the pituitary gland. In this disorder, the pituitary gland produces too much of the hormone responsible for growth, the human growth hormone. Individuals suffering from this disorder can reach great heights. One of the most famous people affected by gigantism is Robert Wadlow, who holds the world record as the tallest man. Mr. Wadlow reached 8 feet, 11.1 inches tall. At his death, he was still growing.

Robert Wadlow died at age 22 from a blood infection. Born in Alton, Illinois in 1918 by the age of six, he was over six feet tall, weighed 160 pounds, and was taller than his father.

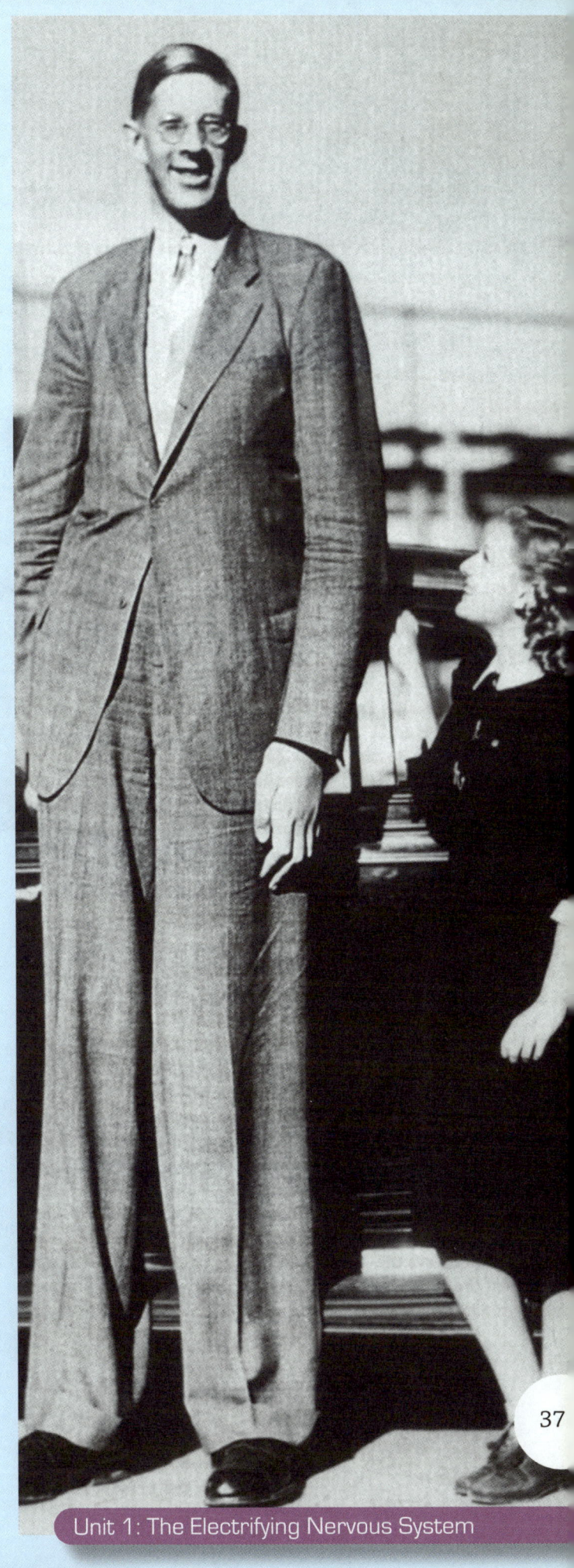

Stay Alert: Mesencephalon

Inferior to (below) the diencephalon is the *mesencephalon* (midbrain). The mesencephalon is critical to sorting through the visual and auditory (what you hear) data that the brain receives. This area maintains alertness. For example, when someone yells, "Foul ball!" at a baseball game, a person's instant reaction may be to close his or her eyes tight and cover his or her head. The midbrain regulates this response.

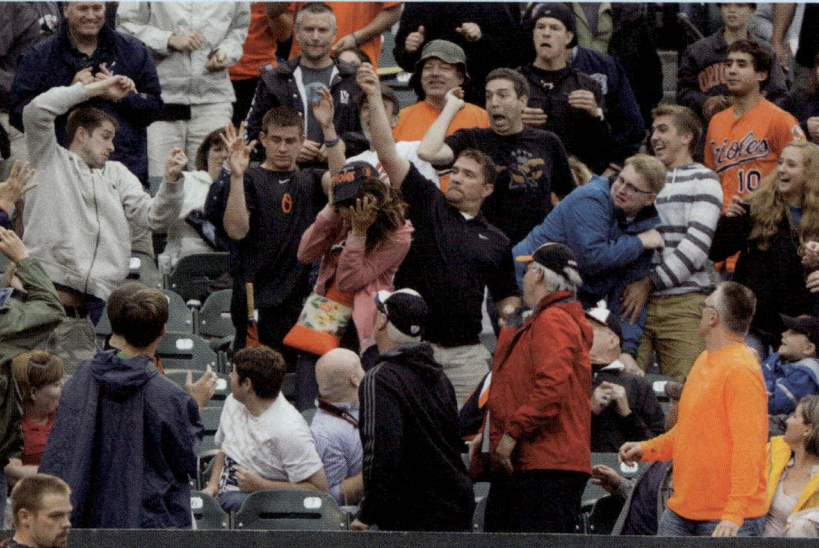

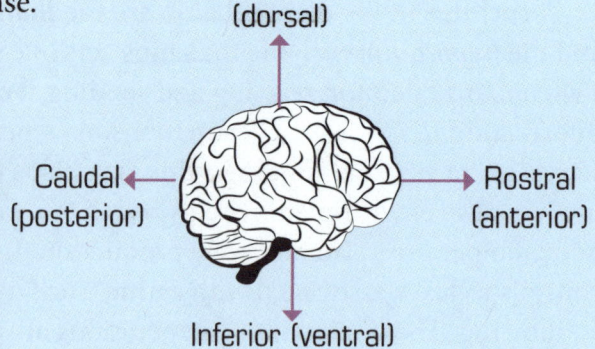

Superior (dorsal)
Caudal (posterior)
Rostral (anterior)
Inferior (ventral)

Another area found farther down the stem is the *pons,* which is Latin for "bridge." The pons is located anterior to (in front of) the cerebellum. It serves as a bridge connecting the cerebellum with the thalamus and helps relay sensory information between the structures.

Mesencephalon

Pons

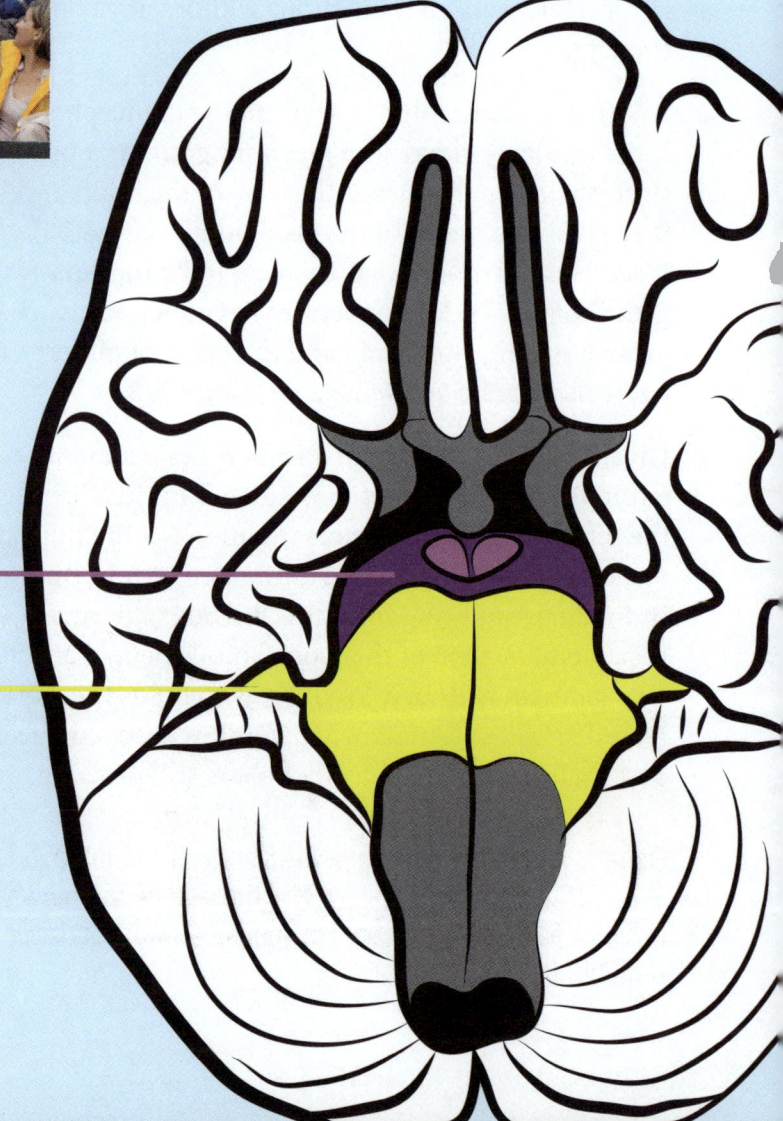

Word Wise!

The use of X-rays for imaging was the "BRAIN CHILD" of Wihelm Röntgen in 1895. The phrase "BRAIN CHILD" refers to creating a unique or original idea. It first appeared in dictionaries in 1881. An earlier variation of that same phrase in 1630 was called "brain brat."

God's Wondrous Machine

A Critical Area: The Medulla Oblongata

The *medulla oblongata* (try saying that a few times fast) is a critical area in the brain that controls the autonomic regulation of the cardiovascular (heart rate and blood pressure), respiratory, and digestive systems.

Do you recall what autonomic means? One can understand many words in medicine and science by breaking these scary, complex names into parts. "Auto-" means self, and "-nomic" means regulated, so putting these two root words together creates a word that means self-regulated. In even simpler terms, the medulla oblongata self-regulates the functions that a person does not have to think about or initiate. How many times a day do you remind yourself to breathe or tell your heart to beat? God has taken these life-sustaining functions out of your conscious thought and given them to the medulla oblongata to handle.

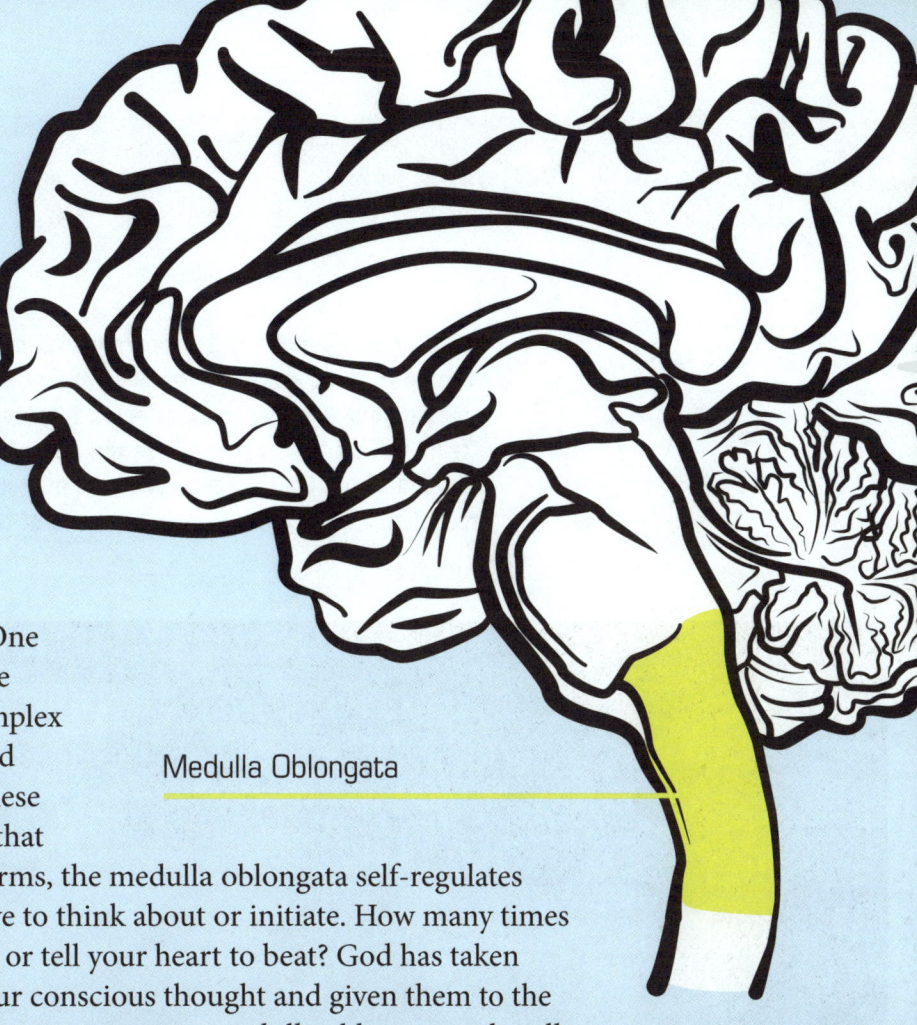

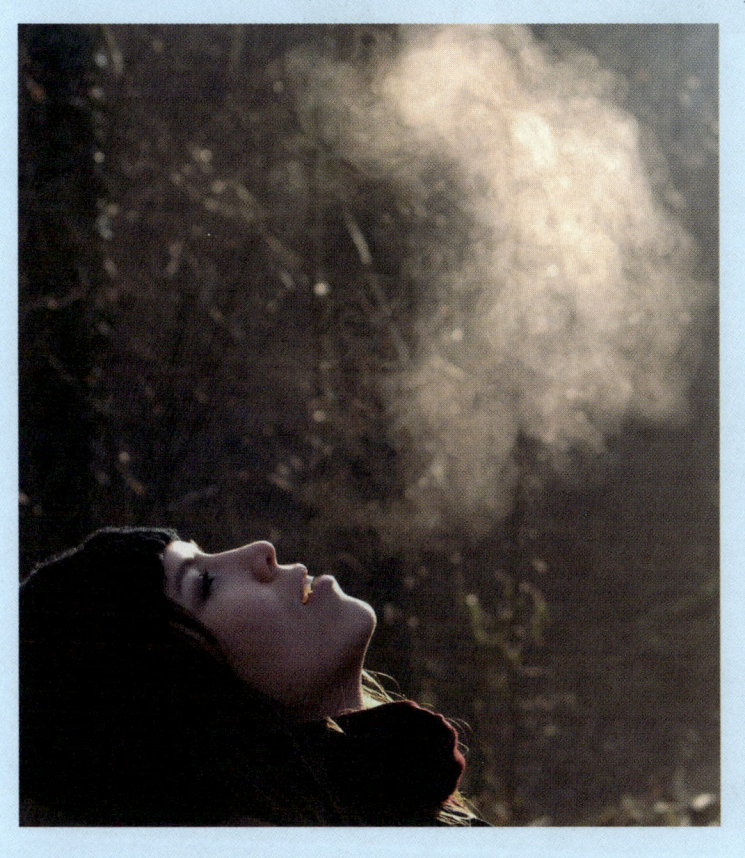

Medulla Oblongata

KNOW IT ALL

Your brain does not feel pain! It can sense and interpret pain in other parts of the body. So what is going on when we have a headache? Well, nerves in the neck and head are able to process the signals for pain - so while your brain isn't hurting, nerves nearby can let you know you have a headache somewhere around your head!

Unit 1: The Electrifying Nervous System

5 The Developing Brain

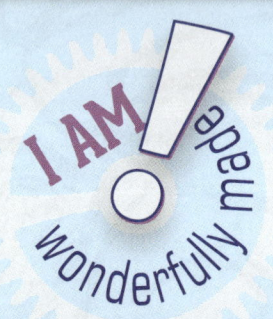

I AM wonderfully made!

PSALM 139:13-16: For you created my inmost being; you knit me together in my mother's womb. I praise you because I am fearfully and wonderfully made; your works are wonderful, I know that full well. My frame was not hidden from you when I was made in the secret place, when I was woven together in the depths of the earth. Your eyes saw my unformed body; all the days ordained for me were written in your book before one of them came to be. (NIV)

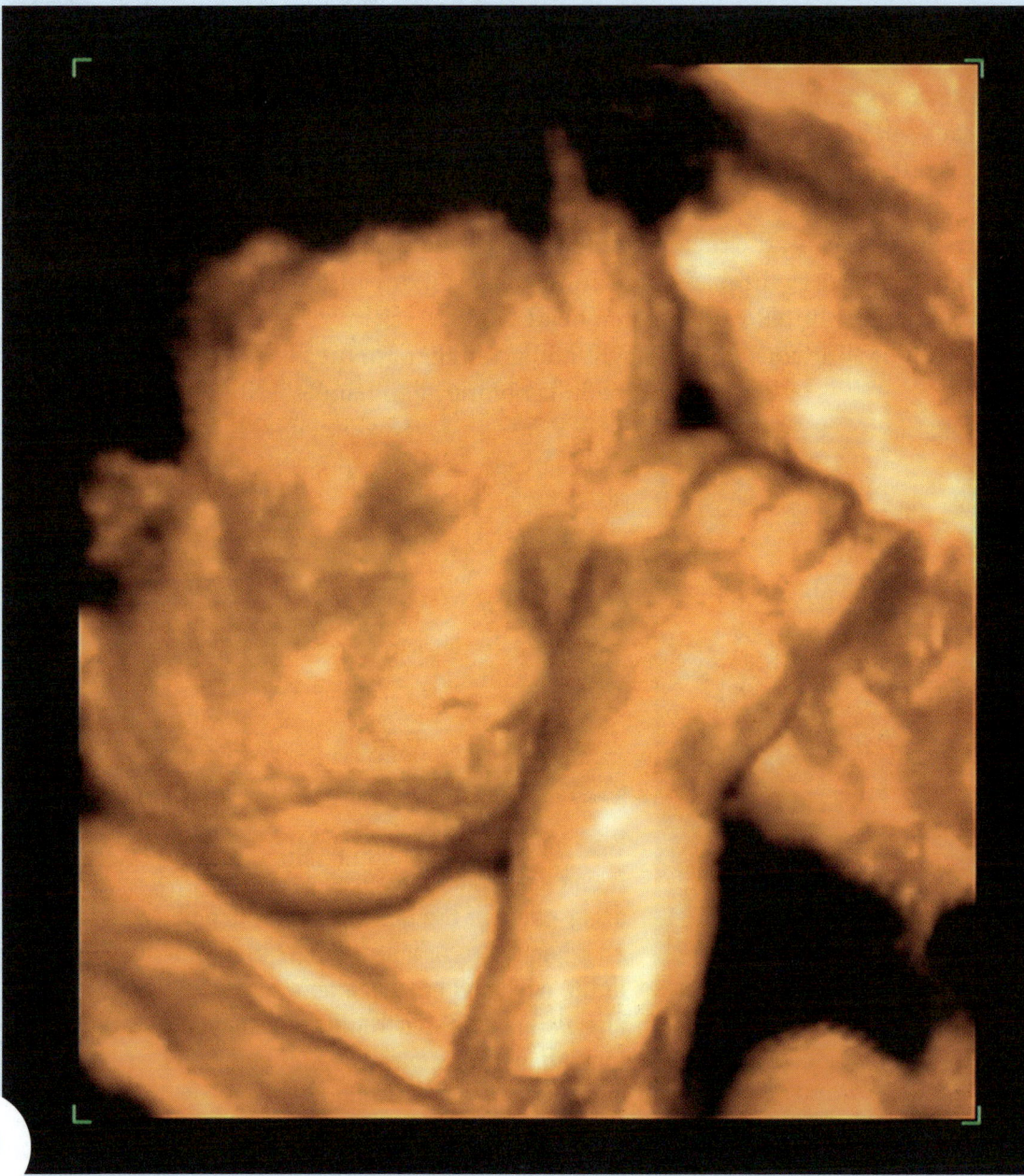

You were once small, very small before you were born. When you were growing inside your mother your brain went through many changes. By the time you were born, your brain weighed less than a pound, around the weight of 3 sticks of butter. That tiny package, your brain, at the time of your birth already contained billions of neurons.

3D Ultra Sound Image

God's Wondrous Machine

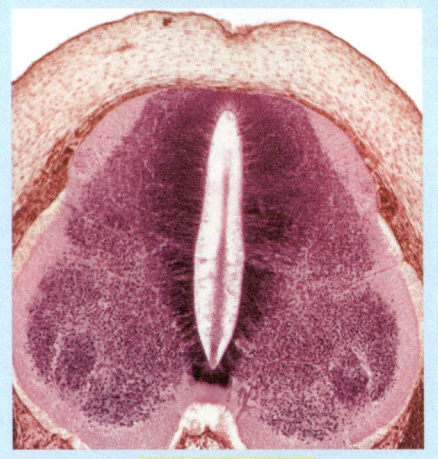

At 3 Weeks

Your central nervous system began to develop when you were 3 weeks old in your mother's womb. Your brain was shaped like a slipper called the neural plate. The edges of the neural plate enlarged and folded to form a tube. This tube is called the neural tube. It is from this one structure that your brain and spinal cord are formed. It is during this stage of life that a forming baby is most sensitive to injury in development. This also happens to be the time frame that most new moms are unaware of a new life developing inside them. At this stage you are the size of a poppy seed! God truly has each of us in His hands.

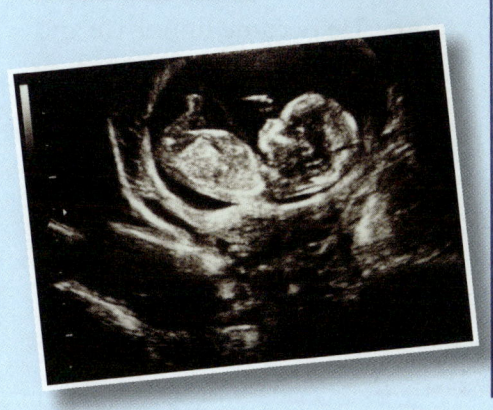

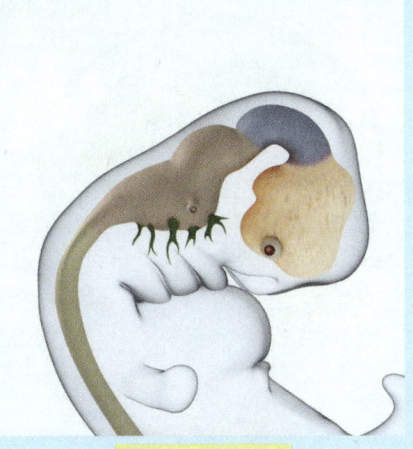

At 7 Weeks

Your brain has developed into five different areas. The cranial nerves, the nerves that originate at the base of the brain begin to develop. By 8 weeks, the brain has become highly developed and composes 43 percent of your total weight. Your growth at this point is proceeding at an exponential rate. The hypothalamus forms at this point. At this stage, you are the size of a blueberry!

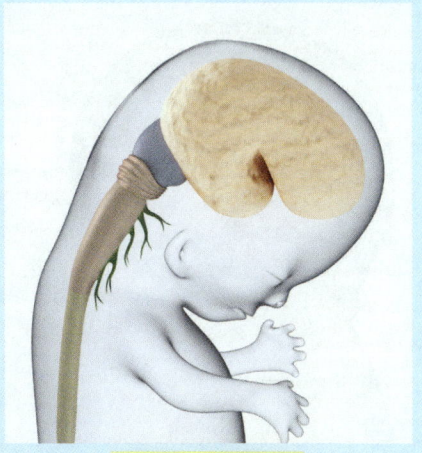

At 11 Weeks

At this point your head is the same size as your body. You are the size of a lime! Your brain is developing at 250,000 nerve cells a minute! You can even swallow and stick out your tongue. Most defects of the spinal cord occur at this time. Spina bifida occurs when the spinal cord and the vertebrae do not close at a particular level in the spine. It may lead to difficulty in walking once the child gets older.

MEDI+MOMENT

MODERN MARVEL: 3D AND 4D ULTRASOUNDS: It is important for mothers to remain healthy during pregnancy — and there are a variety of ways that doctors can check both her health and that of the baby. In some cases where other testing or concerns have hinted at possible problems, 3D ultrasound testing provides three dimensional images of the unborn baby. Essentially, sound waves are sent out, and the returning echoes are processed by computer into an image of the baby. These remarkably detailed scans can help check for any birth defects like spina bifida and to see if the baby's development is occurring as it should. 4D ultrasounds are similar, but they are often real-time and some even show movement of the baby.

Unit 1: The Electrifying Nervous System

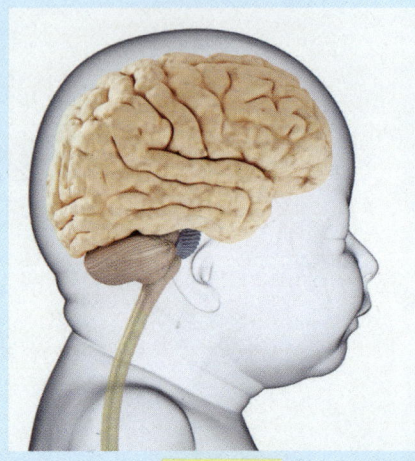

At Birth

Your brain weighs ⅔ to ¾ of a pound and has over a 100 billion neurons. At this point, your brain is fully capable to handling all your basic survival needs and primitive reflexes (see pg. 53).

The nerves in your brain are continuing to grow myelin around the individual neurons, and new neurological connections are being made. This is why a baby is unable to sit up and walk at birth because the brain has not become completely hardwired. When you were born you were able to recognize your mother's voice! This can be seen when a baby is held, the mother stands on one side and someone else on the other side, both call out to the baby simultaneously. The baby will turn its head toward the mother in recognition of her voice. Babies visit the doctor frequently in the first year of life, in order for the doctor to assist the parents in watching and monitoring the child's development.

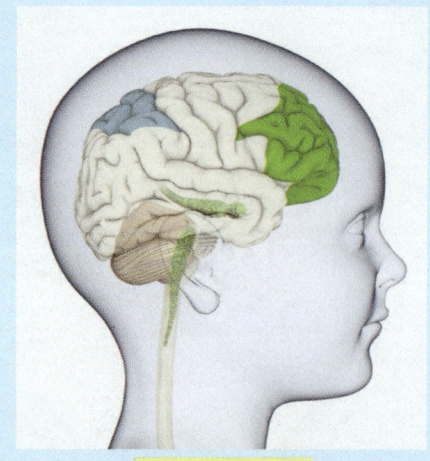

Infant Years

The 0–3 year old period is a time of rapid learning. Synapses — where electrical information can travel from one neuron to the next — are being formed. You travel from being totally dependent and unable to take care of yourself to beginning to establish independence. Many people call this period of development as the "terrible twos" because some children exert their independence and NO becomes a common utterance. Your brain has reached up to 80 percent of the adult volume by the time you were 3 years old.

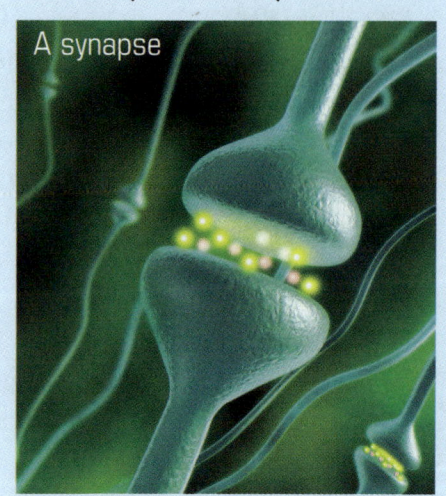

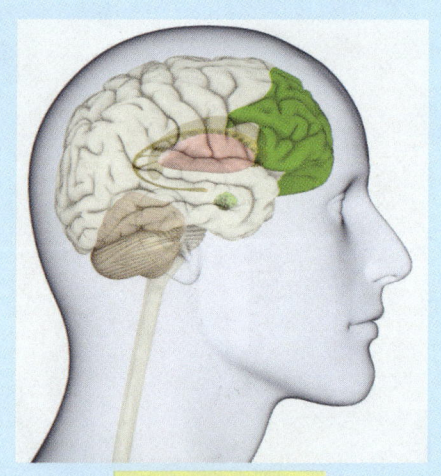

A synapse

Teenage Years

The teenage years are a very unique time in development. The teen looks like an adult in many ways, but brain development continues in these years as the teen transitions to an adult. Teens are far more capable of insight, judging their behaviors, reasoning, and concern for others. The frontal lobe is continuing to develop more myelination and this process is not complete until late adolescence. Some researchers demonstrate that frontal lobe development does not reach maturity until 25 to 30 years of age. Remember Phineas Gage? He had profound damage to his frontal lobe as a result of his injury. He became impulsive and demonstrated poor judgment. The regions in the frontal lobe that are responsible for assessing risk and judgment are the last to finish in development.

God's Wondrous Machine

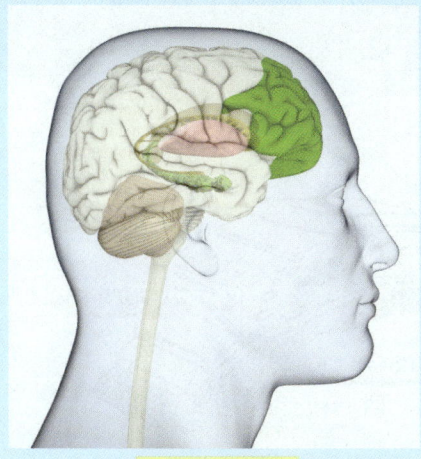

Adult Brain

In the adult brain, synapse formation is much slower. There is an old adage "use or lose it." Synapses in the brain are only formed due to experiences in life. If the brain is not exercised regularly by thinking, reading and challenging your thoughts, it will begin to atrophy, decrease in size. However, a mature brain can continue to grow and people can continue to gain wisdom and insight as they age and continue to keep their brains active.

KNOW IT ALL

A study of taxi drivers in London, England, in 2011 showed that portions of the adult brain tied to memory can get bigger. Basically, the gray matter of the hippocampus increased as drivers memorized thousands of details and street names for a difficult test called "All London" Knowledge over a two-to-four year period!

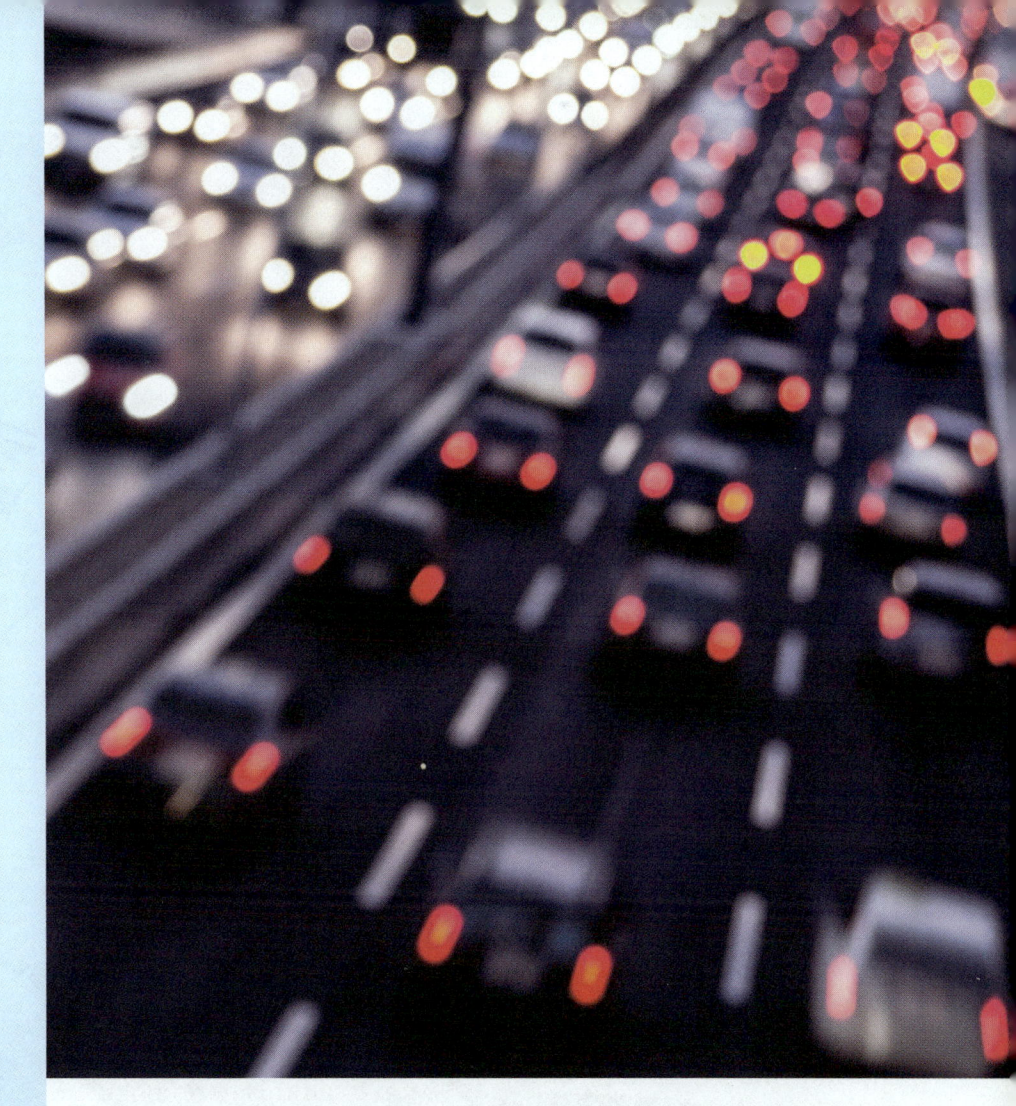

If you ever doubted how amazing your brain may be, think about all the things your brain does while driving — the things that you see and hear that your brain has to process like other cars, signs, specific lanes, changing speeds, signals for turning, someone using their brakes, obstacles in the road, listening to the radio, bad weather, or more! That's a lot of stuff happening every second a driver is behind the wheel!

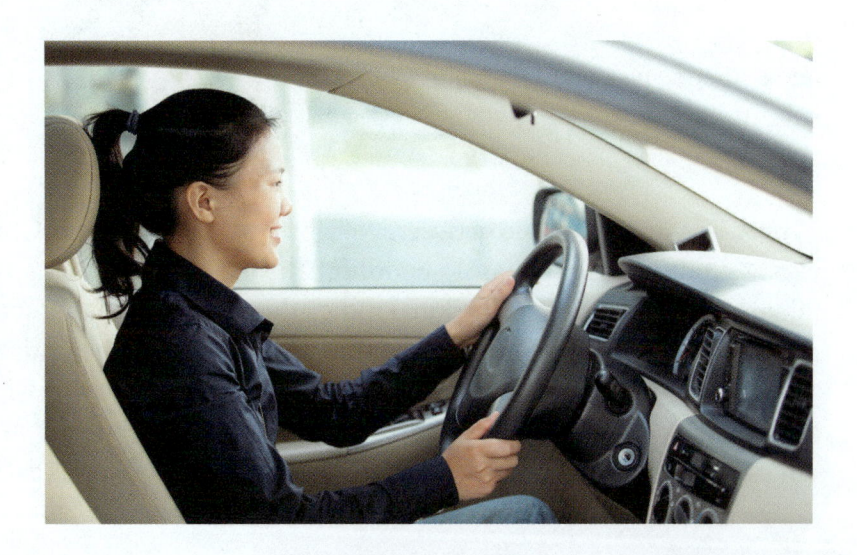

Unit 1: The Electrifying Nervous System

6 A Case for the Brain

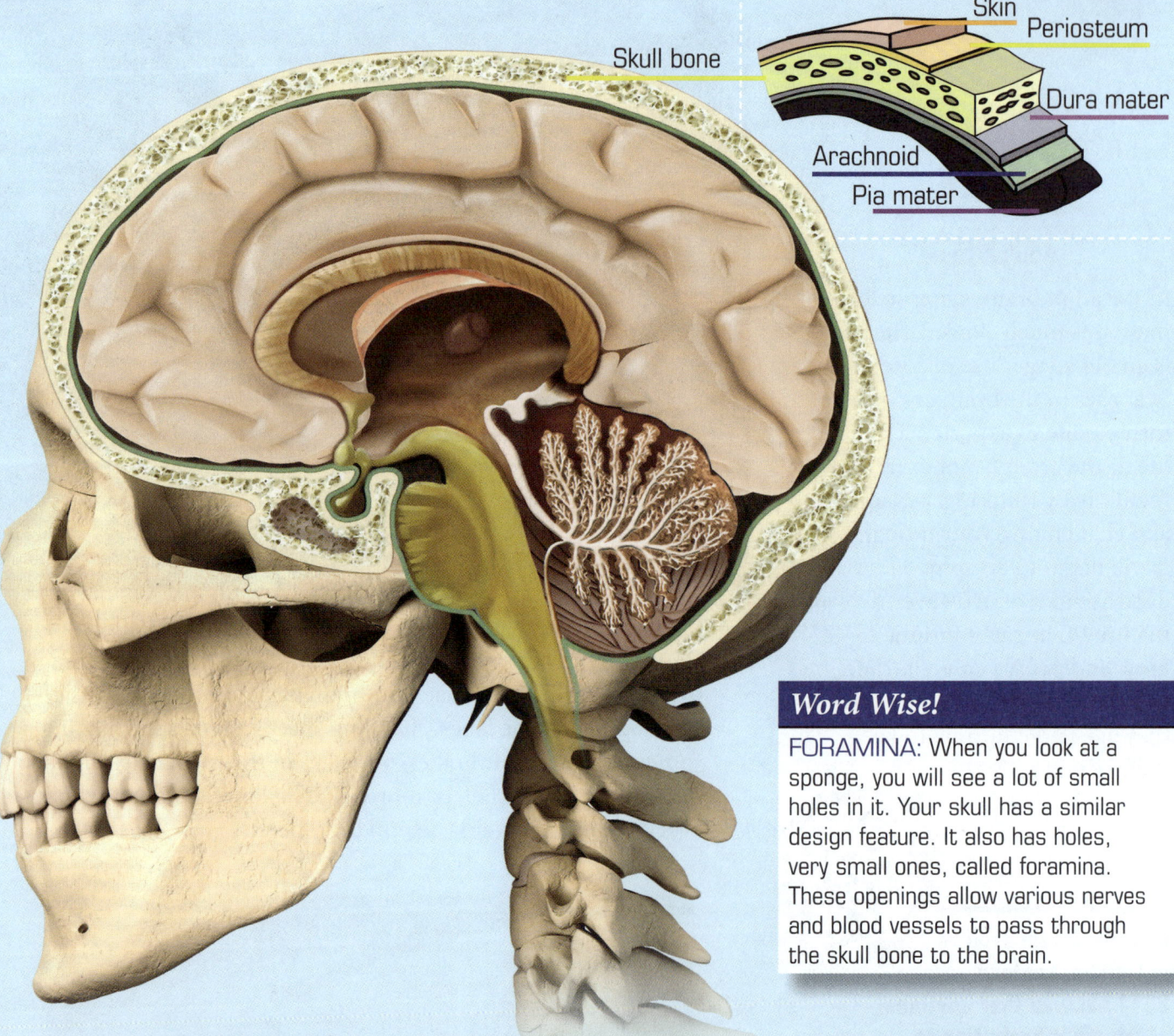

Skull bone
Skin
Periosteum
Dura mater
Arachnoid
Pia mater

Word Wise!

FORAMINA: When you look at a sponge, you will see a lot of small holes in it. Your skull has a similar design feature. It also has holes, very small ones, called foramina. These openings allow various nerves and blood vessels to pass through the skull bone to the brain.

There is very little space between your brain and your skull. Your brain has no padding. The brain floats within the skull. The skull cradles this delicate, sophisticated machine within the *cranial meninges*, which are three layers of tough, fibrous tissue that act like a safety belt to anchor the brain in position. A special fluid — called *cerebrospinal fluid* (CSF) — provides additional protection by keeping the brain bathed and buoyant. The body manufactures *cerebrospinal fluid* (CSF) within the brain's ventricles, which are in the central region of the brain. This lubricant bathes the neural structures and helps transport nutrients, chemical messengers, and waste products.

God's Wondrous Machine

The brain is much like the egg yolk and egg white in an eggshell — they are encased in a hard shell and covered with layers of tough fibrous covering that are also called the *meninges*. When you hard boil an egg and peel away the shell, the thin film that separates the egg white from the shell and egg yolk from the egg white is very similar to the cranial meninges.

Let us consider what happens if you take a raw egg and drop it. The outer shell would hit the floor and stop its forward movement upon contact; however, the yolk would continue its movement and slam against the shell. Just like the yolk, God designed the brain as a delicate structure unable to withstand forceful impacts, therefore it is encased in its hard armor, the skull. This is why so much emphasis is placed on protective headgear when engaging in activities such as bike riding and skateboarding.

The skull is a hard, nonflexible covering over the brain. Between the skull and the brain is a network of blood vessels. An impact to the skull can cause the brain to move within the hard shell, which causes these blood vessels to tear away. These vessels can bleed and cause pressure and damage to the brain. Rupturing blood vessels between the *Dura mater* (the outermost of the three meninges) and the brain is called a *subdural* bleed. The prefix "sub-" means "under;" therefore, subdural means "under the *Dura*."

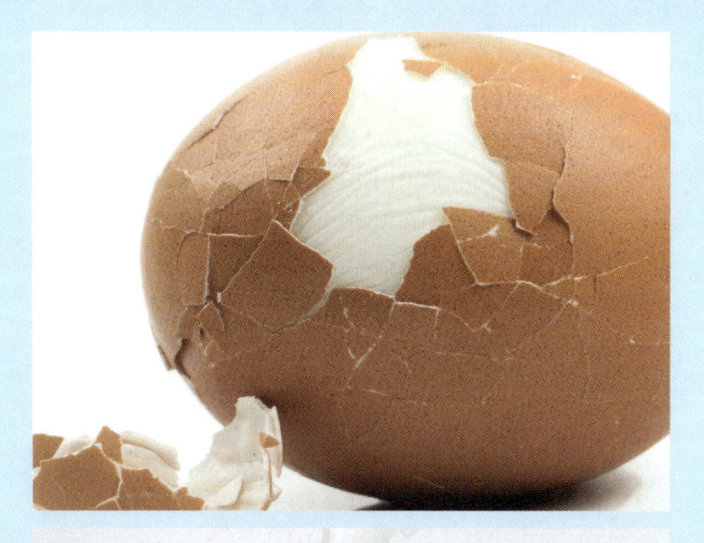

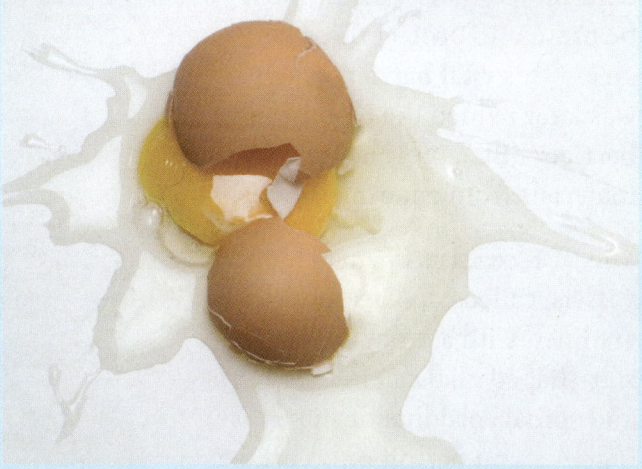

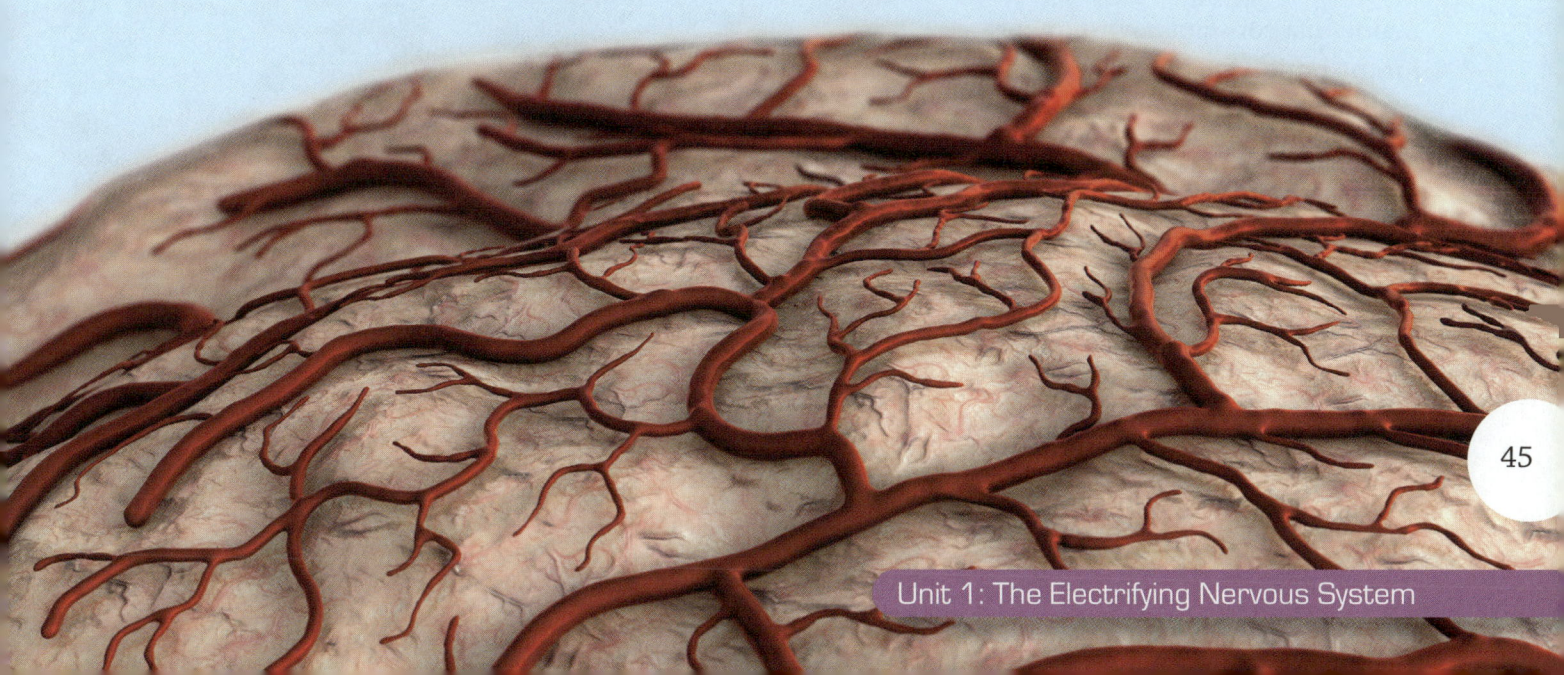

Unit 1: The Electrifying Nervous System

7 The Gate Keeper: The Blood Brain Barrier

A special barrier lies between the brain and the rest of the body. In the late 1800s, Paul Ehrlich discovered that, if an animal's bloodstream was injected with a blue dye and the anatomy of the animal was examined, all of the body's tissues retained the dye except for two key areas: the brain and the spinal cord. After a series of experiments, Mr. Ehrlich determined that a barrier must be present to protect these key areas. This vital barrier, which was later named the blood-brain barrier (BBB), prevents unwanted materials from entering the brain.

The BBB consists of small blood vessels, called capillaries, which are lined with astrocytes, a star-shaped glial cell in the brain and spinal cord that fit snugly together and permit only certain substances to get through. The BBB protects the brain from substances that may damage the brain and helps the body maintain a constant environment for the brain. The brain is very particular: it likes things just so. Many things have the potential to destroy this fortified castle gate to the brain, such as high blood pressure, infections, radiation, and traumatic head injuries.

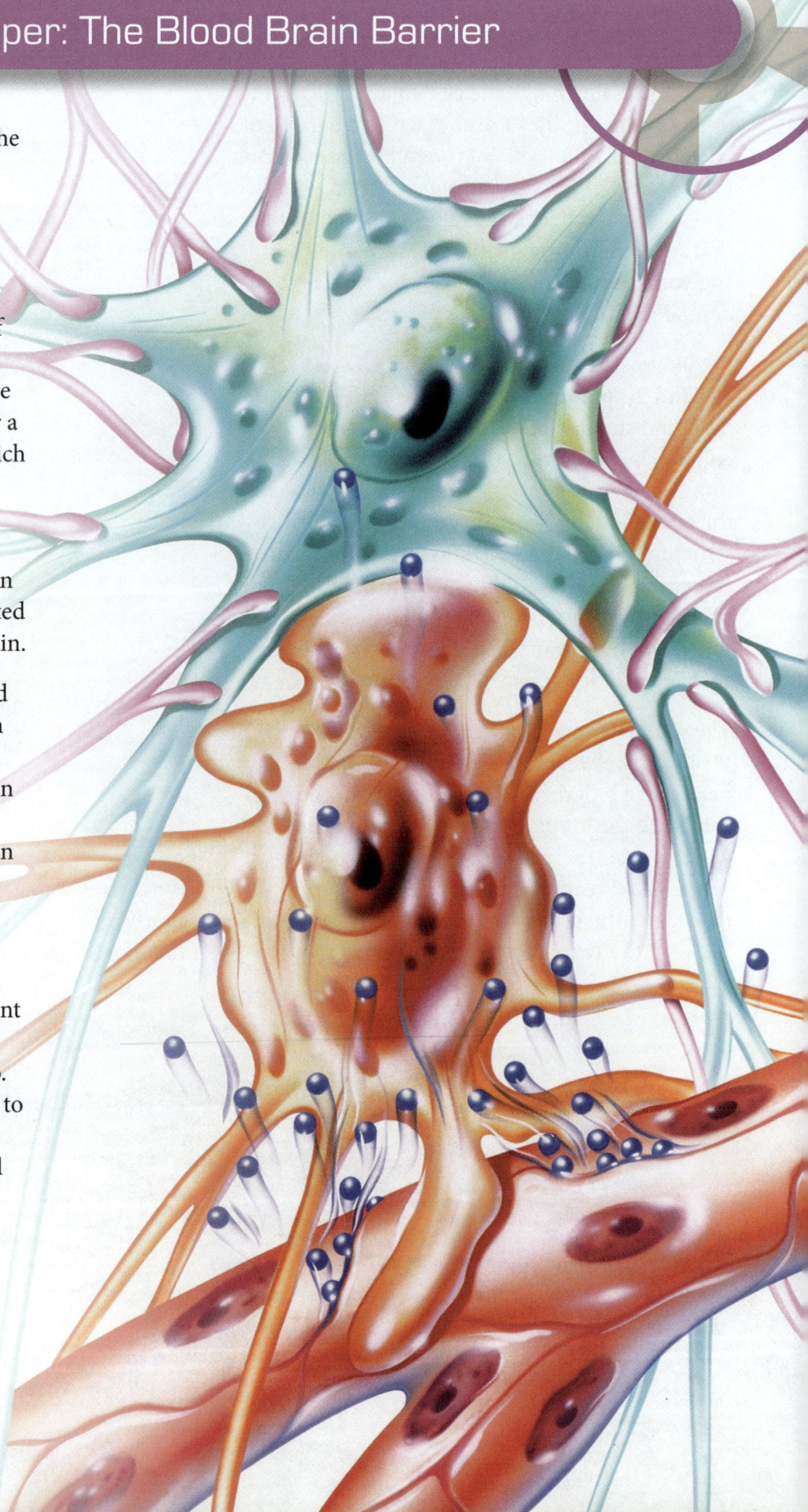

God's Wondrous Machine

Spinal Cord

The spinal cord is a nerve column, like an electrical extension cord, that runs from the base of the brain down through a bony tunnel called the vertebral canal. The cord is a network of nerve fibers that are composed of 31 paired segments. A pair of spinal nerves exits each vertebra in the spine. Your spinal cord connects your brain to the rest of your body. The spinal cord is protected inside your backbone. The spinal cord allows your arms, your legs, and the rest of your body to send information to your brain. As well, it allows your brain to send back information to the rest of your body.

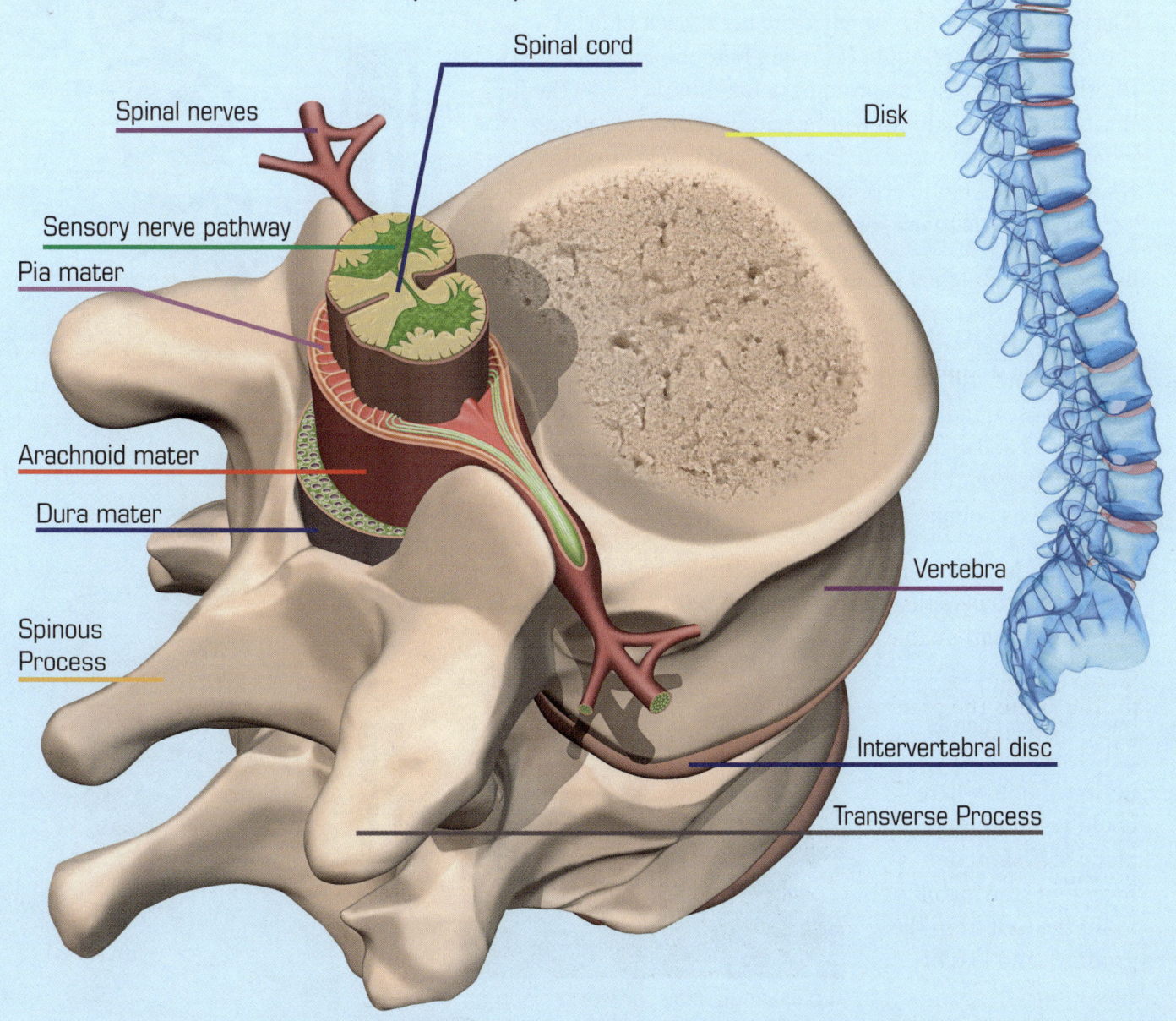

Spinal cord
Spinal nerves
Disk
Sensory nerve pathway
Pia mater
Arachnoid mater
Dura mater
Spinous Process
Vertebra
Intervertebral disc
Transverse Process

Unit 1: The Electrifying Nervous System

8 The Great Stabilizer: The Backbone

"Wow, she really is the backbone of the team!" This is an expression you may hear someone say about the star player for an athletic team. The star player consistently shows up to play hard, is dependable, and is a stabilizing force on the team. Just like this star player, your backbone is a real stabilizing structure in your body. Without your backbone, you would be a bag of skin and organs in one large clump. The spinal column, more commonly called the backbone consists of:

Cervical Area C1-C5: Supplies the neck, back of head, shoulder, and diaphragm. If broken here the injury is life-threatening. The diaphragm (a flat muscle below the lungs that assists in breathing) will be paralyzed and breathing would need to be supported by a special machine called a respirator. A person becomes a quadriplegic. This means the person is unable to use his or her arms or legs.

C5- T1: The Brachial Plexus resides here. If the spine is broken here the person would not need the assistance of a respirator. The person would be able support his or her own breathing but still lose function below that level. This also would cause quadriplegia. Have you have ever injured your leg and needed crutches? If you are not careful and lean on the crutches, your hands will feel numb. This is due to the nerve plexus being compressed.

T2-T12: This area supplies the torso. Injury at this level would lead to paraplegia. This is the inability use one's legs and leaves them unable to walk.

L1-5, S1-S5: Lower back, legs, feet and gluteal region (the bottom). Injury here could result in bowel and bladder dysfunction, a drop foot (the inability to lift the foot from the ground), and loss of sensation.

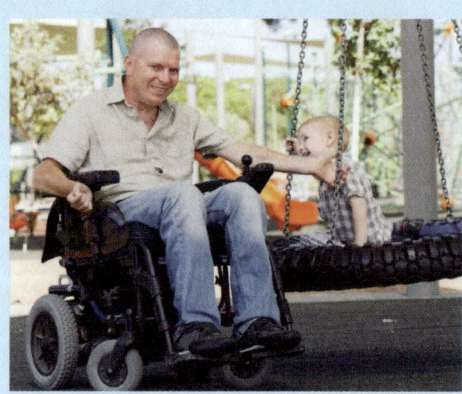

A paraplegic playing with his son on a playground.

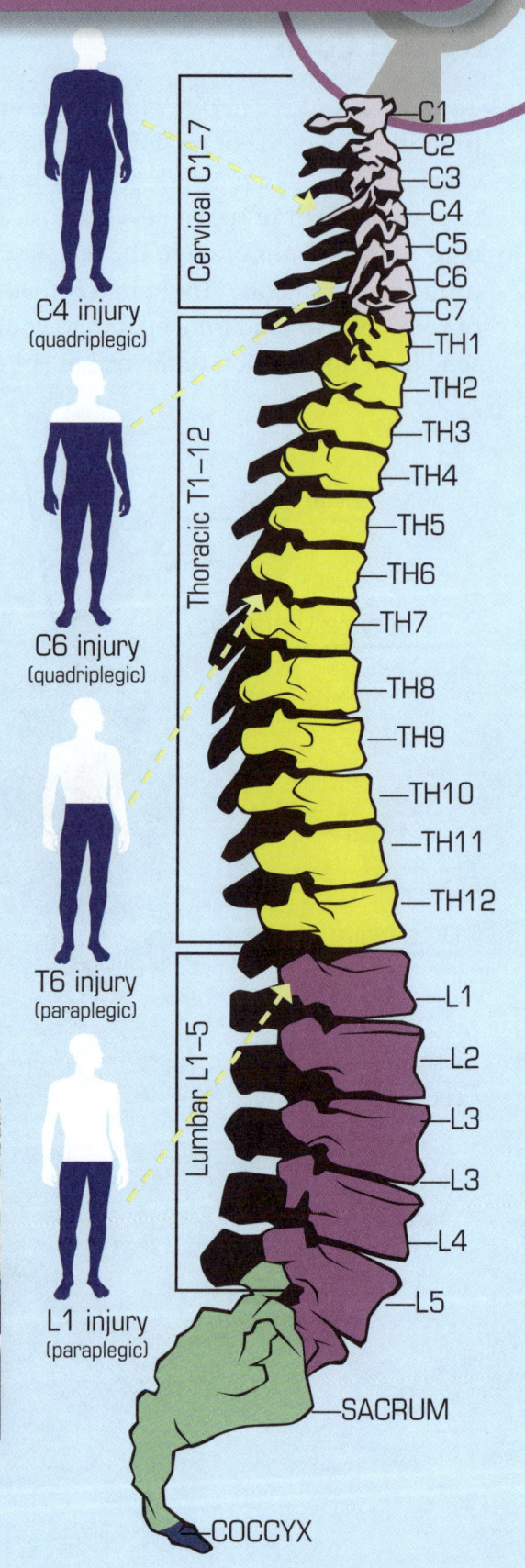

C4 injury (quadriplegic)
C6 injury (quadriplegic)
T6 injury (paraplegic)
L1 injury (paraplegic)

Cervical C1-7: C1, C2, C3, C4, C5, C6, C7
Thoracic T1-12: TH1, TH2, TH3, TH4, TH5, TH6, TH7, TH8, TH9, TH10, TH11, TH12
Lumbar L1-5: L1, L2, L3, L3, L4, L5
SACRUM
COCCYX

48

God's Wondrous Machine

The bony vertebral column that encases the spinal cord has four distinct regions: cervical, thoracic, lumbar, and sacral. A pair of nerves exits each segment and provides the nerve supply to the skin as well as the organs in that region. These nerves permit the skin to receive sensory information about hot, cold, pressure, and touch sensations. An injury to a particular level of the spine will bring dysfunction at that level and below.

The regions of the skin are connected to a pair of separate nerve roots. These regions are called **dermatomes.** An uncomfortable phenomenon relating to the dermatomes is the illness called **shingles**. Shingles is related to the chicken pox virus. Once the virus has infected a person, the virus may go dormant (asleep) after the initial infection and take up residency in a spinal nerve root. At various times, the virus may reactivate and cause problems only in a particular dermatome of that spinal root ganglion. (**Spinal ganglion** are tightly packed groups of nerve cells that lie in a bundle at the site in which the nerve exits the spinal cord. It looks like the bulb of an onion root.)

Cold sores around the mouth are caused by another type of virus that becomes dormant in the nerve roots. It is a small sore that can spontaneously erupt on your skin in times of stress or illness. Seventy to eighty percent of all people are affected by this virus by the time they become adults.

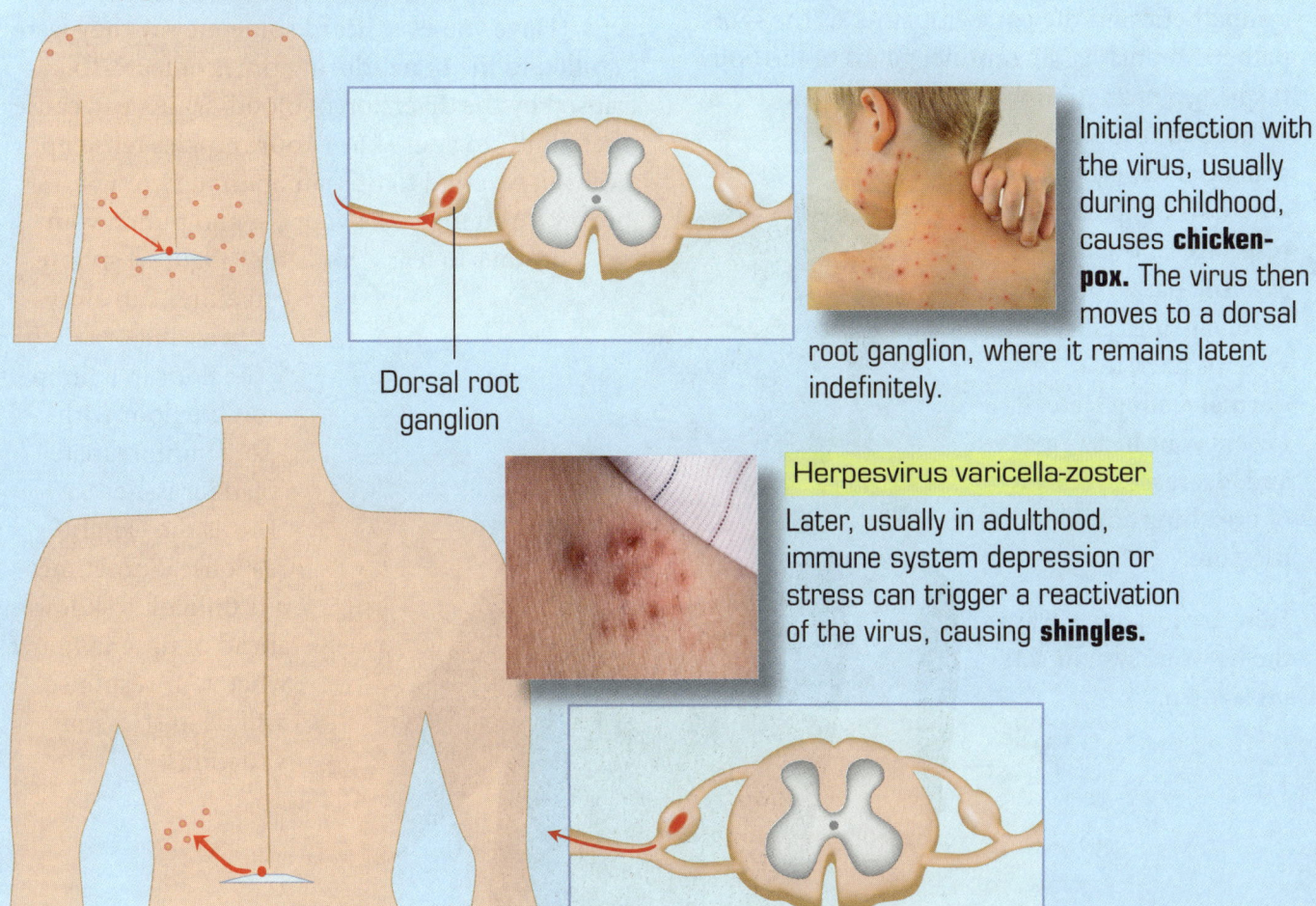

Dorsal root ganglion

Initial infection with the virus, usually during childhood, causes **chicken-pox.** The virus then moves to a dorsal root ganglion, where it remains latent indefinitely.

Herpesvirus varicella-zoster

Later, usually in adulthood, immune system depression or stress can trigger a reactivation of the virus, causing **shingles.**

49

Unit 1: The Electrifying Nervous System

9 It's Simply Automatic

God has designed the nervous system to do a number of things automatically. These automatic responses help people in surprising ways to survive and protect themselves.

The Autonomic System is the part of your nervous system that does not require your conscious attention to control. It controls functions such as heart rate, rate of your breathing, digesting your food and even when you need to urinate or defecate (these are polite terms for going to the bathroom). Isn't it great that you don't need to remember to tell your lungs to breathe or your heart to beat? It would be exhausting to remember all these things.

This independent part of the nervous system can be divided further into two branches, the sympathetic and the parasympathetic. The sympathetic branch is the sentinel guard of the body. It springs into action when you are under stress or need to respond to an emergency situation. One example, is seen in the "fight or flight" response (more on this pg. 51). The parasympathetic branch brings all your systems back to a normal resting state. It lowers your heart rate and, decreases your rate of breathing and blood pressure.

Here are just a few ways the nervous system acts on its own.

FIGHT OR FLIGHT

Let's say, you are walking down the stairs to a dark, damp basement. Straining on your tip toes, you are unable to reach the cord to the overhead light. You feel a bit uneasy being down in the darkness. Suddenly, your calculating devious little brother decides to spring out from behind a wall and yell "Boo!" Instantly, the sympathetic branch of your nervous system is activated. Nervous system impulses are sent to your glands and muscles. Stress hormones (adrenalines) are released. Instantly, your heart rate and blood pressure increase. The pupils in your eyes get wider to allow more light for you to see. The blood vessels in your skin constrict (become smaller) so that precious blood can be diverted to your large muscle groups, like your legs. (Have you ever heard someone say they were "chilled to the bone" during times of fear? This is caused by the diversion of blood, which can cause that "chill" to your skin.) Your muscles tense up. You can respond to this situation in two types of ways. You may take your fist and punch your brother in fear. This is the "Fight" response. You either run away screaming or fall to the floor in a lump on the floor with some unfortunate bladder issue. This is the "Flight" response. Sometimes it is difficult to know ahead of time to know what your response will be in stressful situations.

God's Wondrous Machine

A United States Navy SEAL is a highly trained soldier in the military. They undergo the toughest military training in the world. A key aspect of this training is to learn to override one's natural bodily flight and fearful responses and remain focused on the task at hand.

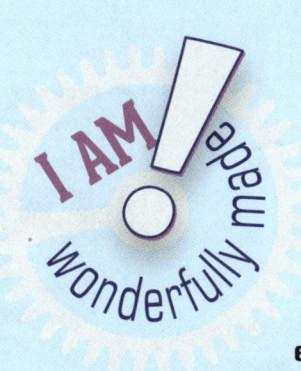

I AM wonderfully made!

God has designed us to have ability to experience this world in many ways through our senses. Have you ever walked into a place and experienced a smell that evoked a strong memory? The area of the brain that controls emotions and memories also houses our sense of smell. This is why smells can be linked to memories.

The FIGHT or FLIGHT Response

THREAT: an attack, harmful event, or threat to survival

BRAIN: the brain processes the signals — beginning in the amydala, and then the hypothalamus

ACTH: pituitary gland secretes adrenocorticotropic hormone

Cortisol released

Adrenaline released

PHYSICAL EFFECTS
- heart rate increased
- bladder relaxation
- tunnel vision
- shaking
- dilated pupils
- flushed face
- dry mouth
- slowed digestion
- hearing loss

Unit 1: The Electrifying Nervous System

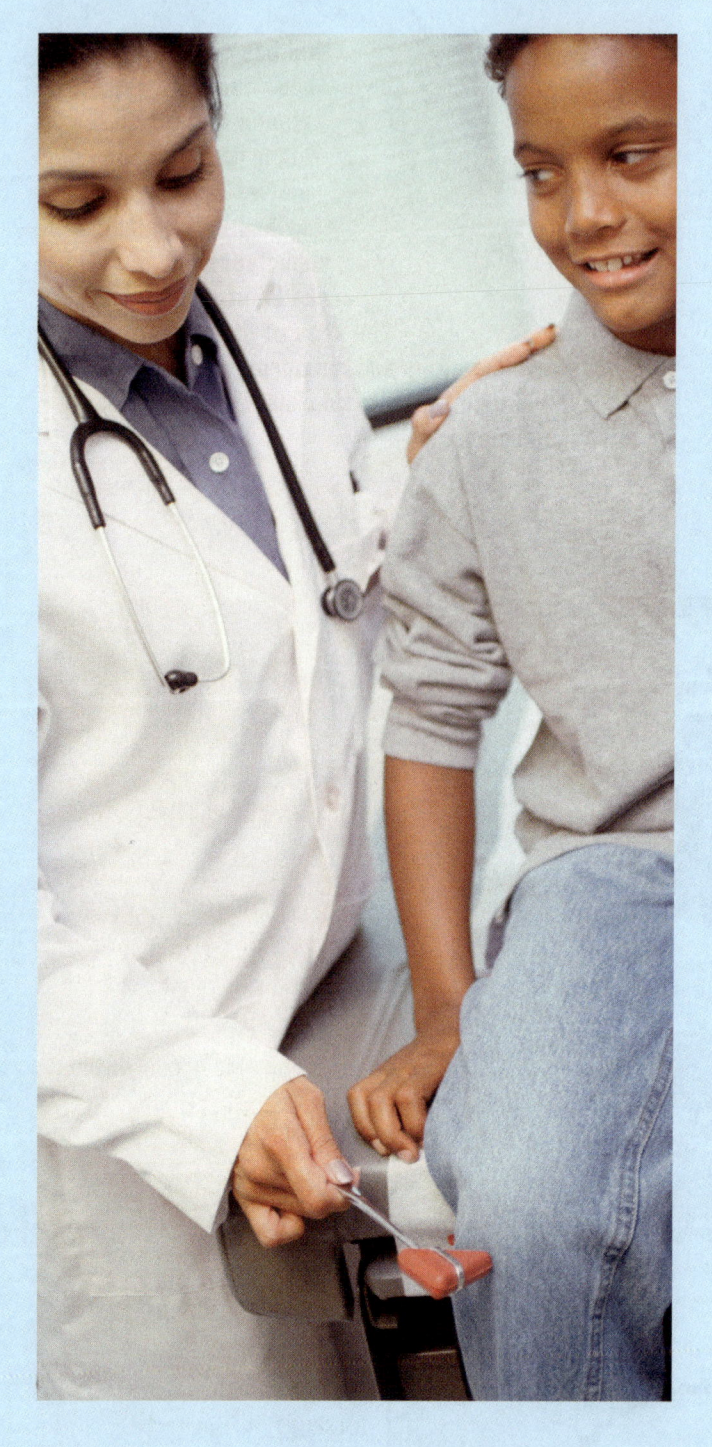

REFLEX ARC

In this incredible design, God has equipped us to respond through our senses when we need to give immediate attention to a situation. When our peripheral nervous system picks up sensory information, it sets our reflexes in action. Reflexes enable us to respond quickly without thinking. For example, if you encounter an irritating stimulus, such as stepping on a nail in your bare feet, your peripheral nervous system activates the receptors in that area of the skin. This sensory stimulus runs to the spinal cord, to the dorsal root (posterior nerve or sensory root). This signal bypasses the brain and immediately sends information to the ventral root (anterior nerve or motor root at the same level) where the muscles react to the unpleasant stimulus. Without thinking, you quickly withdraw your foot, yell "ouch," and hop into the air from the painful nail.

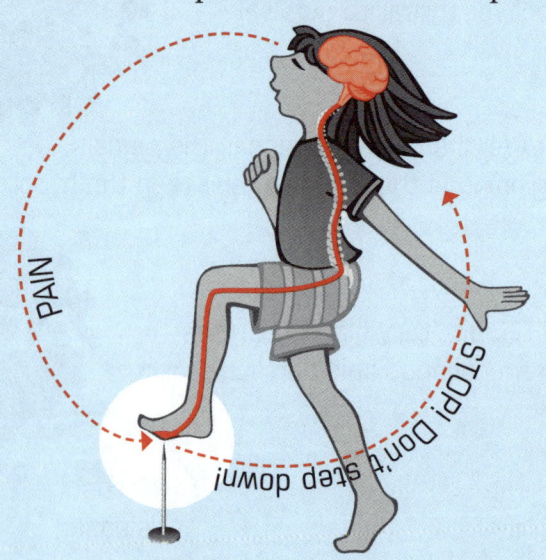

Our bodies possess many reflexes that a doctor can elicit with a reflex hammer to assess whether the nervous system is working properly. For example, if your doctor strikes your knee, your lower leg kicks out. This is a reflex.

God's Wondrous Machine

Step reflex

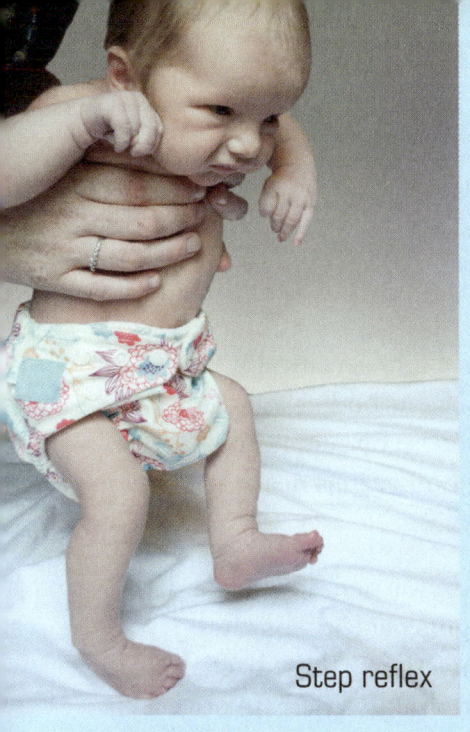

Babies are born with many protective reflexes that disappear as the baby grows older. For example, the rooting reflex is present in a baby to urge them to latch on to their mother's breast to nurse and find nourishment. The rooting reflex is activated when someone rubs a baby's cheek; the baby will turn its head toward the stimulus and open its mouth wide. It is common for babies to try to latch on to anything, including an unsuspecting nose.

The **tonic neck reflex,** or "fencers pose," occurs when a baby is lying on its back with its head turned to one side and its arms take on a characteristic fencing pose. Like a fencer, one arm goes up as the other arm extends out. You can almost hear the baby saying, "En garde."

The **grasp reflex** occurs when the baby reflexively holds onto anything placed in the palm of its hand. The startle or **Moro reflex** occurs when a baby hears a loud noise. The baby startles; both arms fly out in extension; and, many times, the baby will begin to cry.

Some reflexes can also be normal at one point in life and very abnormal later in life, such as the **Babinski reflex.** During infancy, when someone strokes a baby's foot from the heel forward, the baby's toes spread out and big toe extends up. For most babies, this reflex eventually goes away. After infancy, when someone performs this same motion, the toes will curl down. If the Babinski reflex is present later in life, it is a sign of a brain injury.

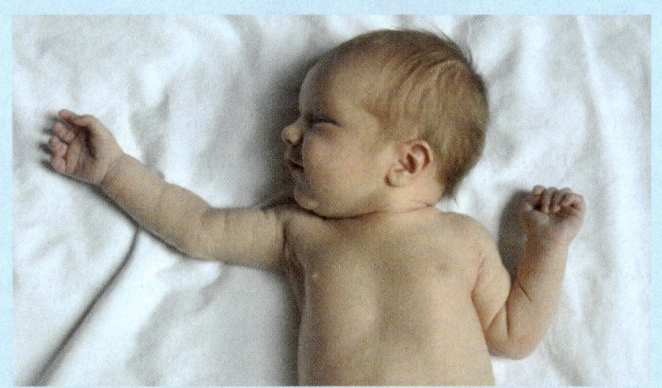

Tonic neck reflex

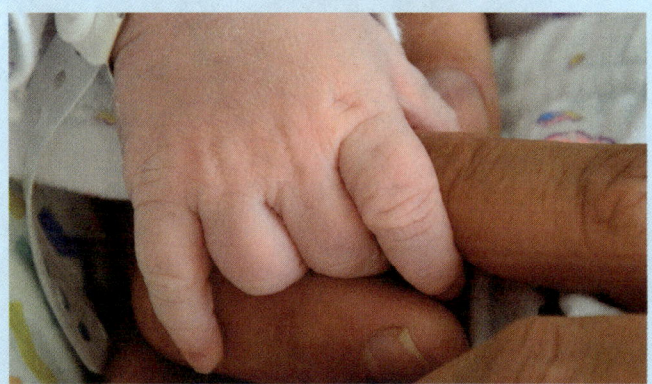

Grasp reflex

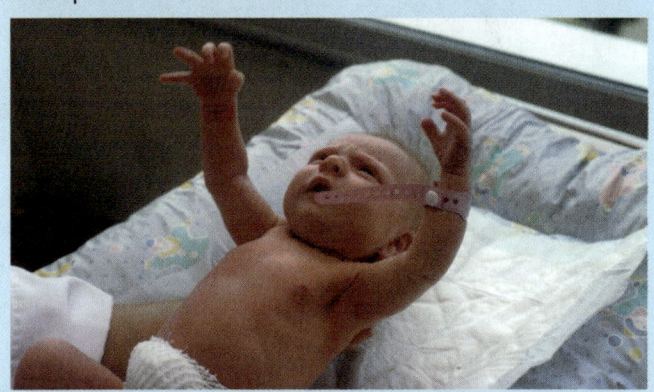

Moro reflex

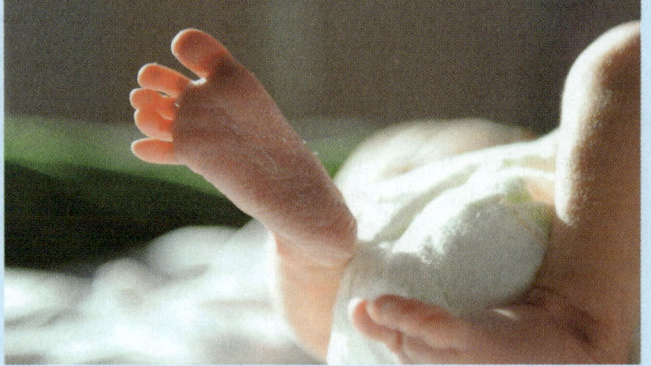

Babinski reflex

Unit 1: The Electrifying Nervous System

10 Take Good Care: Health Facts

Fevers

Our temperature control or thermostat is located in the brain's *diencephalon,* more specifically, the *hypothalamus*. It helps maintain the body's normal temperature. It causes our bodies to heat up by shivering when we are cold. Our shivering muscles help increase our metabolism by generating heat. It also can help cool our bodies down by causing us to sweat. By causing the blood vessels near the skin to enlarge (dilate), the body allows more heat to escape.

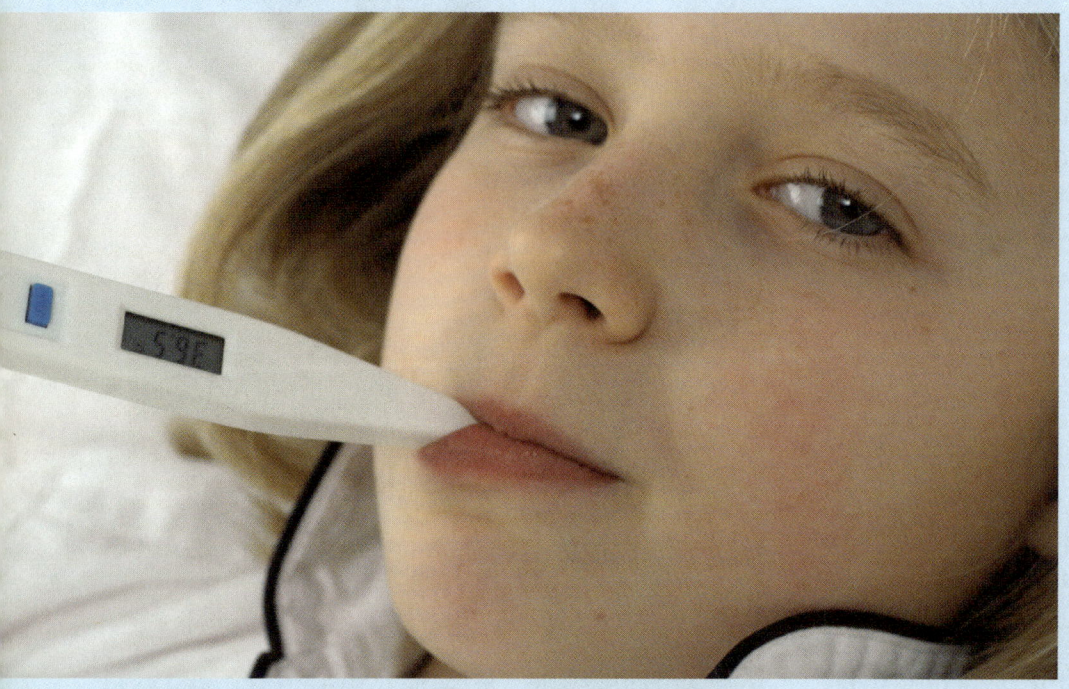

Fever is one way our body fights bacterial or viral infections. These bacterial or viral invaders do not like high temperatures. A fever, also called *pyrexia,* is a higher-than-normal body temperature; normal body temperature is 98.6°F for most people. Fevers are an immune response. The body recognizes the bacteria as alien invaders in the body and releases substances called *pyrogens* that tell the hypothalamus to dial up the thermostat. For example, when your internal thermostat turns up, say to 101°F, your body shivers and you retreat under a pile of blankets in an effort to reach your new higher set point temperature. When your temperature goes down and your hypothalamus resets your temperature back to normal (when your "fever breaks"), you sweat.

Word Wise!

Normally, a human body should have a temperature between 98 and 100 degrees Fahrenheit. The HYPOTHALAMUS is located just above the brain stem. It not only helps to control temperature, but it also houses temperature sensors and helps to trigger sweating and other cooling methods. Hypothalamus comes from the combination of "hypo," meaning under and thalamus "part of the brain where a nerve emerges."

God's Wondrous Machine

Brain Freeze

Sphenopalatine ganglioneuralgia
(sfee-noh-pal-uh-teen-gan-glee-oh-new-ral-juh)

Now that is a mouthful! This gargantuan word is better known as a "brain freeze." Have you ever bitten into a yummy ice cream cone and suddenly clutched your head yelling, "OW!"? Have you ever wondered why this occurs? We all scream for ice cream.

The roof of the mouth, the palate, has nerves and blood vessels that are very sensitive. Cold temperatures on the palate set off an alarm system in those nerves and blood vessels. The nerves control how much blood flows to your head and quickly respond by causing blood vessels in the head to swell. This is the brain's attempt to direct more blood to the area in order to warm it up. This quick swelling causes the head to pound. No damage occurs to the brain; only those vessels react. Fortunately, a brain freeze only lasts 30 seconds or less. The cure for the brain freeze is to eat ice cream slowly, no biting — and keep the ice cream off the roof of your mouth! Just lick it and keep it from contacting the roof of your mouth.

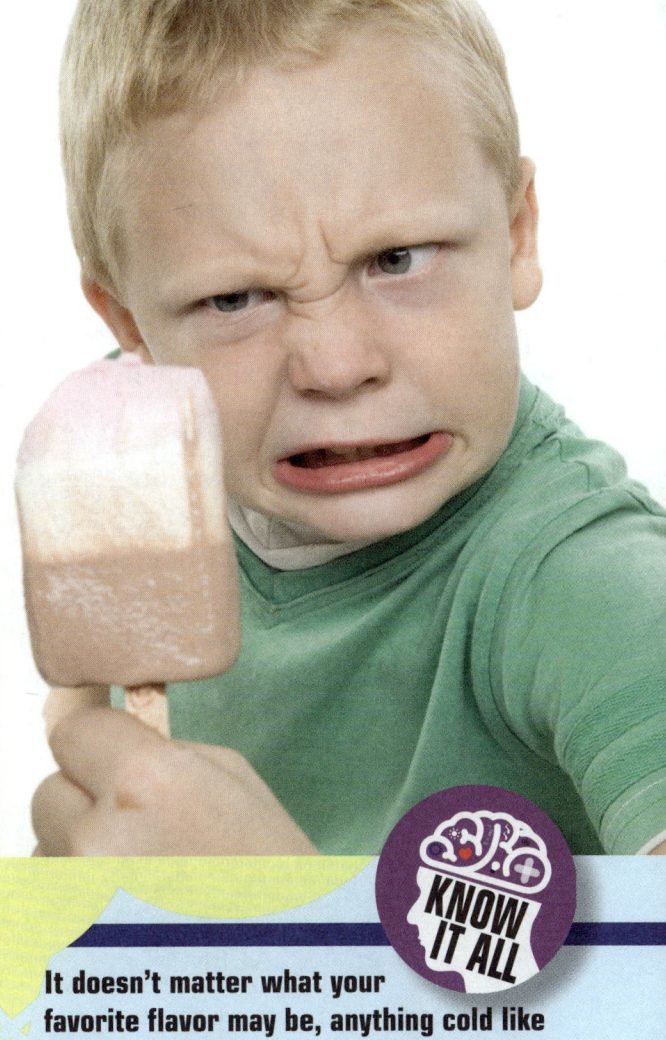

KNOW IT ALL

It doesn't matter what your favorite flavor may be, anything cold like frozen treats or ice cream can be a pain! Though brain freezes don't last long, they definitely hurt. Try tilting your head backward for several seconds, or even pressing your tongue up against the roof of your mouth for a moment. Breathing in warm air to your nasal passages and even drinking something warm can help.

Unit 1: The Electrifying Nervous System

Nite-Nite, Sleep Tight

It has been a long day. You yawn and your eyelids feel heavy. Your eyes begin to flicker shut. Your head bobs up and down as you slowly slip into the first stages of sleep.

Sleep is a huge part of your 24-hour day, and even during sleep, God has designed your body to still be at work. If you add all the time you've spent sleeping by the time you reach 70 years old, you would have slept over 20 years of your life! As you get older, your need for sleep decreases. A newborn baby sleeps 12 to 18 hours a day. School-age children need 10 to 11 hours. Adults require 7 to 9 hours a night. It is during sleep your body does some of its best work! The body uses sleep to repair, grow, and rejuvenate itself. You may have noticed when you are sick or injured you sleep even more.

You will cycle through the various stages of sleep in a night. NREM sleep Stage 1 to Stage 2 to Stage 3 back to Stage 2 and then REM. There are periods in the night in which your sleep is lighter. This is part of the reason a baby will awake several times through the night — not only to feed. Babies, as they grow older, have to learn to self soothe and get back to sleep on their own.

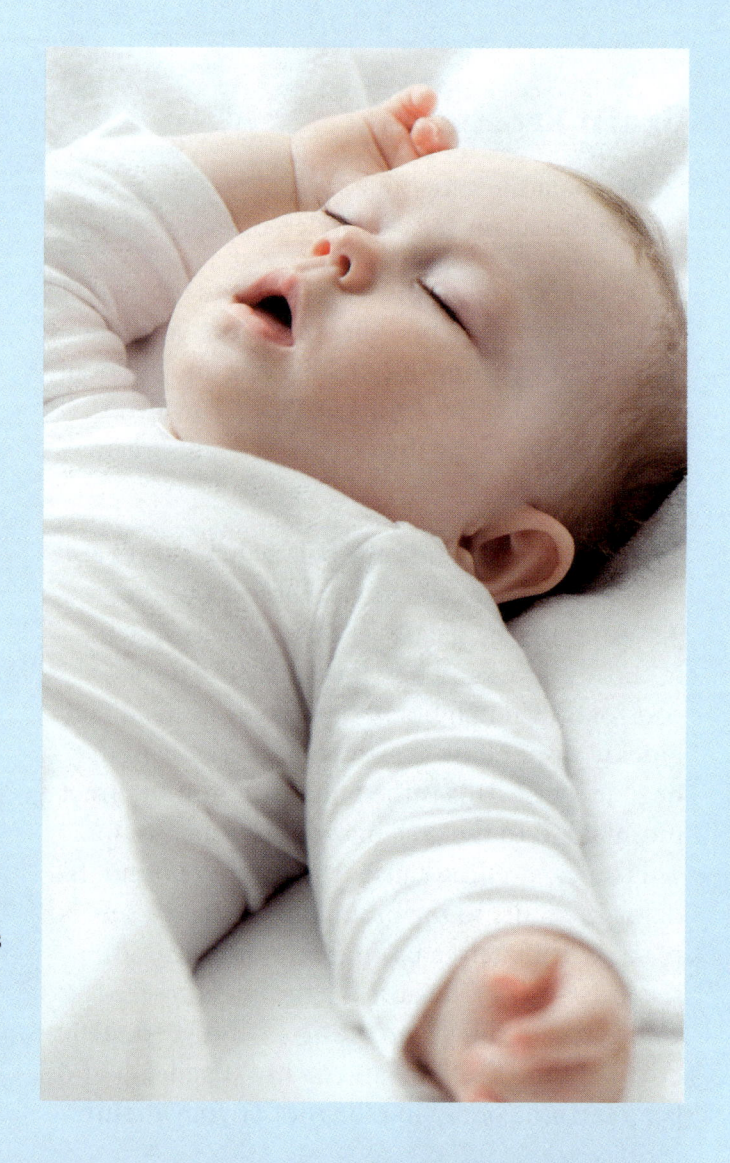

There are two major periods of sleep your body moves through during the night, Rapid Eye Movement Sleep (REM) and Non Rapid Eye Movement Sleep (NREM). Most of your sleeping is NREM, while REM is usually when we are dreaming.

NREM	REM
Sleep is composed of three stages. Stage 1 is when your eyelids feel heavy and you begin to nod off to sleep. It is not uncommon to have sudden twitches or jerks of your body prior to dozing off to sleep. You become a bit harder to awaken during Stage 2 sleep. Stage 3 is when things really slow down. Outside sounds and noises do not disturb your slumber.	The phase of sleep in which you dream. Your brain is as active as if you were awake. You can tell by observing sleeping people when they have entered this stage because their eyes will dart rapidly back and forth under their eyelids. It is also during this stage when you experience a type of paralysis, being unable to move. Your body protects itself through this type of paralysis so that you do not "act" out your dreams.

God's Wondrous Machine

I AM wonderfully made!

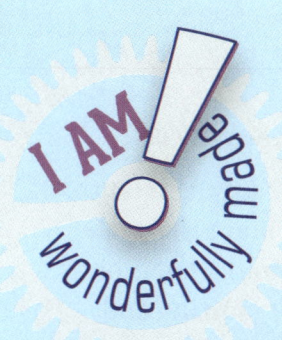

PSALM 4:8 **In peace I will lie down and sleep, for you alone, Lord, make me dwell in safety.**

Many sleep disorders occur during the REM stage of sleep. Two sleep disorders experienced are **Narcolepsy** (NAR-ko-lep-see) and **Cataplexy** (CA-tuh-pleks-ee). Narcolepsy can be very problematic. One moment the person can be laughing and engaged in a lively conversation then suddenly fall deep asleep. People with this disorder can have many sudden episodes of this a day. These episodes of sleep can be as brief as 30 seconds and last up to 30 minutes. You can imagine with the potential of this striking at any moment could place a person in a dangerous situation. People who suffer from Narcolepsy do not go through the stages of sleep but fall directly into REM sleep. Cataplexy is similar to the paralysis that happens during REM sleep.... except the person is awake! These attacks happen at the onset of intense emotion like happiness, fear, or grief. The person will collapse to the ground unable to move while being fully awake. These episodes do not last long.

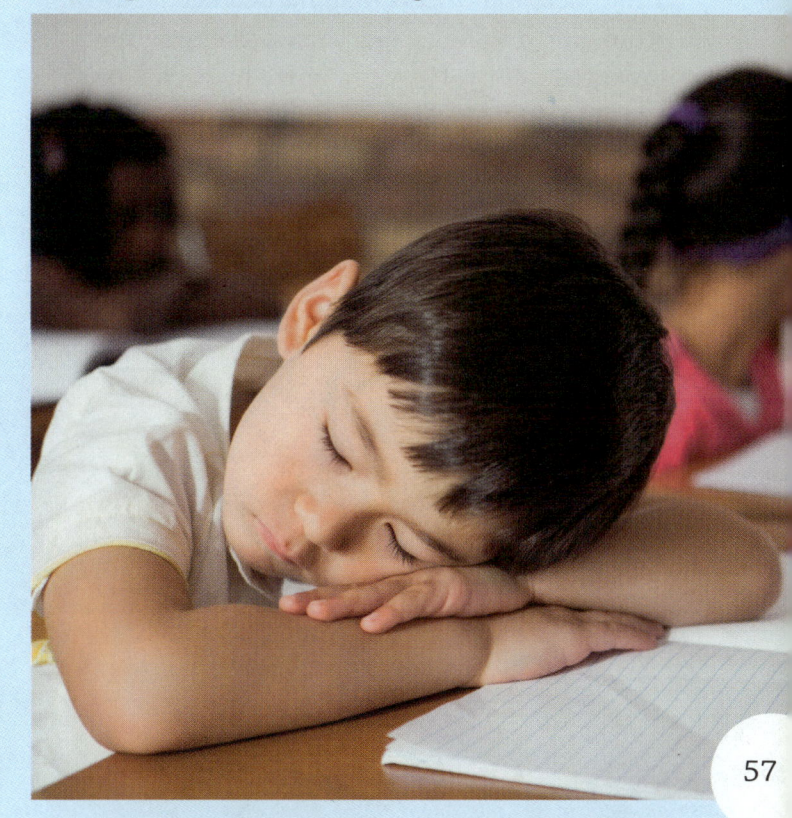

Five Stages of Sleep

Stage 1 (NREM)	When you are barely asleep, almost like daydreaming.
Stage 2 (NREM)	When we are slowly becoming unaware of the sights and sounds around us, more relaxed, breathing rate is normal and regular, and our body temperature starts to drop a little.
Stages 3 and 4 (NREM)	When we are breathing slower, very relaxed muscles, deep and restful sleep, our energy reserves are being re-energized, the muscles are getting more blood, and tissue repair is underway.
Stage 5 (REM)	Our closed eyes are moving back and forth, our muscles are not moving, we are dreaming, and the cycle continues around every 90 minutes after we fall asleep.

Adapted from "What Happens When You Sleep?," National Sleep Foundation, sleepfoundation.org

Unit 1: The Electrifying Nervous System

Sleepwalking

Somnambulism (som-nam'by?-lizm) is the scientific name for sleepwalking. Sleepwalking typically occurs in the first one to three hours after a person falls asleep. Sleepwalkers typically do not remember the incident. The sleepwalker's eyes may be open and appear glassy. In other words, the lights are on, but no one is home. Sleepwalking is most common in children, and many kids will outgrow these episodes by their teen years.

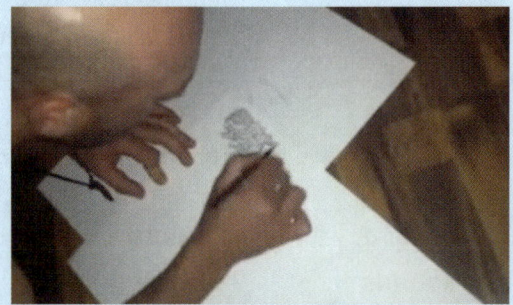

Lee Hardwin drawing in his sleep.

Common factors that may contribute to sleepwalking are fatigue, irregular sleep schedules, some medications, stress, or illness. The condition is not dangerous in itself. However, unusual behaviors have been reported while sleepwalking. A man named Lee Hadwin, from North Wales, experienced sleepwalking quite frequently. He was a nurse by occupation, but at night he became an artist. He would awake from his sleep to find incredible, awe-inspiring works of art. He never remembered drawing these masterpieces, but he soon discovered his hidden talent.

Why Your Brain Is Always Awake!

While you may have to be in bed by a certain time to get enough sleep, your brain is always awake! While you are sleeping and sometimes dreaming, your brain is busy organizing and filing away the things we have learned or seen that day. If something really good or bad happened, then those things can often be a priority for your brain to store as a memory.

Many areas of the brain are awake and active during sleep. However, sleep deprivation, lack of sleep, can have big effects on your body also. The world record holder for the longest period without sleep is up for debate. The most scientifically documented case is held by seventeen-year-old Randy Gardner in 1964. At the time of his record of 11 days continuous without sleep, he was heavily monitored in the Stanford Sleep lab. There have been other accounts of others who have attempted to break this feat. It is said that Maureen Weston of Cambridgeshire, UK, set a record of lack of sleep for 14-18 days during a rocking chair marathon in 1977. It was stated that she suffered from hallucinations, blurred vision, slurred speech, and memory/concentration lapses. All of these symptoms cleared after sleep was returned. *The Guinness Book of World Records* no longer records or recognizes any attempts for voluntary sleep deprivation. The concern is that this practice could be harmful to the record attempter's health.

Word Wise!

SOMNAMBULISM (Som-nam-byuh-liz-uhm) is an abnormal condition of sleep in which motor acts (as walking) are performed

God's Wondrous Machine

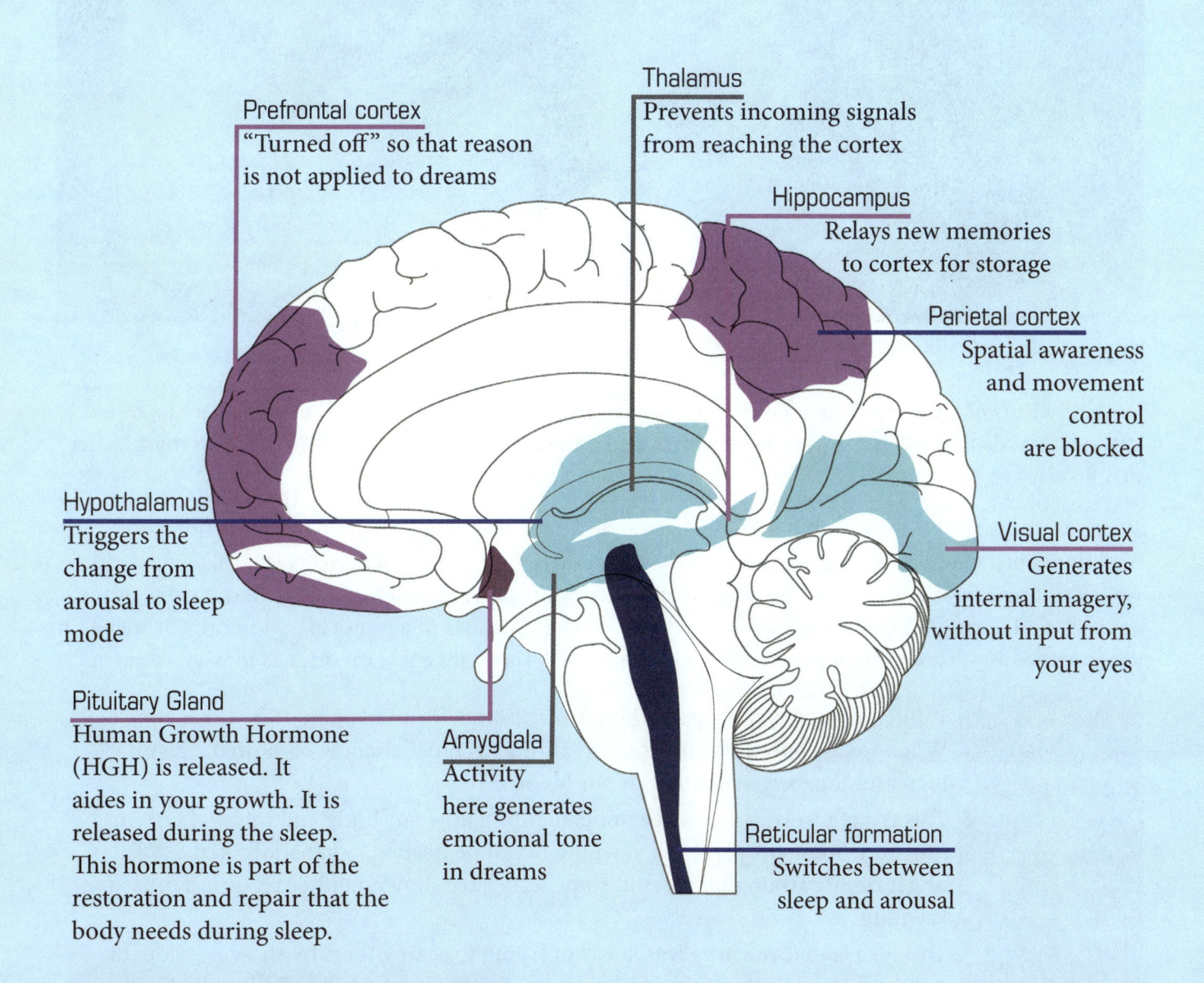

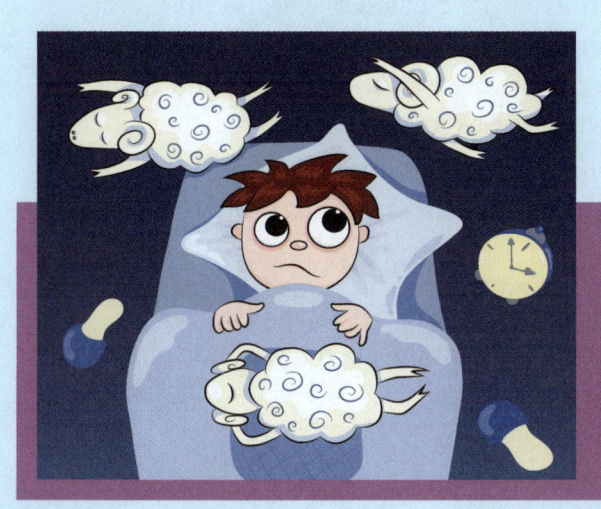

Prefrontal cortex
"Turned off" so that reason is not applied to dreams

Thalamus
Prevents incoming signals from reaching the cortex

Hippocampus
Relays new memories to cortex for storage

Parietal cortex
Spatial awareness and movement control are blocked

Hypothalamus
Triggers the change from arousal to sleep mode

Visual cortex
Generates internal imagery, without input from your eyes

Pituitary Gland
Human Growth Hormone (HGH) is released. It aides in your growth. It is released during the sleep. This hormone is part of the restoration and repair that the body needs during sleep.

Amygdala
Activity here generates emotional tone in dreams

Reticular formation
Switches between sleep and arousal

Ever heard counting sheep helps you sleep? Actually, it's not that effective. According to a study done by Oxford University, expending more mental energy is more effective in helping a person sleep rather than just a repetitive distraction.[1]

Unit 1: The Electrifying Nervous System

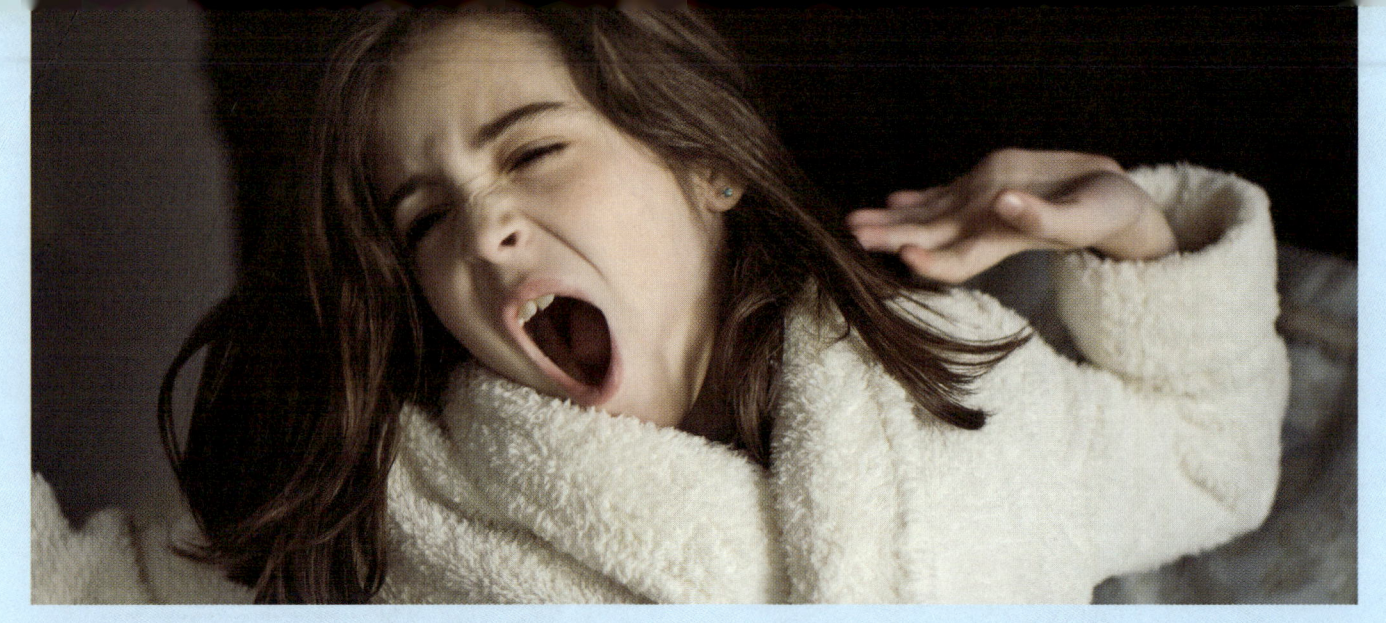

Yawning

First, all kinds of creatures, not just humans, yawn. Dogs, cats, lions, birds, and even fish are included among animals that yawn. So why do we yawn, and why does one person yawning seem to make other people want to yawn too? Try it sometime and see what happens!

We don't know all the answers, but here is what we do know. Yawning is an involuntary action — meaning it just happens without us deliberately planning it. Our mouths start to open really wide and we take a huge breath of air. Our chest muscles expand and contract, and then we blow out some of the air. It could happen because we are sleepy or bored, or even because of a physical condition, but we begin yawning before we are even born, as early as 11 weeks old. There are a few theories as to why we yawn[2]:

Boredom	While yawning can happen when we are bored, it can happen other times too. When we are bored or tired, our breathing becomes shallow or slowed. Yawning increases the oxygen content in our blood.
Physiological	This is a big word referring to understanding how our body and internal systems function. Some people think yawning might be needed to get additional oxygen or get rid of carbon dioxide, but some tests have shown neither really is a cause for yawning.
Evolution	This idea is that yawning was a way of trying to scare others by showing more of our teeth. But, remember how Adam and Eve were created by God in the Garden of Eden — they didn't need to scare anything by showing their teeth. Sometimes when we don't know the answer to something, people use evolution to try and explain it, when in reality — no one really knows what causes it.
Brain cooling	Scientists are studying if yawning happens when our brains are warmer. The idea is that when our brains are cooler, it is clearer and we are more alert. Interesting idea, but again, nothing has been proven yet.

So, while we don't know why we yawn, we do know that one person who yawns can often make someone else yawn too. They seem to be a little contagious! But for humans, you have to be older than four years old before you can "catch" someone else's need to yawn.

God's Wondrous Machine

MEDI+MOMENT

The Human Brain Project began in 2013 and is an effort by European researchers to build a computer that works like our brains do. The biggest challenge — computers haven't been invented that are fast enough. The computer would have to be 1,000 times faster than computers are today. It is estimated that it will take over a billion and a half dollars to create. (Fox News, 10/07/13)

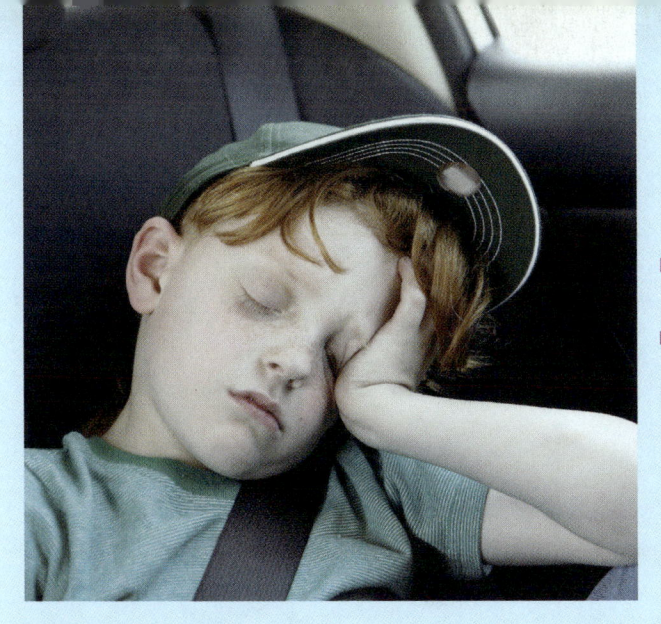

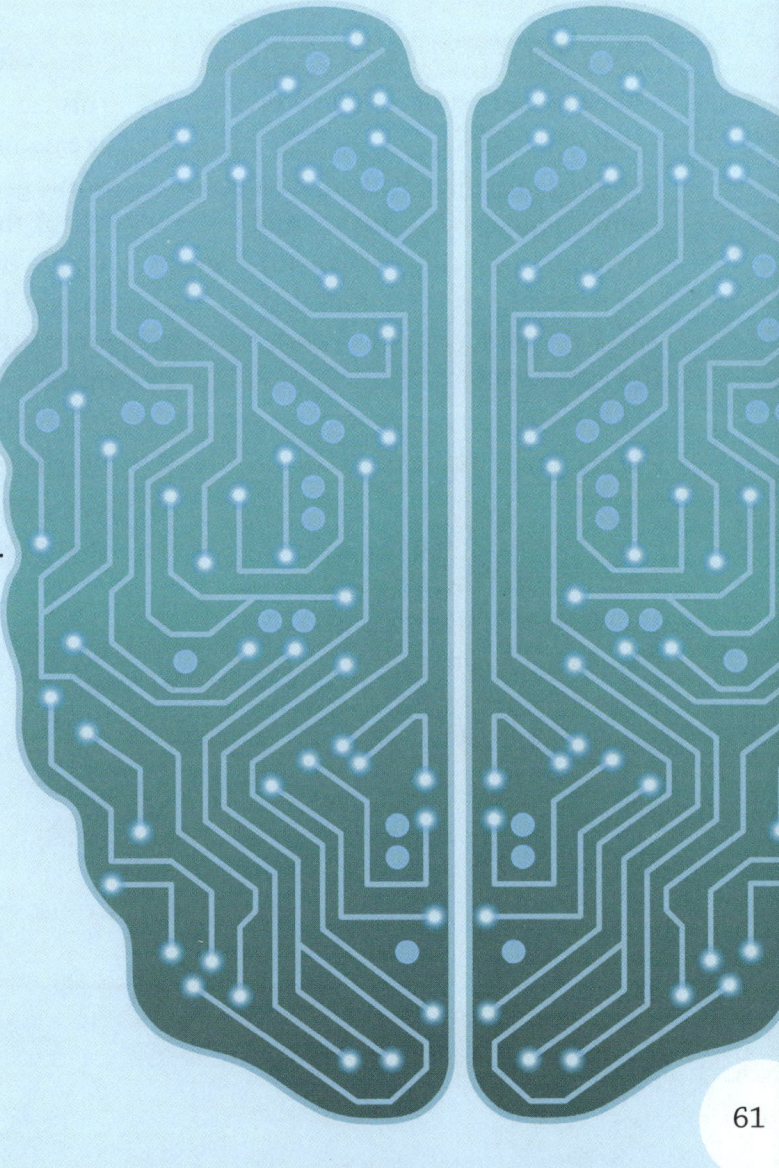

Dreaming[3]

- It may seem you can do anything in your dreams, but apparently, you cannot read or tell what time it is.

- A lot of innovations and inventions have been conceived while dreaming!

- Sometimes people experience a terrifying dream where they are paralyzed or unable to move and there is something scary nearby. This "sleep paralysis" is real and the amygdala region of the brain shows activity when this occurs.

- Dreaming appears to help recharge our creative mental batteries!

- Everyone dreams, but not everyone remembers it.

- People who are blind can dream, usually using other senses, but if they were not born blind, they can dream of seeing things.

- You might only remember one dream, but you can have a number of different dreams the same night.

- We only dream of people's faces that we have already seen.

- And some people don't dream in color, they only dream in black and white.

Adapted from "20 Amazing Facts About Dreams that You Might Not Know About" by Simon Andras, http://www.lifehack.org

Unit 1: The Electrifying Nervous System

BRAIN FOOD

Blueberries, other berries	Pumpkin seeds	Whole grains	Avocados	Tomatoes
WHY?	**WHY?**	**WHY?**	**WHY?**	**WHY?**
They include stuff that will protect your brain, called antioxidants, helping to get rid of free radicals — a by-product of some of the chemical reactions of the brain when converting food into energy — but too many of them can cause damage. Blueberries can also help improve your memory!	Full of zinc, which can help make your memory better and help with your thinking!	This can be things like oatmeal or whole grain bread (check the label), but are usually brown. These help provide fuel for the brain in the form of glucose, which can help keep you alert and focused!	These contain a lot of Vitamin E, which can help prevent damage to the brain from aging, and could possibly even delay some of the effects of dementia and Alzheimer's.	Not only do they taste good, but they also contain lycopene. This and other antioxidants are important to your health — not just for your brain, but also are being studied in how they can help prevent cancer and heart disease.

God's Wondrous Machine

Nuts	Broccoli, cauliflower, or brussels sprouts	Oily, fatty fish	Chocolate	Water
WHY?	**WHY?**	**WHY?**	**WHY?**	**WHY?**
These are another great source for Vitamin E, which in addition to being good for your brain can also help your immune system, and even prevent blood clotting.	These and other veggies contain Vitamin K, another brain health and memory booster!	Salmon, sardines, and even albacore tuna contain omega-3 fatty acids (um…yum?), which don't sound tasty, but they do help the brain cells transmit signals to one another. Remember, too much of something may not be good for you — fish can sometimes contain exposure to mercury, which is bad for you, so it's important to limit how much you eat!	Oh, yeah! Chocolate! The dark kind is best because it contains flavonoids, another kind of antioxidant. And chocolate tastes really good! Apples, purple and red grapes, tea, and even onion — yeah, onions — contain flavonoids.	Our body has to have water — it's an important part of what helps the body to function as it should. The brain is 75 percent water, and it is important to keep water in your system. At least six glasses a day, please!

Unit 1: The Electrifying Nervous System

MED+MOMENT

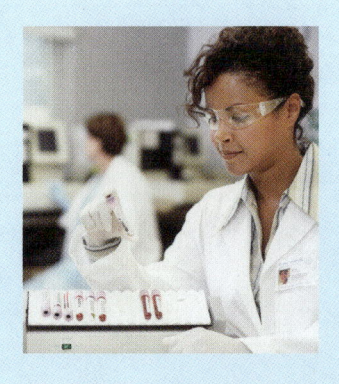

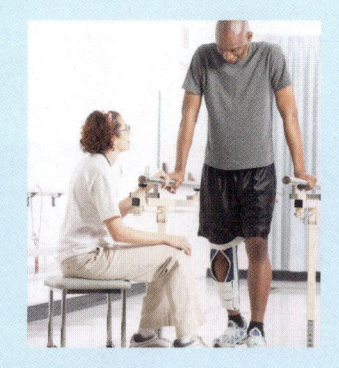

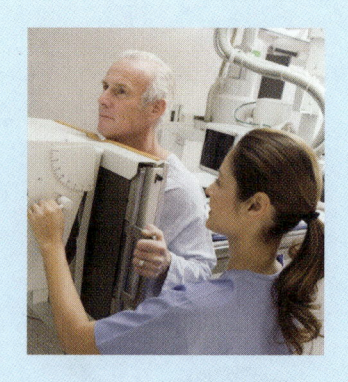

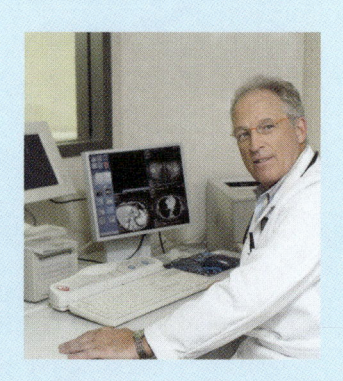

Careers in Neuroscience Medical careers can include a lot of different kinds of jobs, including many focused on the brain. Here are just a few:

Neurochemist	they study the chemical processes of the central nervous system
Neurologist	doctor who specializes in the treatment of the nervous system from headaches to seizures and much more
Educational psychologist	works to treat learning disabilities in children
Occupational therapist	works with people who have a variety of disabilities or injuries and helps them learn to function as independently as they can
Neuroimmunologist	people who focus on studying the immune system of the body and its interaction with the nervous system
Speech therapy	helping to diagnose and treat speech problems or conditions that affect swallowing
Neuropharmacologist	creates medicines to try and fix chemical problems with the brain
Neuroscience Nurse	works with doctors and assists people who have injuries or conditions related to the nervous system and brain
Psychiatrist	a doctor who treats mental conditions and disorders
Neuroanatomist	a person who is studying the anatomy, or structure, of the central nervous system
Neurosurgeons	surgeons who specialize in doing repairs or procedures on the brain
Electroneurodiagnostic Technician	the person who operates the equipment to record the brain's electrical activity
Neuropathologist	a person who studies all the diseases in the nervous system
Neuroradiologist	they use CT scans, x-rays, and other imagining techniques to help diagnose diseases of the brain and nervous system

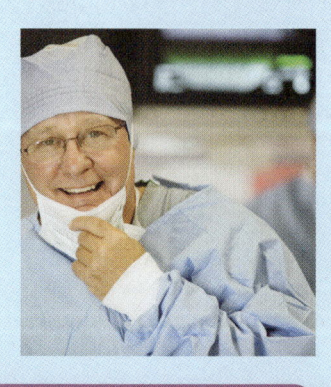

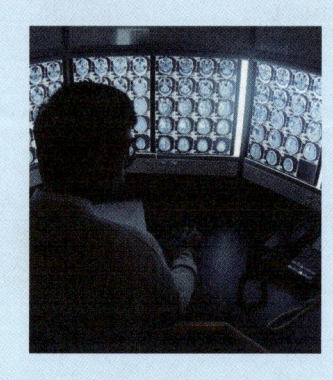

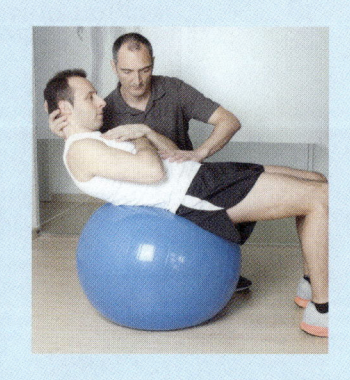

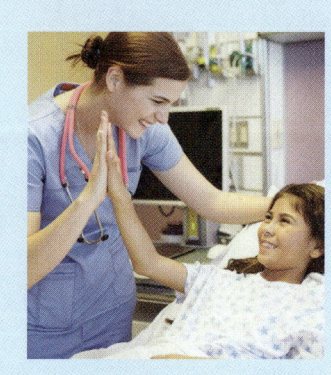

God's Wondrous Machine

Puzzle Power!

Puzzles can be a fun and interesting way to exercise your brain! They can be an important part of cognitive (learning, understanding, thinking, remembering, knowing) development for children. When a child is given a puzzle to solve, the brain gets to work, trying to figure out what it should look like, and then how it can be put together the way it should. Then the brain tells the hands how to pick it up and then turn or position the puzzle piece so that it fits. Many puzzles also contain words, colors, or shapes, which is another opportunity to help train or exercise your brain.

For adults, puzzles can also be beneficial in helping to keep your brain active and giving your memory a workout. But other activities can also be helpful — learning new things, a new language, logic exercises, reading, physical exercise, Sudoku puzzles, chess, trying to solve mysteries, and more!

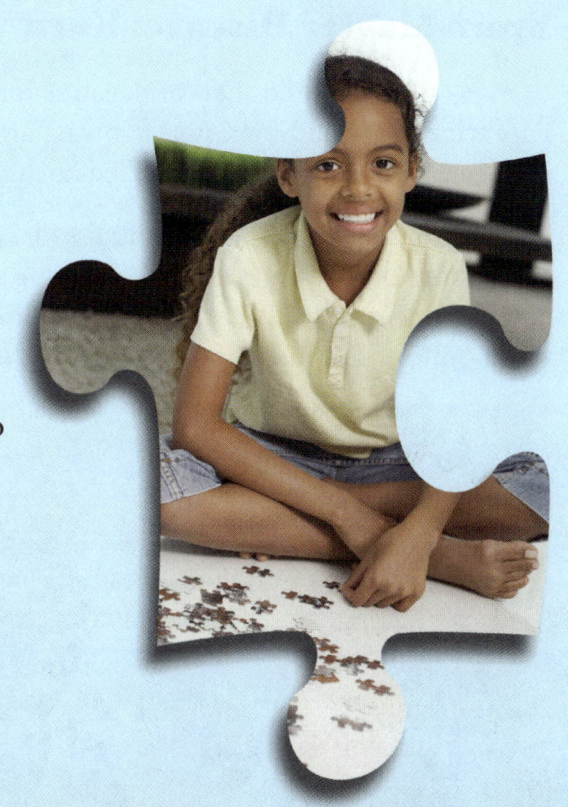

Final Thoughts (The End ...But Not Really!)

God's design of the brain is far more complex than any other human design. It has to work with all the systems of your body! Even the most complex computer made by man cannot hold up to God's mightily designed brain. Many mysteries still exist surrounding the functions of the brain that are waiting to be unraveled. The instructions of the Bible are clear. In Romans 12:2 it says, "Do not conform any longer to the pattern of this world but be transformed by the renewing of your mind . . ." (NIV). The brain is a powerful tool in understanding God's Word. By studying, reflecting, and applying His Word to our hearts, we strive to be transformed. Transformation of our minds is not just grasping some intellectual knowledge base but striving to understand how all the aspects of our lives can be fully surrendered to God.

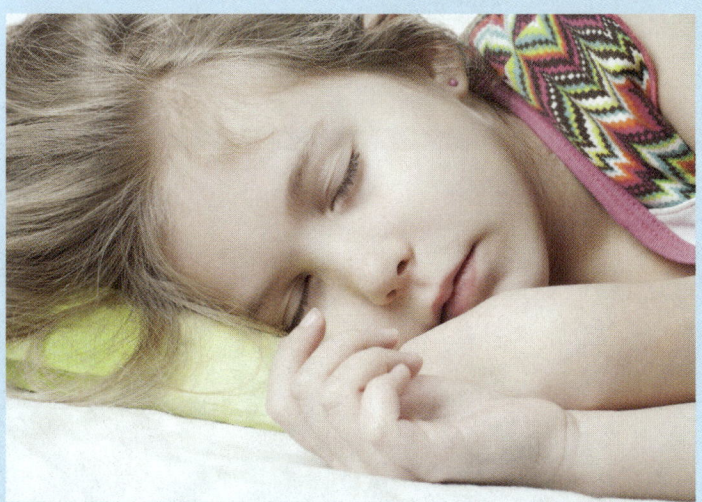

Unit 1: The Electrifying Nervous System

11 Facts: The Wacky, the Weird and Wow

Brain Matter Disease: Kuru

In many places around the world, eating animal brains is a common event. But for the Fore tribe in Papua New Guinea, it was cannibalism, eating human body parts including the brain, that led to an outbreak of a disease called kuru. An epidemic of kuru in the 1960s led to over 1100 deaths.

Initial symptoms include unsteadiness, decreasing muscle control, slurred speech, emotional instability, and tremors. By the end of the disease's progression, sufferers are unable to sit up, cannot speak and have trouble swallowing, and are unresponsive to their surroundings. Death usually occurs within a few months to 2 years of the onset of the disease.

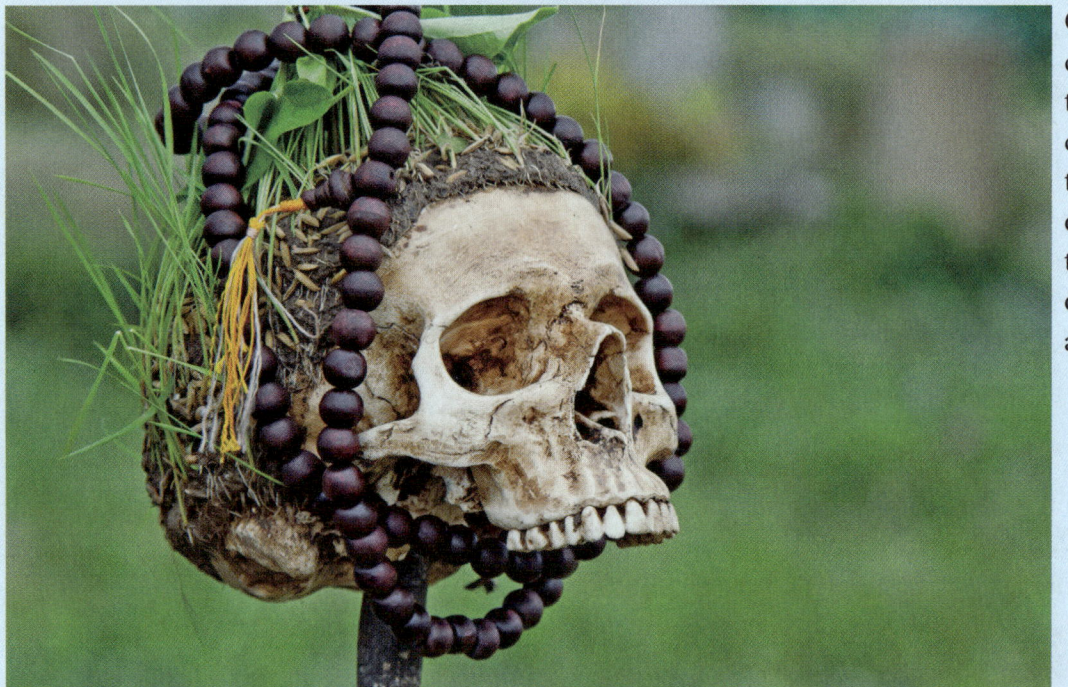

Outlawing the practice of cannibalism helped to lead to the decline of kuru, though cases of it still appear from time to time because it can incubate over a period of decades. In this section, you will discover other weird, wacky, and really amazing brain stories!

Beef brains can be a delicacy, but there is a danger. Mad cow disease can be transmitted through eating infected tissue. Many hunters also do not eat the brains of wild animals in North America because of fears over chronic wasting disease being transmitted.

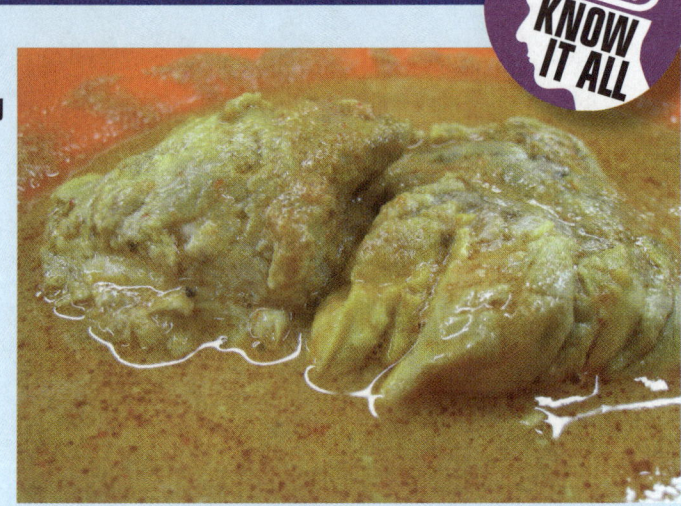

God's Wondrous Machine

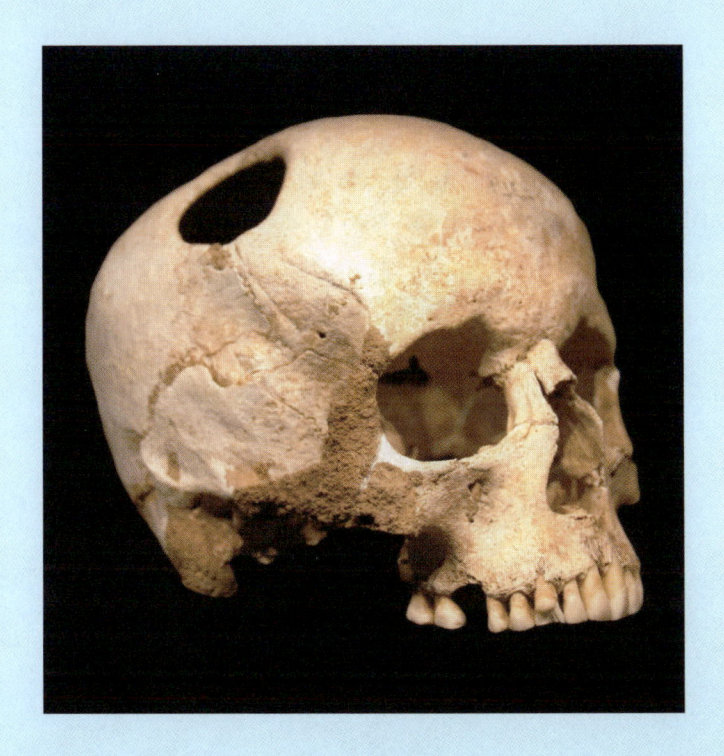

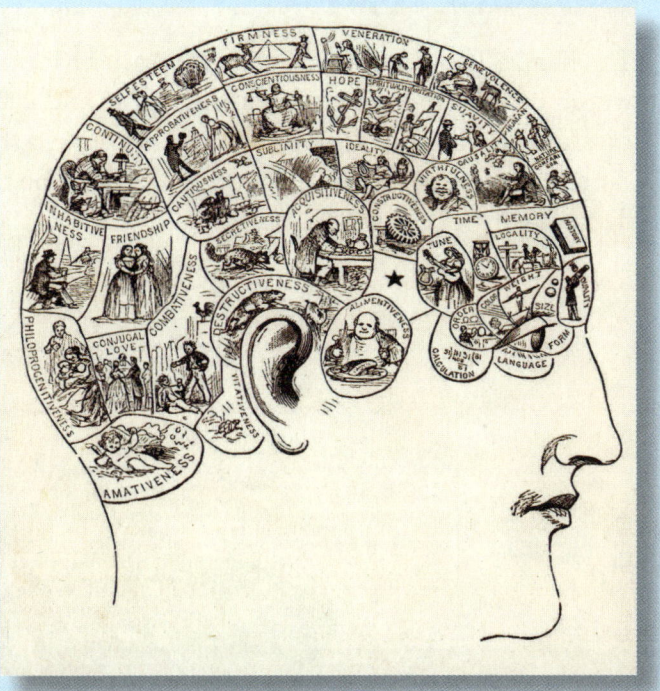

An 1883 phrenology chart

The Cure

During the dark ages, the "cure" for a throbbing headache was a hole in the head. This barbaric, potentially lethal medical procedure was called trephining or trepanning. Historians believe that the process entailed chipping or hacking a hole in the sufferer's head with a rock or an axe. The patient was most likely alive, based on the case evidence obtained from archaeological digs, which have demonstrated that some skulls with holes had bone regrowth in the margins of the orifice or hole. This practice gives new meaning to being "open-minded."

Lump in the Head

In Europe and America, from the 18th century to the middle of the 19th century, scientists practiced the "science" of phrenology. They believed they could analyze one's character by studying the shape and bumps on the skull. Those bumps were supposed to be excellent predictors of a person's personality. They surmised that a bump identified an area of the brain that was more developed, though it didn't really work.

Prize Winner

The ruler of Seville, Spain, from 1042 to 1069 — 'Abb ad al-mu'tadid — had an unusual collection. He collected unique souvenirs from his conquests. His greatest trophies were the skulls of his dead enemies, which he used as planters for flowers. What a "lovely" way to brighten the décor of a drab castle.

Unit 1: The Electrifying Nervous System

Shrunken Treasure

The Jivaros (he-var-ohs) tribe in the Andes Mountains practiced the sport of head hunting. They would capture their enemies during battle and claim their trophies — the heads of the losers. After carefully pulling the skin off a head, they boiled the skin in herbs and then placed stones and heated sand in it. They smoked the head overnight. The result was a shrunken head that they could display decoratively for all to admire.

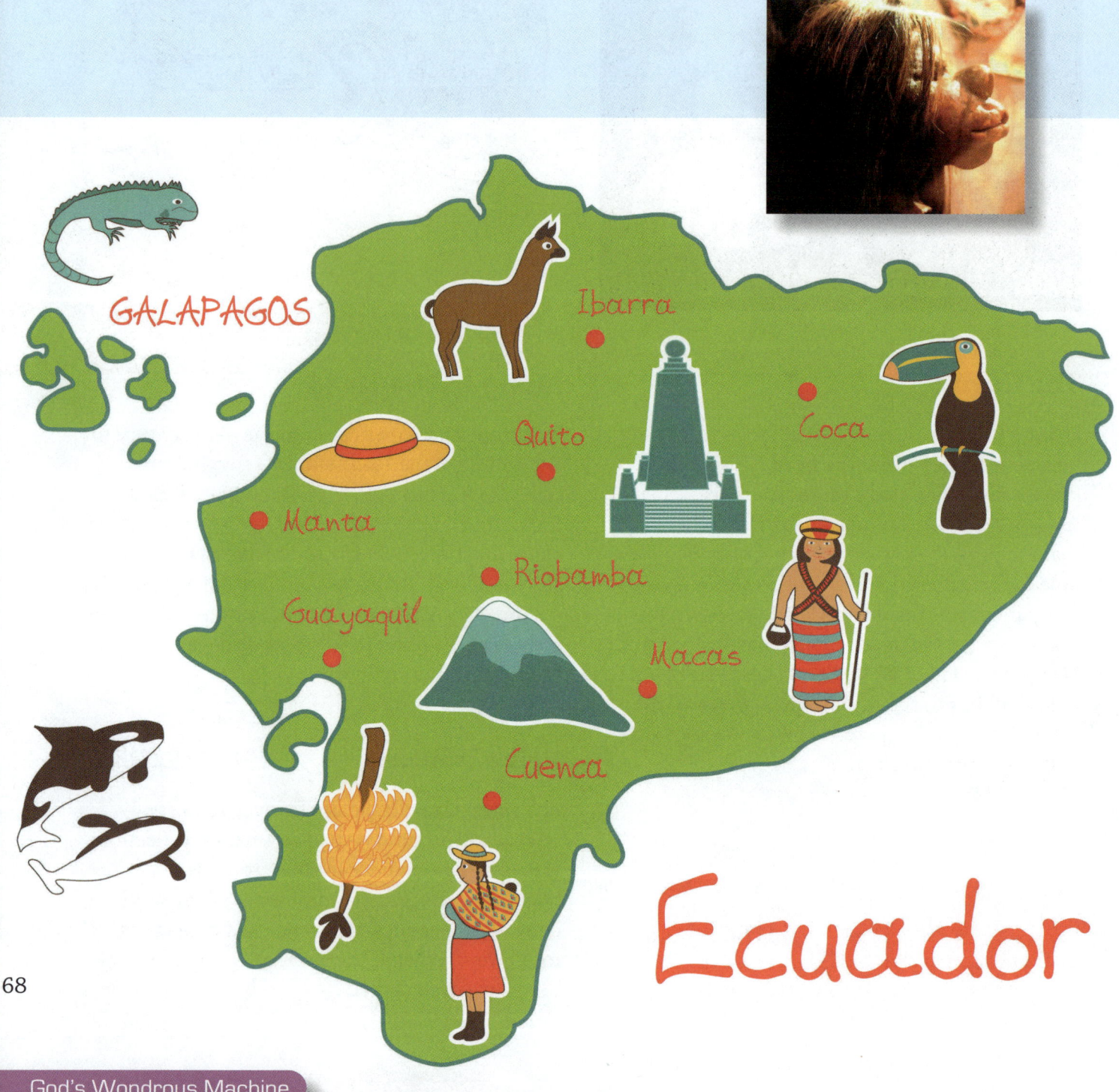

Ecuador

GALAPAGOS

Ibarra
Quito
Coca
Manta
Riobamba
Guayaquil
Macas
Cuenca

God's Wondrous Machine

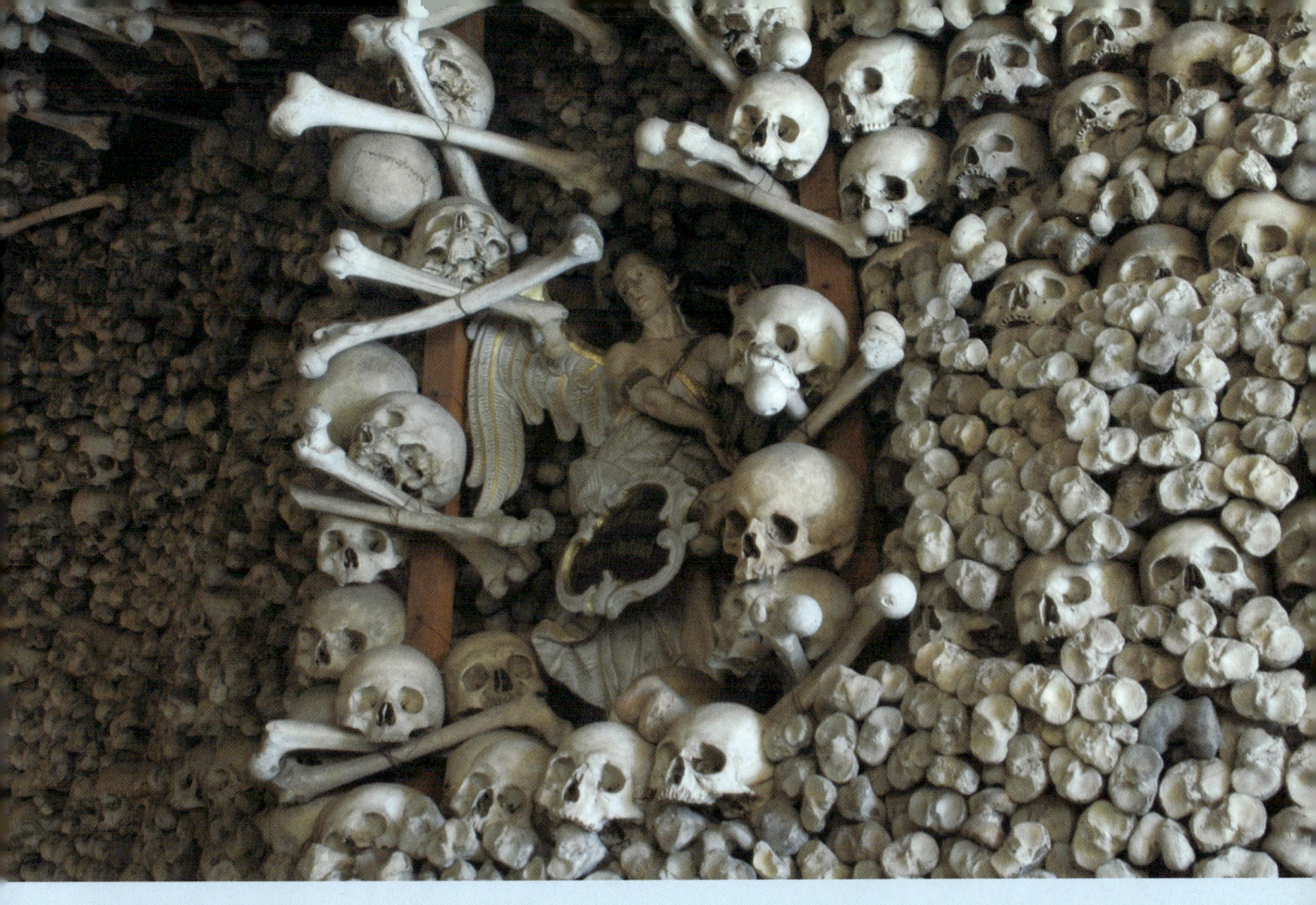

Bone Chapels

There are some amazing examples of architecture built or decorated with human skulls and other bones. These places are called ossuaries, and were sometimes used when there was not enough room for burials, and with this method, a lot of remains could be stored in a smaller area. There are a number of churches in Europe that contain large collections of bones, many of which have been displayed in special ways. Often underground passageways, called catacombs, were also used for storing bones.

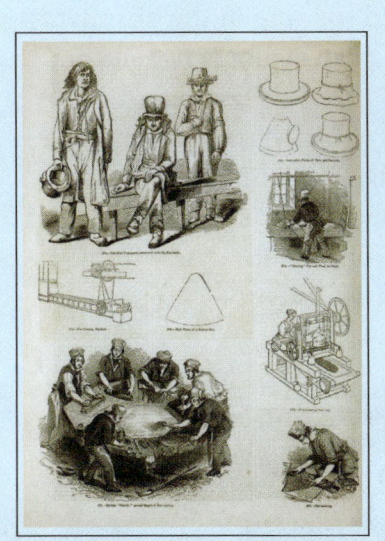

Mad as a Hatter

The unfortunate character in *Alice of Wonderland,* the Mad Hatter, may have suffered from an ailment that befell artisans of the hat-making industry. In the 19th century, people who made hats frequently displayed neurological disturbances because of mercury poisoning. Mercury and nitrate were sprayed onto the felt to make the hat shiny. These unknowing hat makers experienced symptoms such as difficulty in thinking and twitching hands, which led to the expression "mad as a hatter."

Unit 1: The Electrifying Nervous System

Telemedicine – Medical Advances for the Future

Medicine has an interesting history and perhaps an even more exciting future. As technology is developed to help us learn more about the human body, there are also efforts to improve healthcare in both rural areas of developed countries and that of developing areas around the globe.

Often these are the areas that face a shortage of doctors, medical specialists, hospitals, and even some of the more advanced testing and diagnostic equipment. There are a variety of solutions — mobile medical teams and equipment, efforts to attract new doctors to areas that need them, and international organizations specializing in special clinical or surgical technique.

Telemedicine is an emerging field that holds promise to improving medical care in isolated or rural populations. Telemedicine is basically where doctors and health professionals use satellites, the internet, and other communication techniques to link doctors and patients for care. This can be for testing, assessments, diagnoses, check-ups, reviews, and even arranging medicine. It can even be used in emergency situations, consultations among medical staff in diverse facilities, and even in rehabilitation programs. There are three main categories of telemedicine:

INTERACTIVE: This means testing can be done in one location while the doctor in another region or area of the country and is watching the test and able to communicate with the patient while it is ongoing.

REMOTE MONITORING: This is where patients are monitored electronically, but results appear in a different facility and are watched by medical personnel.

STORE-AND-FORWARD: A process in which imagery or test data is taken and then transmitted to another site or facility for review by medical staff at a future time.

Computers, webcams, smart phones, and more are just a few of the modern tools for telemedicine. Stroke Telemedicine, telestroke, is used to evaluate someone who has experienced a stroke. (A stroke occurs when the blood flow to a part of the brain is interrupted.) Neurologists, doctors with advanced training in the disorders of the nervous system, can evaluate patients in remote emergency rooms. Performing a prompt neurological evaluation and making an accurate diagnosis decreases the possibility of suffering from lifelong debilitation or death. It represents a promising and exciting new frontier for medical professionals.

God's Wondrous Machine

You've Got to Be Kidding

What does a brain do when it sees a friend across the street?	It gives a brain wave.
What kind of fish performs brain operations?	A neurosturgeon.
What do you get when you cross a thought with a light bulb?	A bright idea.
What works even after it is fired?	A neuron.
What do you get when you cross a bad idea that has fur with 100 billion neurons?	A hare-brained idea.
What happens when you bother the parietal lobe?	It gets touchy.
What is a brain's favorite kind of boat?	A cranial blood vessel.
Why is the left cerebral cortex always wrong?	Because it is never the "right" hemisphere.
What did the doctor say to the man who had an elephant sitting on his brain?	"Looks like you have a lot on your mind."
Why didn't the brain want to take a bath?	It didn't want to be brainwashed.
What did the parietal say to the frontal?	I lobe you.
When does it rain brains?	During a brainstorm.
Why was the neuron sent to the principal's office?	It had trouble controlling its impulses.
When does a brain get afraid?	When it loses its nerve.

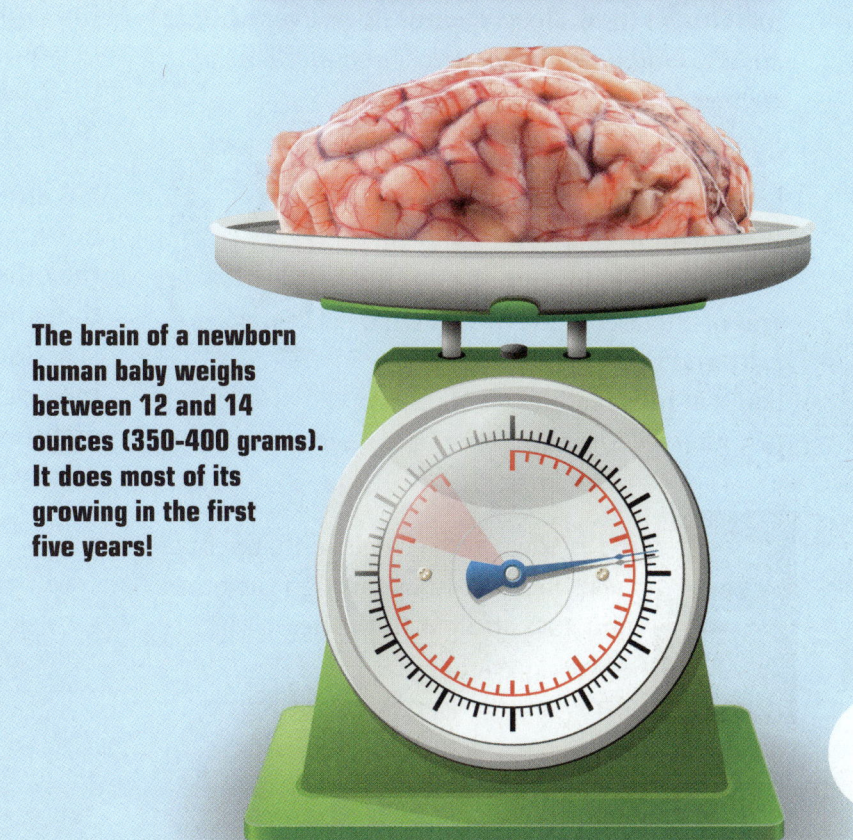

The brain of a newborn human baby weighs between 12 and 14 ounces (350-400 grams). It does most of its growing in the first five years!

Unit 1: The Electrifying Nervous System

Brain Quotes – What Do They Mean?

Our brain is made up of a number of physical structures as we have seen, but it is more than simply an organ. It is the place where our memories are stored, our creativity is found, and our imaginations run wild within its limitless boundaries. It controls our body, it sparks our dreams, and it is the tool we use to try and understand important ideas, articulate opinions, and develop understanding of important questions as we form our worldview. Here are some quotes from accomplished writers and scientists that talk about the aspects and qualities of the brain:

"There will one day spring from the brain of science a machine or force so fearful in its potentialities, so absolutely terrifying, that even man, the fighter, who will dare torture and death in order to inflict torture and death, will be appalled, and so abandon war forever." *Thomas A. Edison, American inventor*

"I do not think there is any thrill that can go through the human heart like that felt by the inventor as he sees some creation of the brain unfolding to success… such emotions make a man forget food, sleep, friends, love, everything." *Nikola Tesla inventor, electrical and mechanical engineer*

"I like nonsense, it wakes up the brain cells. Fantasy is a necessary ingredient in living, it's a way of looking at life through the wrong end of a telescope. Which is what I do, and that enables you to laugh at life's realities." *Dr. Seuss, pen name of Theodor Seuss Geisel, writer and cartoonist*

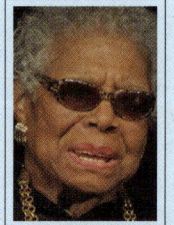

"The idea is to write it so that people hear it and it slides through the brain and goes straight to the heart." *Maya Angelou, African-American poet and actress*

"Tears come from the heart and not from the brain." *Leonardo da Vinci, painter, sculptor, engineer, anatomist, and inventor*

"The chief function of the body is to carry the brain around." *Thomas A. Edison, inventor*

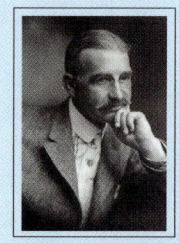

"I can't give you a brain, but I can give you a diploma." *L. Frank Baum, author of* The Wonderful Wizard of Oz

"I do not feel obliged to believe that the same God who has endowed us with sense, reason, and intellect has intended us to forgo their use." *Galileo Galilei, astronomer, mathematician, engineer, and philosopher*

"A strange thing is memory, and hope; one looks backward, and the other forward; one is of today, the other of tomorrow. Memory is history recorded in our brain, memory is a painter, it paints pictures of the past and of the day." *Grandma Moses, folk artist*

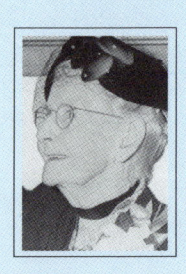

"Toleration is the greatest gift of the mind; it requires the same effort of the brain that it takes to balance oneself on a bicycle." *Helen Keller, a blind author, lecturer, and activist*

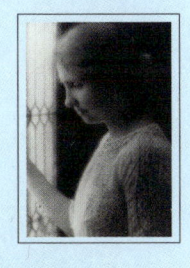

"The brain is wider than the sky." *Emily Dickinson, poet*

"God gave you a brain. Do the best you can with it. And you don't have to be Einstein, but Einstein was mentally tough. He believed what he believed. And he worked out things. And he argued with people who disagreed with him. But I'm sure he didn't call everybody jerks." *Clint Eastwood, actor and director*

"A great architect is not made by way of a brain nearly so much as he is made by way of a cultivated, enriched heart." *Frank Lloyd Wright, architect, writer, and educator*

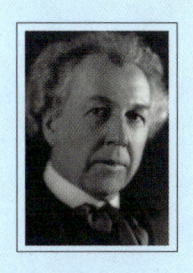

"I consider that a man's brain originally is like a little empty attic, and you have to stock it with such furniture as you choose." *Sir Arthur Conan Doyle, Scottish physician and writer/creator of detective Sherlock Holmes*

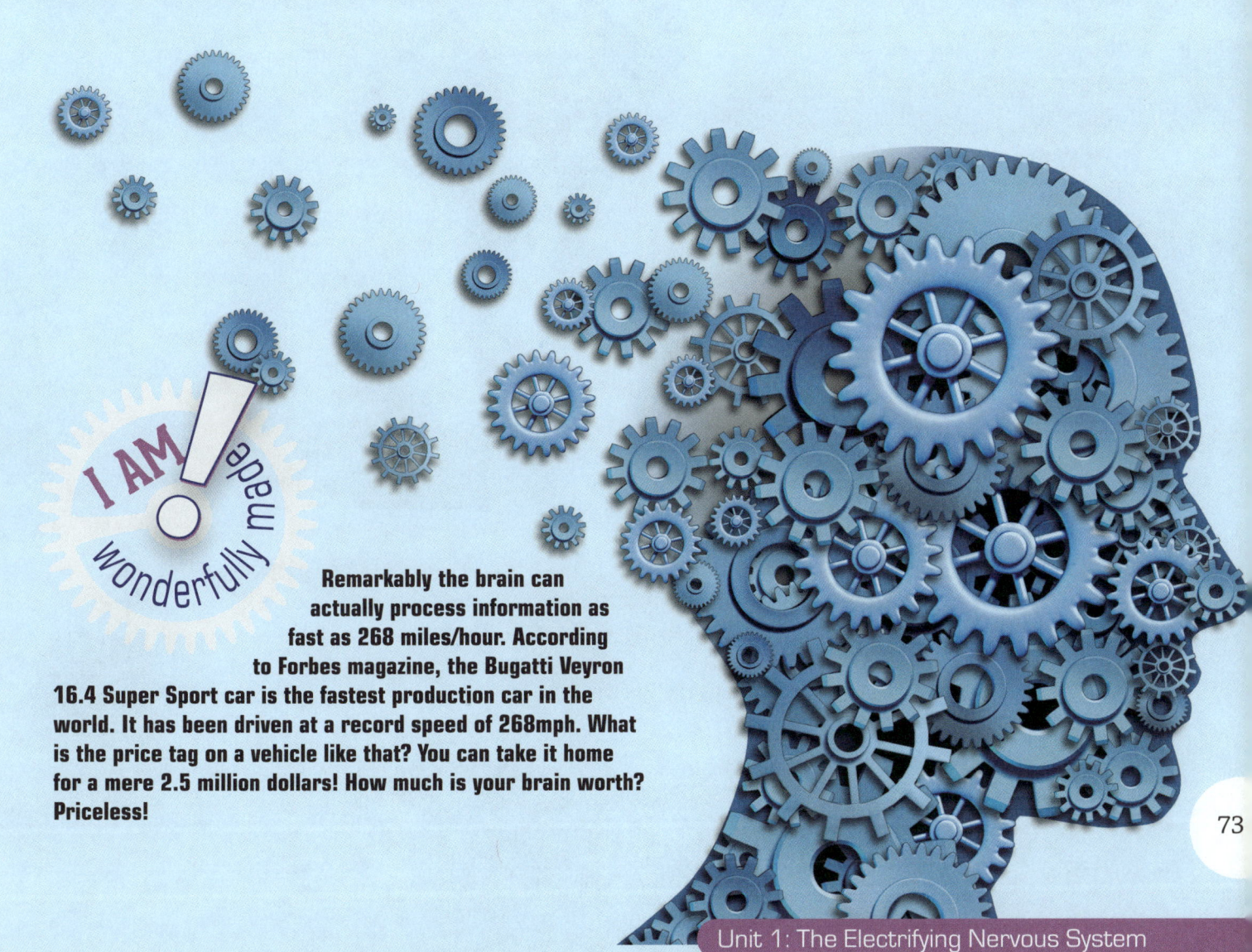

I AM wonderfully made!

Remarkably the brain can actually process information as fast as 268 miles/hour. According to Forbes magazine, the Bugatti Veyron 16.4 Super Sport car is the fastest production car in the world. It has been driven at a record speed of 268mph. What is the price tag on a vehicle like that? You can take it home for a mere 2.5 million dollars! How much is your brain worth? Priceless!

Unit 1: The Electrifying Nervous System

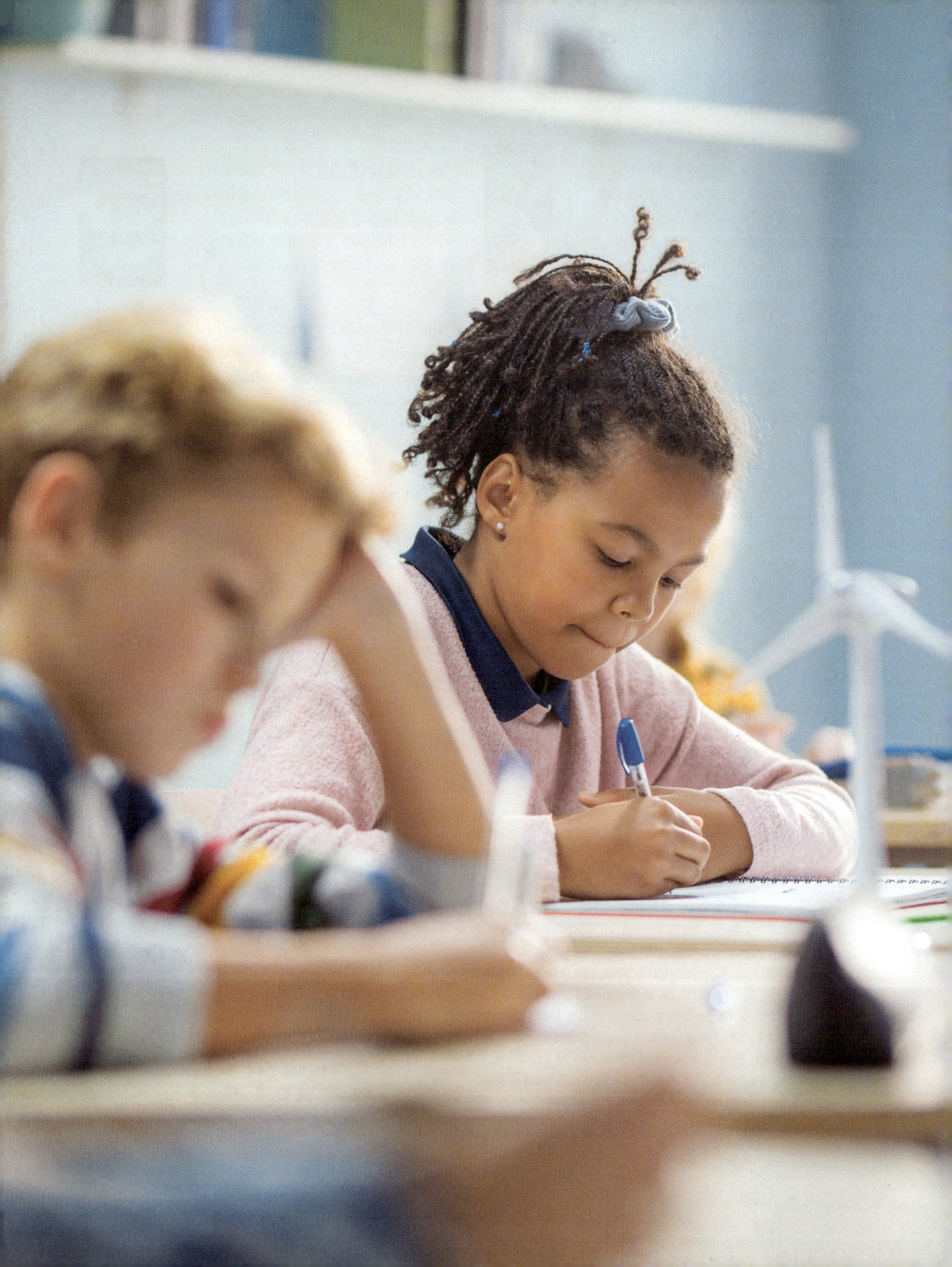

GOD'S
WONDROUS MACHINE

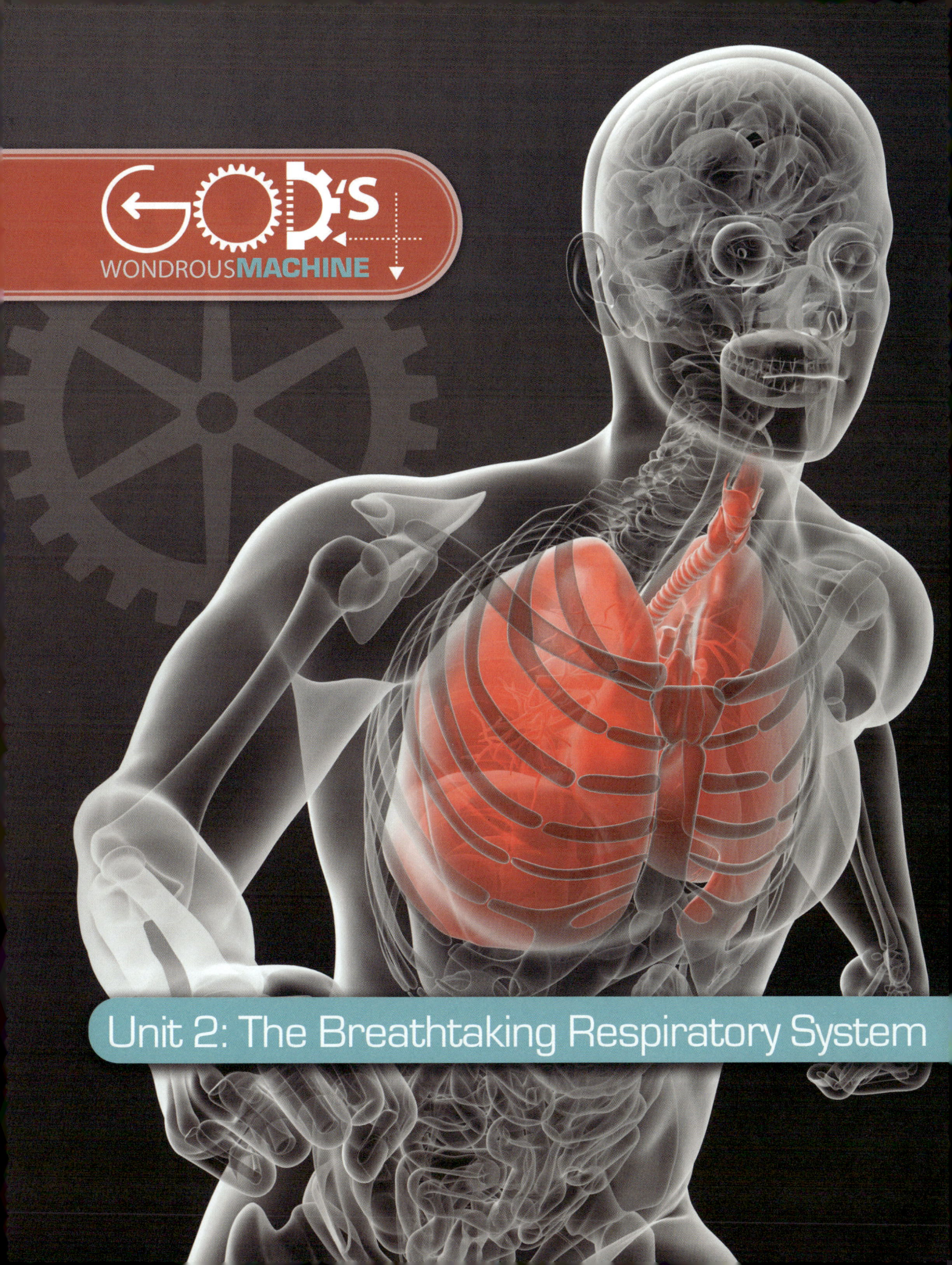

Unit 2: The Breathtaking Respiratory System

VOCABULARY LEVELS

Choose the word list based on your skill level. Every student should be able to master Level 1 words. Add words from Levels 2 and 3 as needed. More proficient students should be able to learn all three levels.

Level 1 Vocabulary

- Allergy
- Inhale
- Stethoscope
- Alveoli
- Larynx
- Upper Respiratory Tract
- Asthma
- Lower Respiratory Tract
- Virus
- Bacteria
- Mucus
- Vocal Cords
- Bronchi
- Nares
- Carbon Dioxide
- Pharynx
- Cilia
- Exhale

Level 2 Vocabulary

Review and Know Level 1 Vocabulary

- Allergens
- Influenza
- Trachea
- Anosmia
- Iron Lung
- Ventilation
- Antiseptic
- Laryngitis
- Bronchioles
- Pandemic
- Cystic Fibrosis
- Physiologist
- Diffusion
- Pleura Sac
- Epidemic
- Polio
- Epiglottis
- Sinuses

Level 3 Vocabulary

Review and Know Level 1 and 2 Vocabulary

- Apneustic Center
- Chemoreceptors
- Cribriform Plate
- Epithelium
- Gestation
- Goblet Cells
- Nasal Turbinate
- Organogenesis
- Pneumotaxic Center
- Surfactant
- Tracheostomy

on the nose.

The surface area of the lungs is roughly the same size as a tennis court. God's amazing design of the lungs means that you use this large surface area for the diffusion of oxygen and carbon dioxide for breathing!

God's Wondrous Machine

See It, Say It, Know It!

- Level 1 Vocabulary
- Level 2 Vocabulary
- Level 3 Vocabulary

Word [Pronunciation]	Definition
Allergens al·ler·gen (al´er-jen)	A foreign substance, such as mites in house dust or animal dander, that, when inhaled, causes the airways to narrow and produces symptoms of asthma
Allergy al·ler·gy (al´er-je)	An abnormally high, acquired sensitivity to certain substances, such as drugs, pollens, or microorganisms, that may include such symptoms as sneezing, itching, and skin rashes
Alveolus al·ve´o·lus Alveoli alve´oli (plural form)	Small air sacs or cavities in the lung that give the tissue a honeycomb appearance and expand its surface area for the exchange of oxygen and carbon dioxide
Anosmia an·os·mi·a	Loss of the sense of smell
Antiseptic an·ti·sep·tic	Capable of preventing infection by inhibiting the growth of bacteria
Apneustic Center app·new·stik sen·ter	The neurons in the brain stem controlling normal respiration
Asthma asth·ma	A common inflammatory disease of the lungs characterized by episodic airway obstruction caused by extensive narrowing of the bronchi and bronchioles. Common symptoms of asthma include wheezing, coughing, and shortness of breath.
Bacteria bac·te·ri·a	Organisms not able to be seen except under a microscope, found in rotting matter, in air, in soil, and in living bodies, some being the germs of disease
Bronchi bronc-i	The two branches of the trachea that extend into the lungs
Bronchioles bron·chi·ole	Any of the small, thin-walled tubes that branch from a bronchus and end in the alveolar sacs of the lung
Carbon Dioxide car·bon di·ox·ide	A colorless, odorless, incombustible gas, CO_2, formed during respiration, combustion, and organic decomposition and used in food refrigeration, carbonated beverages, inert atmospheres, fire extinguishers, and aerosols
Chemoreceptors che·mo·re·cep·tor	A sensory nerve stimulated by chemical means
Cilia cil·i·a	Short, hairlike, rhythmically beating organelles on the surface of certain cells that provide mobility, as in protozoans, or move fluids and particles along ducts in multicellular forms

Unit 2: The Breathtaking Respiratory System

Word [Pronunciation]	Definition
Cribriform Plate crib-i-form plate	Located in the ethmoid bone of the skull in the nasal cavity where the nerve endings of the sense of smell are found
Cystic Fibrosis cys'tic fibro'sis	An inherited disorder of the exocrine glands, usually developing during early childhood and affecting mainly the pancreas, respiratory system, and sweat glands. It is marked by the production of abnormally thick mucus by the affected glands, usually resulting in chronic respiratory infections and impaired pancreatic function.
Diffusion dif·fu·sion	The movement of atoms or molecules from an area of higher concentration to an area of lower concentration. Atoms and small molecules can move across a cell membrane by diffusion.
Epidemic ep·i·dem·ic	An outbreak of a disease or illness that spreads rapidly among individuals in an area or population at the same time
Epiglottis ep·i·glot·tis	The thin elastic cartilaginous structure located at the root of the tongue that folds over the glottis to prevent food and liquid from entering the trachea during the act of swallowing
Epithelium ep·i·the·li·um	Any tissue layer covering body surfaces or lining the internal surfaces of body cavities, tubes, and hollow organs
Exhale ex·hale	To breathe out
Gestation ges·ta·tion	The period during which unborn young are "carried" inside the womb
Goblet Cells Gob·let cells	Cells in the respiratory tract that produce mucus
Influenza in·flu·en·za	A highly contagious and often epidemic viral disease characterized by fever, tiredness, muscular aches and pains, and inflammation of the respiratory passages
Inhale in·hale	To breathe in; inspire
Iron Lung i'ron lung	An airtight metal cylinder enclosing the entire body up to the neck and providing artificial respiration when the respiratory muscles are paralyzed, as by poliomyelitis
Laryngitis lar·yn·gi·tis	Inflammation of the larynx, often with accompanying sore throat, hoarseness or loss of voice, and dry cough

| Level 1 Vocabulary |
| Level 2 Vocabulary |
| Level 3 Vocabulary |

Word [Pronunciation]	Definition
Larynx lar·ynx	The upper part of the trachea in most vertebrate animals, containing the vocal cords. The walls of the larynx are made of cartilage. Sound is produced by air passing through the larynx on the way to the lungs, causing the walls of the larynx to vibrate. The pitch of the sound that is produced can be altered by the pull of muscles, which changes the tension of the vocal cords. Also called voice box.
Lower Respiratory Tract lo·wer res·pir·a·tory tract	Consisting of all the structures in the respiratory tract lying below the larynx. The lower respiratory tract is composed of the trachea and lungs. The lungs include the bronchi, respiratory bronchioles, alveolar ducts, alveolar sacs, and alveoli.
Mucus mu·cus	The slimy, viscous substance secreted as a protective lubricant by mucous membranes. Mucus is composed chiefly of large glycoproteins called mucins and inorganic salts suspended in water.
Nares nar·is	An external opening in the nasal cavity of a vertebrate; a nostril
Nasal Turbinate Na·sal tur·bi·nate	Any of the scrolled spongy bones of the nasal passages in man and other vertebrates
Organogenesis or·gan·o·gen·e·sis	The development of bodily organs
Pandemic Pan·dem·ic	An epidemic that spreads over a very wide area, such as an entire country or continent
Pharynx phar·ynx	The passage that leads from the cavities of the nose and mouth to the larynx (voice box) and esophagus. Air passes through the pharynx on the way to the lungs, and food enters the esophagus from the pharynx.
Physiologist phys·i·ol·o·gist	Biologist specializing in physiology (the biological study of the functions of living organisms and their parts)
Pleura Sac pleu·ra sac	A membrane that encloses each lung and lines the chest cavity
Pneumotaxic Center pneu·mo·tax·ic sen·ter	A nerve center in the upper pons of the brain stem that rhythmically inhibits inspiration
Polio po·li·o	Poliomyelitis, an acute viral disease marked by inflammation of nerve cells of the brain stem and spinal cord that can affect the ability to walk and breathe

Word [Pronunciation]	Definition
Sinuses si·nus·es	A cavity or hollow space in a bone of the skull, especially one that connects with the nose
Stethoscope steth·o·scope	An instrument for listening to the sounds made within the body, typically consisting of a hollow disc that transmits the sound through hollow tubes to earpieces
Surfactant sur·fac·tant	Surfactant reduces the surface tension of fluid in the lungs and helps make the small air sacs in the lungs (alveoli) more stable.
Trachea tra·che·a	A thin-walled, cartilaginous tube descending from the larynx to the bronchi and carrying air to the lungs; also called windpipe
Tracheostomy tra·che·os·to·my	Surgical construction of an opening in the trachea, usually by making an incision in the front of the neck, for the insertion of a catheter or tube to facilitate breathing
Upper Respiratory Tract up·per res·puh·rah·tow·ree tract	Composed of the parts of the upper respiratory system: the nose, sinuses, pharynx, and larynx
Ventilation ven·ti·la·tion	The exchange of air between the lungs and the environment, including inhalation and exhalation
Virus vi·rus	Any of various extremely small, often disease-causing agents consisting of a particle (the virion), containing a segment of RNA or DNA within a protein coat known as a capsid. Viruses are not technically considered living organisms because they cannot carry out biological processes.
Vocal Cords vo'·cal cords	The two folded pairs of membranes in the larynx (voice box) that vibrate when air that is exhaled passes through them, producing sound

*Most pronunciation keys from: http://medical-dictionary.thefreedictionary.com

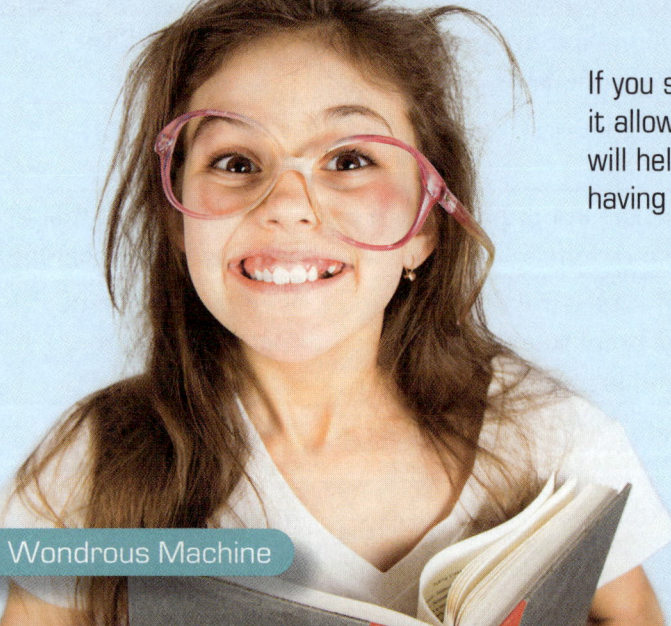

If you sit up straight while reading a book out loud, it allows you to use more of your lung capacity. This will help keep you from getting short of breath or having to gasp for air in the middle of a sentence!

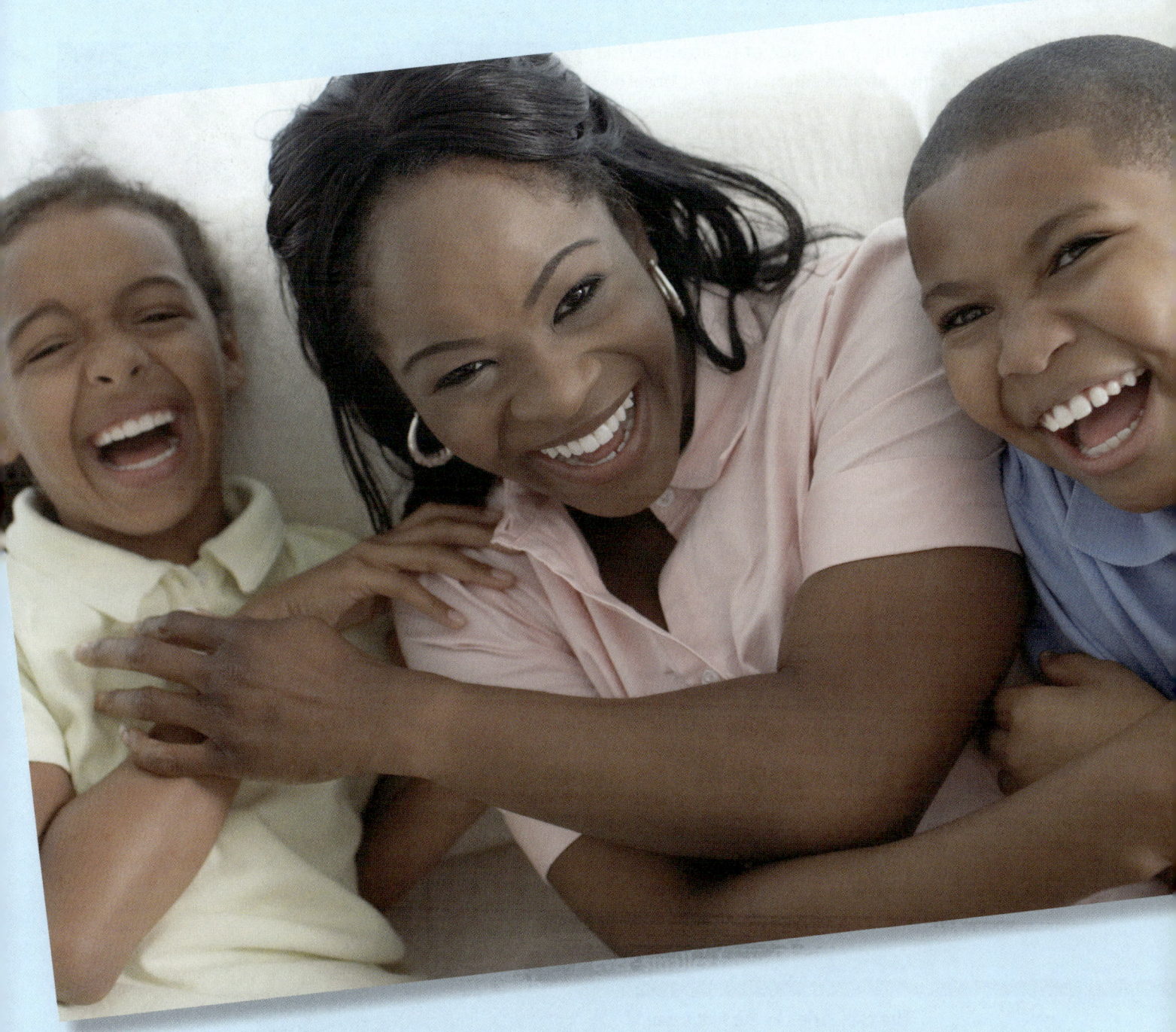

When you laugh, the muscles in your chest and your diaphragm contract, pushing air out of the lungs in a quick rush that makes your larynx vibrate to make the sound of laughter — ha ha! It has been observed that the average young child laughs nearly 300 times in a day. Adults, on average, laugh 15 to 100 times a day.

Laughter is good medicine! It helps to reduce pain and blood sugar levels. Proverbs 17:22 says, "A cheerful heart is good medicine, but a crushed spirit dries up the bones."

Unit 2: The Breathtaking Respiratory System

1 Introduction: Why Do We Breathe?

With a loud-piercing wail, each of us entered this world as a crying baby taking in our first breath of air. That breath ushers in a new independent life outside the mother's womb. Created from the dust on the ground and with the breath God breathed into his lungs, Adam took his first breath. This life-giving force originates from none other than God: the giver of life and breath. The respiratory system is yet another demonstration of God's provision, our human frailty, and our complete dependence on Him.

Why do we breathe? We breathe because we eat. Okay, that sounds a bit ridiculous. But it makes sense when we look at our bodies as an incredible engine. For an engine to carry out all of its processes, it needs energy. Oxygen is needed to burn and utilize the fuel we eat. The billions of cells in our bodies grab the oxygen we breathe from the red blood cells that travel by and utilize it to perform all of its complicated actions. The cells throw out the garbage from their day's work in the form of a gas called carbon dioxide. The lungs inhale oxygen and exhale carbon dioxide.

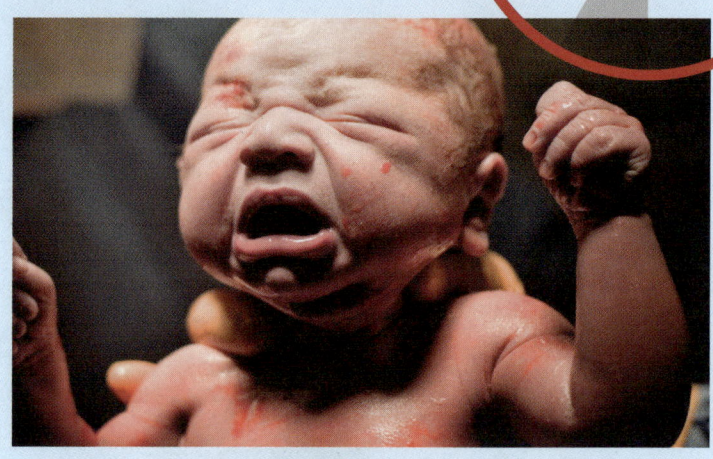

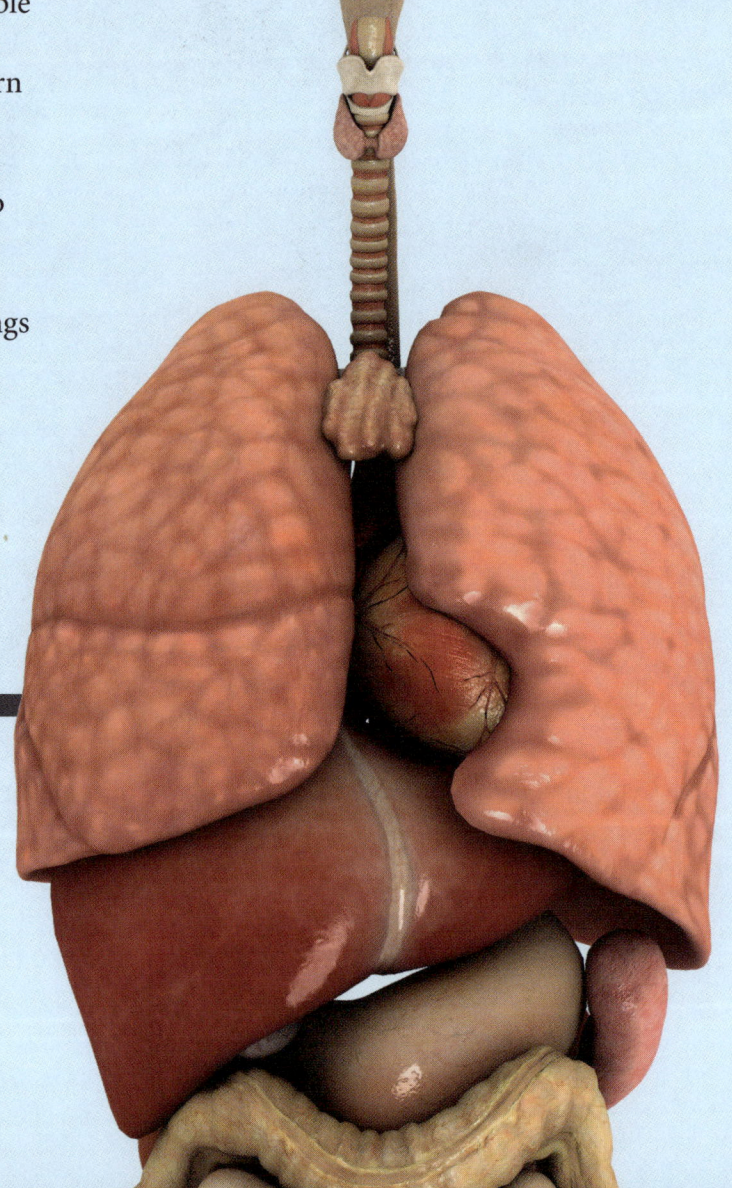

on the nose.

The capillaries in the lungs would extend 1,600 kilometers, almost 995 miles, if placed end to end. That is just slightly shorter than the distance between New York City and Tampa, Florida or almost equal to the distance between Chicago and Denver.

God's Wondrous Machine

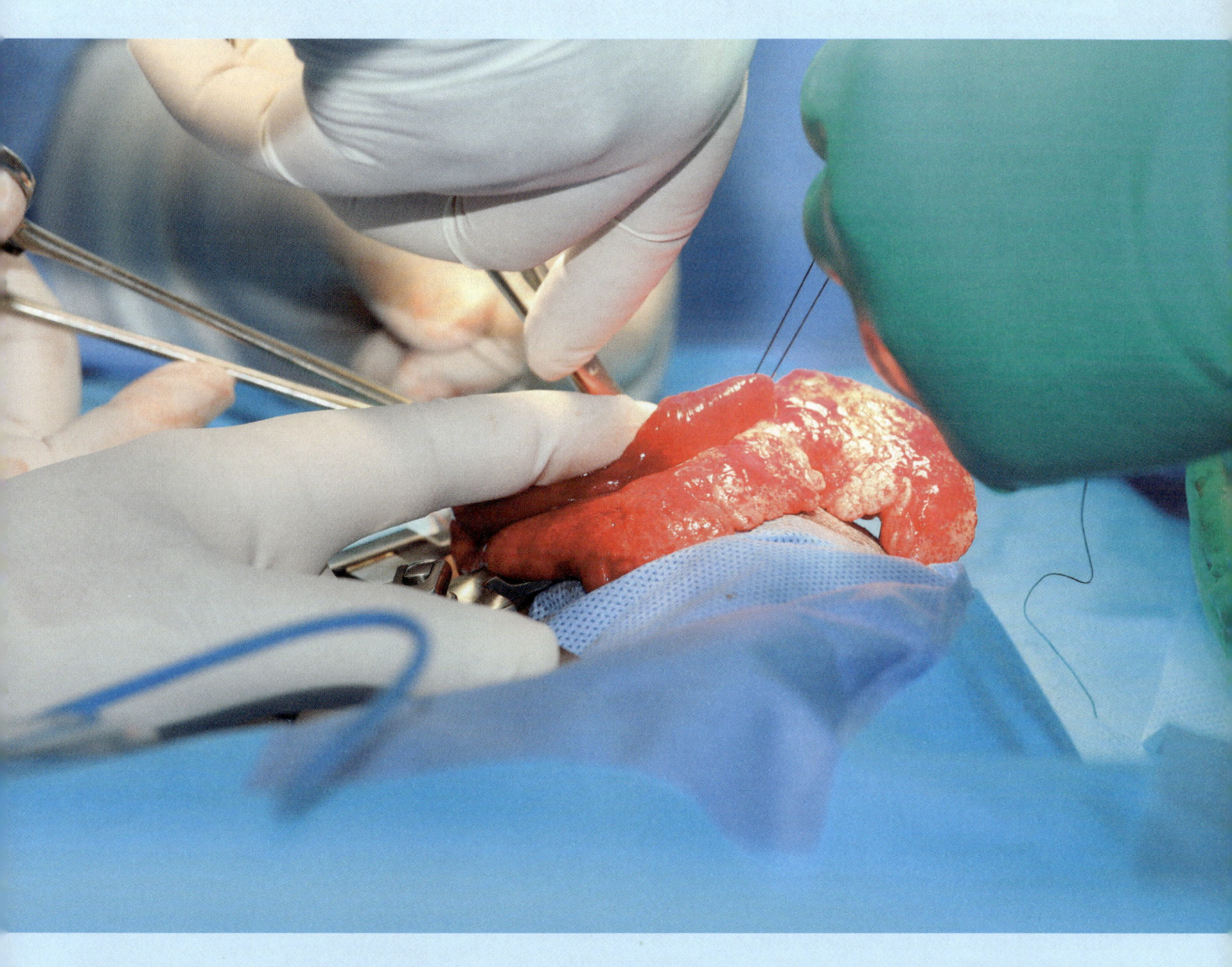

Sit back and breathe in. Come, as we embark on a captivating voyage through the wind tunnels of the body, and be prepared to be amazed. At the first stop on our journey, we will peer into the Bible and see what God's Word says about this life force. We will then take a look back in the pages of time and learn about discoveries that have helped shape our understanding of the respiratory system today. We will learn about the anatomy and physiology of this inverted tree-like structure called the lungs.

Discover remarkable things about your soft, spongy lungs. Did you know it is the only organ in your body that can actually float on water? The surface area of the alveoli (the small air sacs of the lungs) alone could cover the surface of an entire tennis court! Breeze in and witness this incredible expanse of God's Wondrous Machine. It will take your breath away!

Unit 2: The Breathtaking Respiratory System

2 Respiratory History Timeline: A Walk Back in Time

But isn't history just about a bunch of dead people? Why should it matter to me? How important is medical history for a particular system of the body? The dates and events are meaningless to our lives, right? Wrong. As you dive into "God's Wondrous Machine," you will see how these events have shaped what we understand to be true today. We encounter real problems in life. It is through those problems that we acquire new knowledge and original ways to solve those problems. History connects the past with the present and the future. When we study history, we can observe how things change over time and understand the situations and life circumstances that generate the necessity of innovation and invention. As you read, observe the frailty of our being and how God has given us each unique minds to help impact the world in which we live. You will see that the knowledge base that you now bring to the table far exceeds the knowledge of people from yesterday. We are confronted with new problems. The hope is that you will play a part in creating real solutions to the problems we encounter today to impact the advances of tomorrow.

Let's set sail through the pages of time and see how the various discoveries have provided a platform for future breakthroughs.

500 B.C.
Anaximenes, of ancient Greece, believed that all things were made of air. He called it *pneuma* which means "breath" in Greek. The Greeks believed everything was alive and breathing.

470 B.C.
Empedocles, the Greek philosopher, taught that all things were made of four elements — earth, air, fire, and water.

350 B.C.
Aristotle thought the heart was on fire. Breathing in cooled the fire and kept it from burning up the whole body.

1660
Marcello Malpighi, born in Crevalcore, Italy, March 10, 1628, showed that the lungs consist of many small air pockets and a complex system of blood vessels by observing capillaries through a microscope. He described the circulation of blood.

1765
John Morgan founded the first medical school in America at the College of Pennsylvania.

1772-1774
Joseph Priestley discovered nitrous oxide and is credited with the discovery of oxygen.

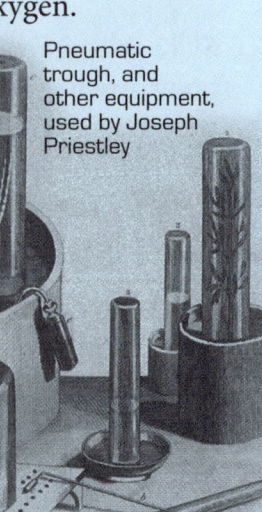

Pneumatic trough, and other equipment, used by Joseph Priestley

God's Wondrous Machine

da Vinci anatomy drawings

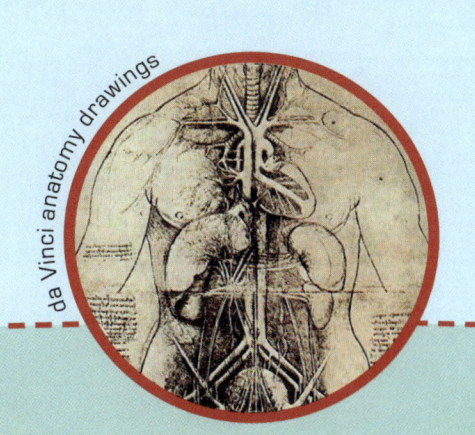

280–271 B.C.
Greek physician Erasistratus came very close to recognizing the circulation of the blood, especially by noting the relationship of the lungs to the circulating system.

A.D. 170
Galen taught that the secret of life was a spirit or *pneuma* that came from the air.

1500
Leonardo da Vinci, Italian painter and inventor, suggested that air was not made from one element but a combination of two gases.

1643
Evangelista Torricelli proved that air had weight and took up space.

1660
Robert Hooke, an Englishman, found that parts of the body act like pumps. Our ribs help pump air in and out of the lungs.

Re-enactment of the first operation under anesthesia

1779
Thomas Beddoes and Humphry Davy recognized nitrous oxide's anesthetizing effects, but did not think to use it to take away pain.

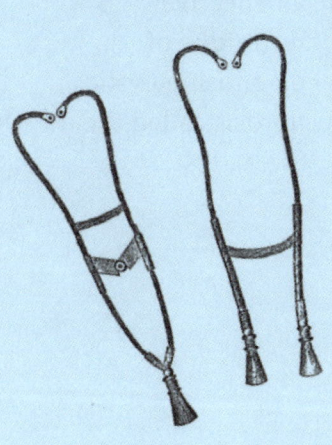

1779
Lavoisier proposed the name "oxygen" for the part of air that is breathed and responsible for combustion. He discovered that air was composed mainly of two components — oxygen and nitrogen.

1819
Treatise on Diagnosis by Listening to Sounds by physician Theophile René Laennec was written in which he demonstrated the use of a tube for investigating the lungs and heart sounds.

Early flexible stethoscopes

1845
Anesthetic inhaler invented. *Anesthetic* comes from the Greek word meaning "loss of feeling." Prior to the invention of anesthesia, patients were strapped down and held by strong individuals as the surgeon speedily worked.

1845
William Morton, an American doctor, used ether to extract a tooth from a patient. A sealed glass jar with an air valve containing several ether-soaked sponges was used, with a long rubber tube as a mouthpiece.

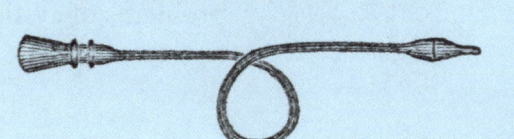

Unit 2: The Breathtaking Respiratory System

85

1847
Chloroform came into use. It was found that it was particularly useful in childbirth by James Young Simpson. This met a great deal of criticism — it was believed that it was always a woman's fate to suffer pain during childbirth. Queen Victoria popularized its use when she used it during the birth of her seventh child, Leopold.

1855
George Phillip Cammann, an American doctor, took Laennec's idea and developed the stethoscope we know today.

1882
Robert Koch discovers the bacterium that causes tuberculosis, the first definite association of a germ with a specific human disease.

1904
The National Association for the Study and Prevention of Tuberculosis was founded. This organization later became the American Lung Association.

1906
Jules Bordet discovered *Bordetella pertussis*, the bacterium that causes whooping cough.

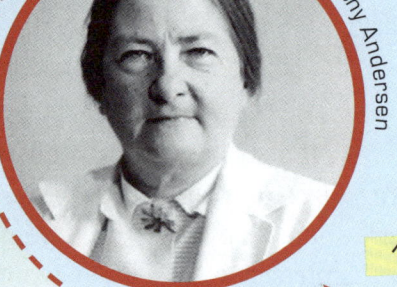

1938
Dr. Dorothy Andersen, a pathologist at Columbia-Presbyterian Babies and Children's Hospital in New York, was the first to document and observe the problems of cystic fibrosis, a genetic disease.

1953
Dr. Paul di Sant'Agnese developed an effective technique of diagnosing cystic fibrosis called the Sweat Test.

Jules Bordet

Dr. Dorothy Andersen

Queen Victoria, with the Princess Royal

86

God's Wondrous Machine

1927
Phillip Drinker developed the "iron lung," a mechanical metal device that encased a patient to help him breathe.

1938
Corneille Heymans of Belgium won the Nobel Prize for physiology or medicine for his discoveries in respiratory regulation.

1938
The National Foundation for Infantile Paralysis was established by Franklin D. Roosevelt. This organization's name was later changed to the March of Dimes.

Franklin D. Roosevelt

Thousands send dimes to aid the Infantile Paralysis Foundation

Dr. Jonas Salk

1955
Dr. Jonas Salk, an American medical researcher, developed an injectable polio vaccine based upon a live weakened polio virus.

1957
Dr. Albert Sabin, a Polish American microbiologist, developed an oral (taken by mouth) vaccine that used a live weakened version of the polio virus.

1989
The gene responsible for cystic fibrosis was identified, giving hopes of a cure one day by gene therapy.

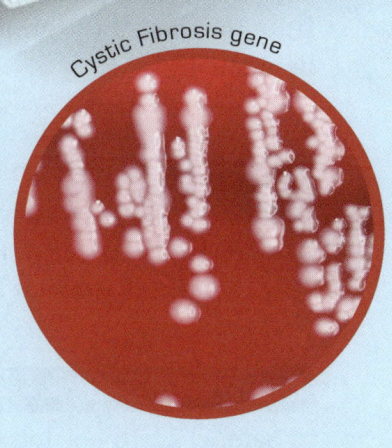

Cystic Fibrosis gene

Unit 2: The Breathtaking Respiratory System

Joseph Priestley: The Dissenter Discovers Oxygen

Joseph Priestley (1733–1804) was born on March 13, 1733, in Fieldhead, England. Joseph's father died shortly after his birth. Joseph's mother was a devout religious woman who taught Joseph about God. As Joseph grew, he had a ravenous appetite for the Bible and learning. Faith and religion were central parts of daily life in England. England's official church was the Anglican Church, or the Church of England. It was a powerful organization and controlled many aspects of daily life. As Joseph matured in his faith, his views changed from the views held by the Anglican Church. Joseph became a dissenter. Dissenters were a diverse group that included Baptists, Lutherans, Methodists, Presbyterians, and Quakers that disagreed with the Church of England and broke away. Dissenters had limited rights in England. They could not attend the large universities, like Oxford and Cambridge. Nonetheless, Joseph pursued his passion for learning and God. He became an instructor at a local academy, a scientist, and was ordained as a Dissenting minister.

Priestley published six volumes of *Experiments and Observations on Different Kinds of Air* between 1772 and 1790. He detailed his experiments on gases or "airs." He is credited for the discovery of several gases: nitrogen dioxide, ammonia, nitrous oxide (laughing gas), nitrogen, and oxygen. The success that Priestley experienced as a scientist is credited to his keen mind and his ability to design ingenious contraptions to study gases he discovered.

The Breath of Life

Breathing is essential to life. Without the air that rushes into your lungs you would cease to exist. The Bible makes many references to breathing. Our Heavenly Father is the giver of life and through His breath He calls all creatures into existence. In Genesis 2:7 it says, "Then the Lord God formed a man from the dust of the ground and breathed into his nostrils the breath of life, and the man became a living being."

There is no evidence here of man being formed from an evolutionary process, but rather being formed from the actual loving hands of God. Job, through all his adversity, knew where his life force came from. In Job 33:4 he states, "The Spirit of God has made me; the breath of the Almighty gives me life." Remember, as Psalm 150:6 states, "Let everything that has breath praise the Lord. Praise the Lord."

Biblical References:			
2 Samuel 22:16	Job 4:9	John 20:22	Acts 17:25
Isaiah 11:4	Ezekiel 37:5–10	Isaiah 30:28	

I AM wonderfully made

God's Wondrous Machine

The Haldanes and Their Bad Gas

Today, scientific research is heavily managed and monitored. In the 1970s, the Food and Drug Administration (FDA) developed laws to protect human subjects taking part in clinical trials. Clinical trials are research studies that determine how well new medical approaches work in people.

Prior to this time, there was no standard on how things were tested on people. Many doctors and scientists would do unsafe practices on themselves or others in order to observe and learn new medical advances. There are two such scientists, father and son, who used themselves as human guinea pigs. (Guinea pigs have been commonly used in laboratory studies.) John and Jack Haldane utilized their bodies for scientific exploration. They made many contributions to our understanding of the respiratory system and the nature of gases.

John Haldane was a Scottish physiologist born in the late 1800s. A physiologist is a type of scientist that strives to understand how body systems work. Mr. Haldane demonstrated an insatiable thirst for knowledge. He would conduct experiments on himself. He would check the quality of air by locking himself in closed chambers and inhaling potentially deadly gases. He would then record the effects it had on his body and mind. John's son, Jack, was quick to get into the act. Jack began his own experimentation at three years of age when he gladly allowed his father to take a small amount of his blood for study. At the ripe old age of four years, Jack started breathing "bad air" in the underground railway and mines, and at 13 years he dove into the ocean in a leaky diving suit. Jack was a child scientist by his father's side.

On many occasions, the Haldanes felt the ill effects of their experiments. They suffered from headaches, vomiting, passing out, and on some occasions even turned blue. John was able to show that most of these ill effects were not due to a lack of oxygen but a build-up of carbon dioxide in their bloodstream.

They did many crazy things. It is not surprising that the family motto of the Haldane family was just one word — "suffer." They inhaled many mixtures of gases and studied the effects on their bodies. They were one of the first to identify that breathing was controlled by the blood-brain barrier that transported gases to a sensitive area of the brain. They were the experts on the hazards of breathing bad air. Their discoveries revolutionized and protected the jobs of miners, soldiers, deep sea divers, and submarine dwellers. They unlocked the mysteries of respiration and the gases that affect us.

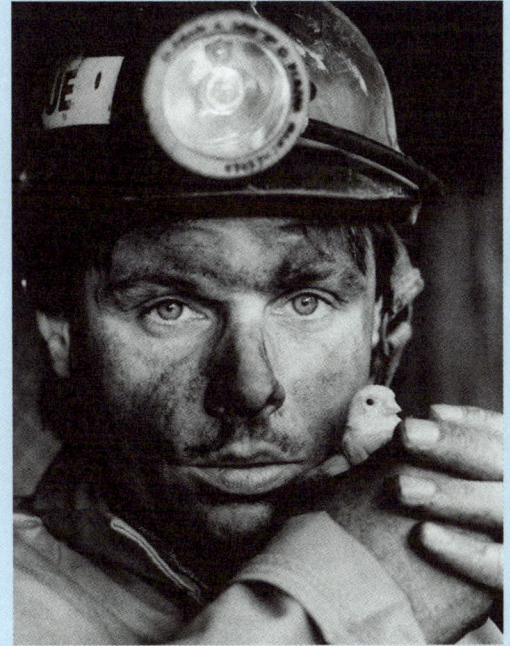

John Haldane came up with the idea of using canaries as an early warning system. The miners carried a caged canary into the coal mine and if dangerous gases like carbon monoxide were present they would kill the canary before the miners felt the ill effects.

Unit 2: The Breathtaking Respiratory System

3 The Structure of the Respiratory Tract

The breathtaking respiratory system can be divided into two general parts: the upper respiratory tract and the lower respiratory tract. The upper respiratory tract is more like a tunnel system that propels the air downward. The air cannot be used by the lungs until it arrives at the lower respiratory tract.

If the actual spongy tissues of the lungs were removed and the respiratory tunnels were left, it would resemble an upside-down tree. The respiratory tree originates at the trachea (the trunk) and spreads, dividing to smaller and smaller branches called the bronchioles. Let's take a closer look at the different parts, starting with the upper respiratory tract.

Upper Respiratory Tract

The main function of the upper respiratory tract, is to be the passageway for air to the lungs. The air rushes in and is propelled down the tract. From top to bottom, the parts of the upper respiratory tract are as follows:

1. Nose
2. Sinuses
3. Pharynx
4. Larynx

Your nose is really cool! At the top of the nasal cavity there is a space the size of a postage stamp that has some 10 million small receptor cells. Your nose doesn't only just help you breathe and smell stuff; it's also connected to your sense of taste. That's why it's hard to taste your food when you have a stopped-up nose!

- Nasal cavity
- Nostril
- Epiglottis
- Larynx
- Trachea

Word Wise!

NOSTHYRL means "nose hole" in old English. From this came the word "nostril" that we know today!

God's Wondrous Machine

Mucus: A Bat in the Cave

A bat in the cave, snot, phlegm, and loogie are just a few terms people use when referring to the wonderful substance of mucus. Before starting our downward journey through the tract, let's take a look at this natural multipurpose lubricant called mucus. Most people find the discussion of mucus a bit gross. It is actually a wonderful invention by our Heavenly Father. What is that? You say that it has never been part of your prayers when thanking God for His many provisions? There are so many things we take for granted in our bodies until they malfunction. Step up as we take an appreciative look at mucus.

Mucus is a lubricant. A lubricant is something that is slimy and cuts down friction on surfaces as things slide past. It has many functions aside from just being slimy. Mucus can be as thick and sticky as maple syrup. This stickiness allows it to trap bits and pieces of dust and dirt. In addition, it traps unwanted visitors into our bodies like nasty, germy bacteria. Mucus keeps things nice and moist, preventing the lining of our nose, stomach, and intestines from drying out. It also has antiseptic enzymes within its goo. These antiseptic enzymes act on bacteria and decrease the incidence of infections. The mucus traps these particles and other potentially harmful substances and whisks them off to the pharynx to be swallowed and demolished by digestive juices in the stomach.

Way back in the Middle Ages, it was believed the body was composed of four humors, or fluids. Phlegm, or mucus, was one of these mistaken humors. If a person's body was off balance and not well, the fault was attributed to one of the humors. If you felt sluggish and emotionally up and down, this was most likely due to being "phlegmatic." In other words, too much phlegm or mucus within your body was upsetting your healthy balance.

There are cells in your body called goblet cells that make this hard-working substance of mucus. Mucus is composed of mucopolysaccharides (mew-kow-pol-ee-sack-ah-rides). The recipe for mucus is 95% water, 2% mucin, and 2–3% salt. The mucin gives the mucus its slimy goodness and sticky composition. The average person produces about one quart of mucus a day! A quart is the size of the container in which milk, mayo, and motor oil are usually purchased.

Eeeewwwww!

Sometimes when your nose starts to itch on the inside, you have an overwhelming urge to sneeze. In one sneeze, thousands of tiny droplets of snot and other bacteria hitchhikers sail out of your nose like a rocket into the air space surrounding you. Anyone within three to five feet may be pelted by the aerosol. There has been long debate about how fast a snot rocket can be ejected. Some have stated that it can hit speeds up to 100 miles an hour. In the show *Mythbusters*, Jamie Hyneman and Adam Savage set up high-speed cameras to be eyewitnesses to the physics of mucoid propulsion. They sniffed items that would cause forceful sneezing. Taking turns as great scientists, they recorded their results. Adam clocked a speed of 35 mph and Jamie rocketed at 39 mph.

The average person produces about one quart of snot a day!

on the nose.

Unit 2: The Breathtaking Respiratory System

The Nose

The nose is one of the top producers of mucus. The nose's function is to warm and filter the air. It is the passageway for air where it is humidified (water is added to it) and moistened. Inside your nose, there are thousands of hairs. These hairs partner with the mucus to provide a trap for dust. Once tickled, the hairs can trigger a sneeze to expel any unwanted items.

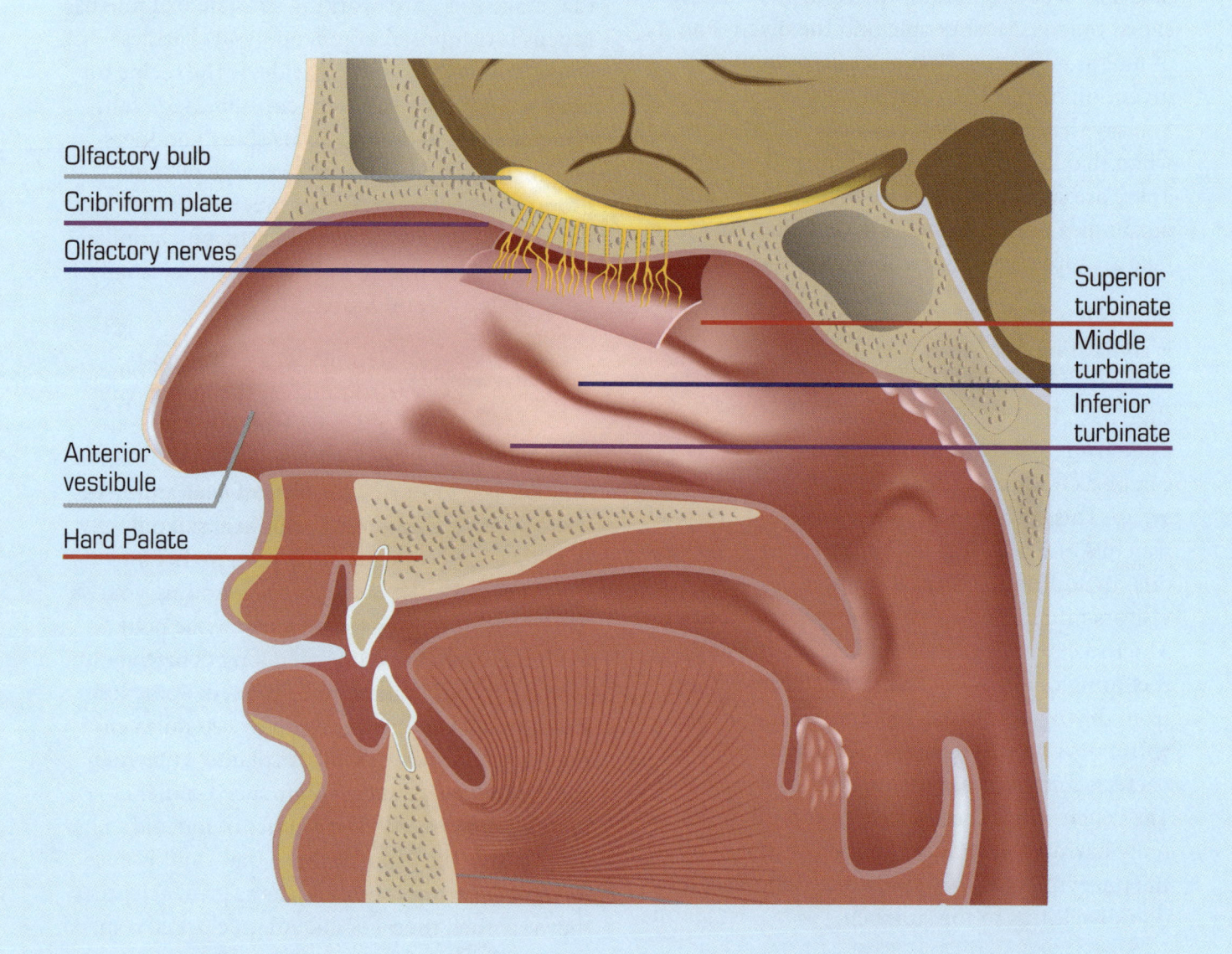

- Olfactory bulb
- Cribriform plate
- Olfactory nerves
- Anterior vestibule
- Hard Palate
- Superior turbinate
- Middle turbinate
- Inferior turbinate

Parts of the Nose

Air enters the nose at the nostrils. These two openings enter at the anterior vestibule. The anterior vestibule is the area in which most nose bleeds occur. Many kids and adults alike may from time to time engage in attempts to extract a hardened mucoid fragment from their nose — a booger. The nose has many blood vessels that are close to the lining on the inside. It is through

God's Wondrous Machine

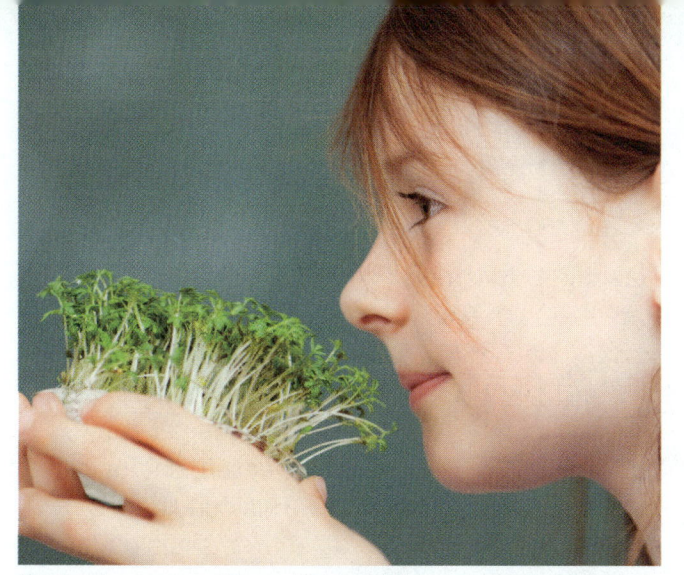

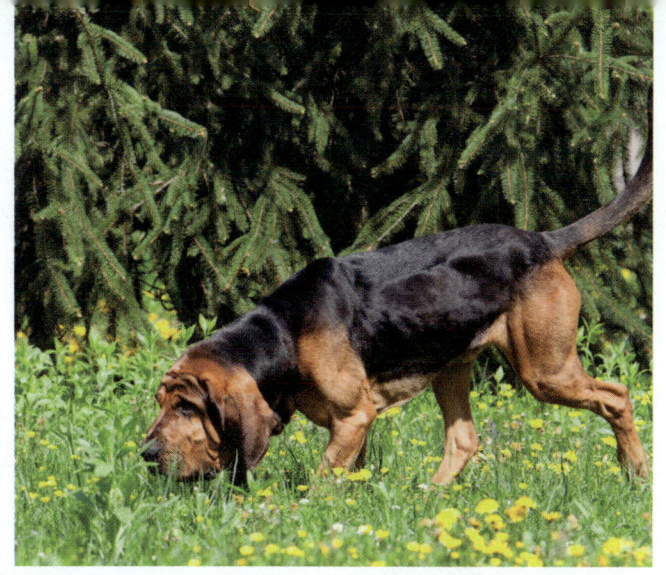

God gave us an incredible ability to smell. We can enjoy the fragrances of flowers, good food, and even the rain as it falls. Most people can distinguish over 10,000 different odors, and women have a better sense of smell than men. Dogs are still better at smelling than we are! They can detect the tiniest traces of an odor and can even smell the chemicals that come with emotions like fear or sadness.

these vessels that warm blood flows, assisting in warming the air that you inhale. A scrape in this area can cause a nosebleed. The art of nose picking is greatly frowned upon in modern-day society. In the 1500s, it was considered acceptable behavior. There was even a code of etiquette on how to pick your nose while in the company of others.

Next in line is the nasal turbinate or concha. There are three bony plates on each side of the nose, covered with the nasal lining. These nooks and crannies serve to increase the surface area of the nasal cavity and cause the air to be more turbulent in flow. This turbulence and surface area further aids the nose to filter, cleanse, warm, and moisten the air you breathe. The right and the left sides of your nasal cavity are divided by the septum.

The cribriform plate lies at the top of the nasal cavity. It is the part of the skull that separates the brain from the nasal cavity. There is a special nerve network that emerges at this site. The olfactory bulb sends nerve endings through openings in this region. Olfactory nerves deal with our sense of smell. A skull fracture in this area can potentially damage these nerves and cause anosmia (an-OHZ-me-uh), a loss of the ability to smell.

We take our sense of smell for granted. Your sense of smell helps you to taste foods. It helps you to smell the light fragrance of a rose. Most importantly, it helps you to sense smells that could be dangerous to you like the smell of rancid milk. You smell the milk and know instantly it is something you do not want to drink.

Animals like bloodhound dogs have an exquisite sense of smell. Bloodhounds have approximately 230 million olfactory cells! That is 40 times greater than we humans have. It is amazing to watch these dogs happily at work. Bloodhounds can sniff an article of clothing and obtain the unique odor of a person. This smell sticks to the dog's scent receptors in its nose. The odor serves like a smell photograph of the person to the dog. The dog's instincts take over and it can track the scent of an individual for miles.

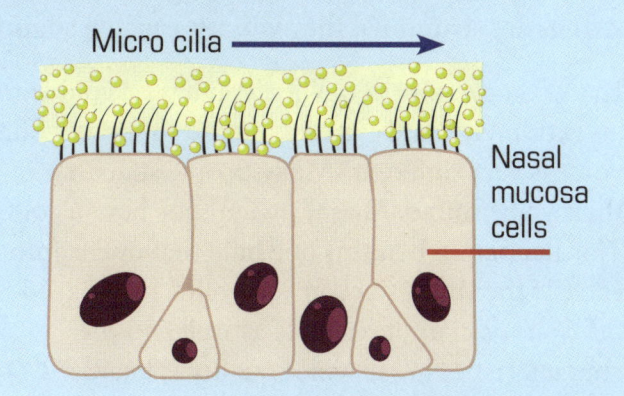

Micro cilia

Nasal mucosa cells

Unit 2: The Breathtaking Respiratory System

Healthy | Inflamed

- Frontal sinus
- Ethmoid sinus
- Sphenoid sinus
- Maxillary sinus

Sinusitis: Sometimes the tissues that line the hollow spaces of the sinuses get red, swollen, and painful. This condition is called sinusitis, and is often caused by allergies or an infection. The redness, swelling and pain are by-products of your body trying to heal itself.

Sinuses

Within the confines of your facial bones lie four pairs of hollow spaces. These spaces are called the sinuses. The names of the four pairs are (1) frontal, (2) sphenoid, (3) ethmoid, and (4) maxillary.

Their function is to assist in warming and moistening the air that you inhale. It provides a hollow space that acts like a resonance chamber for speech production. A resonance chamber is a completely enclosed space aside one hole that allows sound to enter. Sound waves enter through the hole and are amplified (made louder). For example, in stringed instruments like the guitar or violin, the hollow body is this type of chamber. The sound hole lies below the strings. As the strings are strummed they vibrate, causing sound.

Have you ever noticed when you have a cold with an extremely "stuffy" nose that the sound of your voice is very different? Many people state that their voice sounds "nasal" when they have a cold. This happens when this one hole that opens into each of the sinuses becomes swollen or plugged off. Sounds cannot resonate as well and the characteristic "nasal" voice quality is heard.

The hollow sinuses allow the skull to weigh less. They also produce mucus to trap and get rid of unwanted materials that enter. The mucus in the sinuses drains through their hole into the nasal cavity. In the nasal cavity, there are nasal hairs near the entrance of the nose. Germ droplets that aren't caught in the nose hairs may enter the sinuses. The sinuses will become irritated and swollen. This swelling will block off the drainage of the sinuses. The sinuses become a closed container of mucus and germy critters. The space becomes like a stagnant pool. These germs love warm, dark, and moist environments. There they grow, multiply, and have a party. The result is a sinus infection or sinusitis. (*Sinu:* hollow cavity, *-itis:* inflammation.) The face or forehead over the infected area of the sinus can become swollen and red.

Word Wise!

"RHINITIS" is what we doctors call inflamed (swollen) nasal membranes. It's commonly known as having a stuffy or runny nose!

God's Wondrous Machine

Your sinuses aren't fully developed after birth. The frontal sinuses and sphenoid sinuses don't begin to develop until a child reaches his or her second birthday. The actual cavities cannot be seen by x-ray imaging until the child is at least five or six years old. Your sinuses continue to grow until your teenage years.

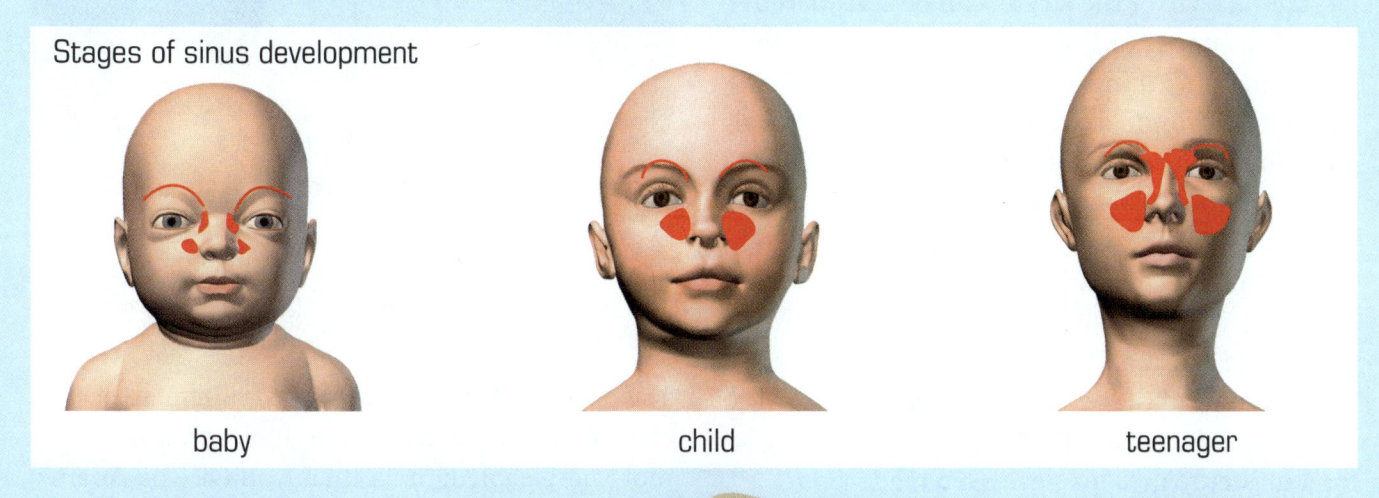

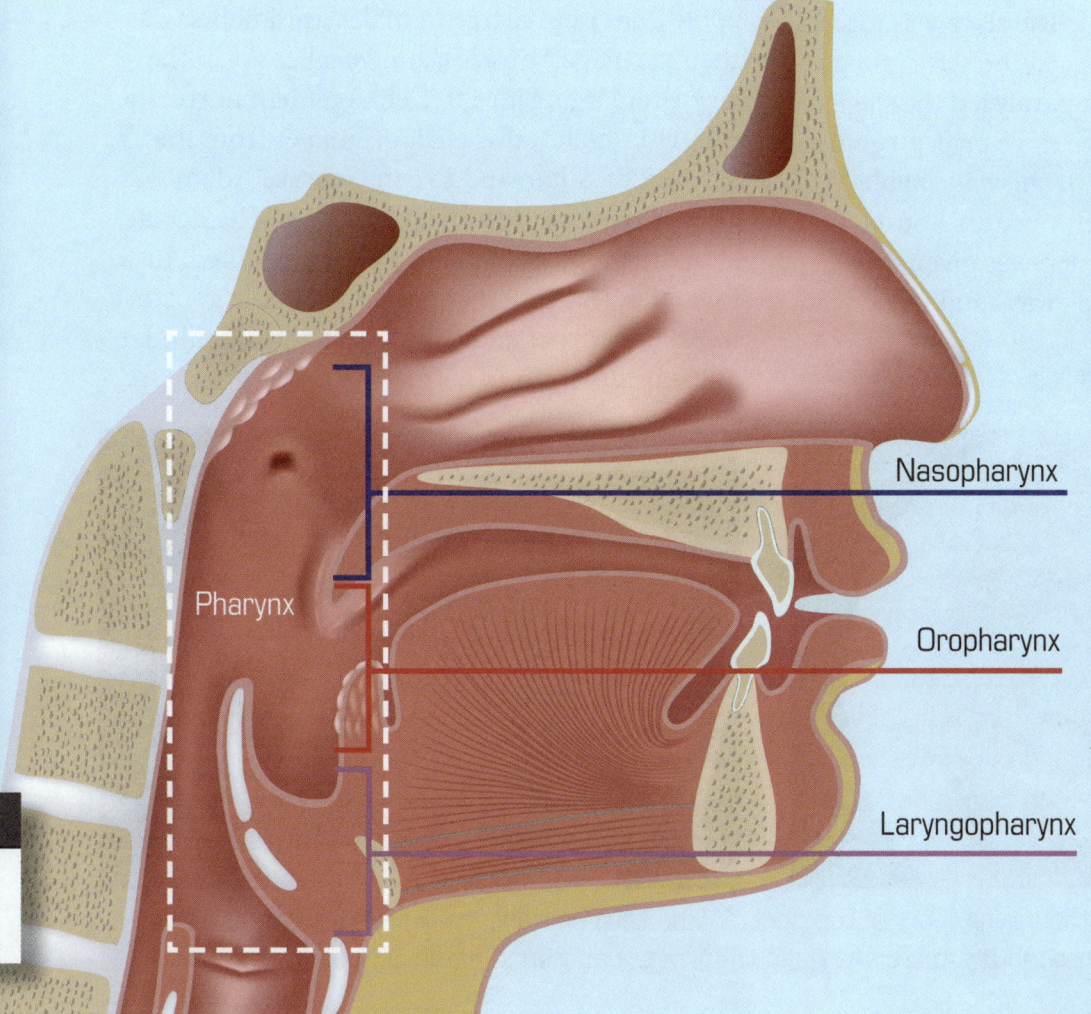

Stages of sinus development

baby | child | teenager

Pharynx

Air enters the nose and travels down to the pharynx. The pharynx is the back of your throat. Your oral cavity, the inside of your mouth, and your nasal cavity both open up in the back to join together at the pharynx. The area directly behind the nasal cavity is called the nasopharynx. The area directly behind your oral cavity is called the oropharynx. See the pattern? We use very specific terms in Anatomy in order to effectively communicate with precision.

Nasopharynx
Oropharynx
Laryngopharynx
Pharynx

Unit 2: The Breathtaking Respiratory System

95

The Larynx

The pharynx meets up with the larynx. The area where the pharynx and larynx meet is called the laryngopharynx. (The larynx can be considered part of the upper or lower respiratory tract.) This whole anatomy thing is a piece of cake, right? The larynx is the home of your vocal cords. The vocal cords are like the reed of a wind instrument. When air goes by them they vibrate and produce sound. Kids' voices are much different from adult voices. In males, at puberty, the larynx and vocal cords grow larger. The vocal cords also become longer and thicker. These changes are what cause a man's voice to deepen. Speaking of vocal cords, during Roman times, it was not uncommon for a master to give his slave a tea made from dieffenbachia (dumb plant). The slave was forced to drink the tea. The tea caused the slave's tongue and mouth to swell. It even paralyzed the slave's throat. This was given to the slave prior to going to the market to ensure he or she was unable to speak and gossip about their master's household. As you can image, if too much was given, the swelling would cut off the airways and could lead to death.

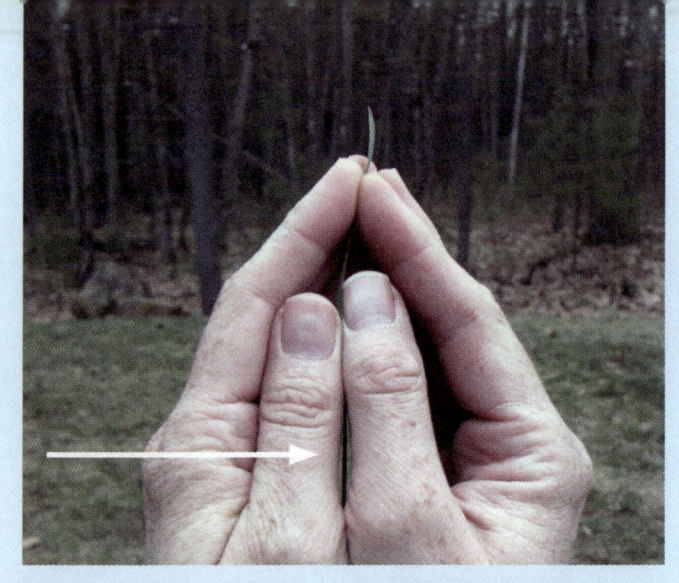

In the summer, it is fun to take a blade of grass, stretch it taut, grasp it tightly between your thumbs, and blow forcefully. A loud whistling noise can be heard as the blade of grass vibrates in the rushing air much like your vocal cords.

The outside of the throat is a prominent area commonly called the Adam's apple. This area is more noticeable in men than women. The Adam's apple does not enlarge in males until puberty as their cartilage, muscles, and vocal cords in the larynx enlarge. Since this enlargement normally occurs in males, this term originates from the account of Adam and Eve in Genesis. Adam was offered the forbidden fruit from Eve. The debate about the type of fruit has been questioned. In folk tales, it is said that part of the apple got stuck in Adam's throat and continues to be a reminder of his original sin.

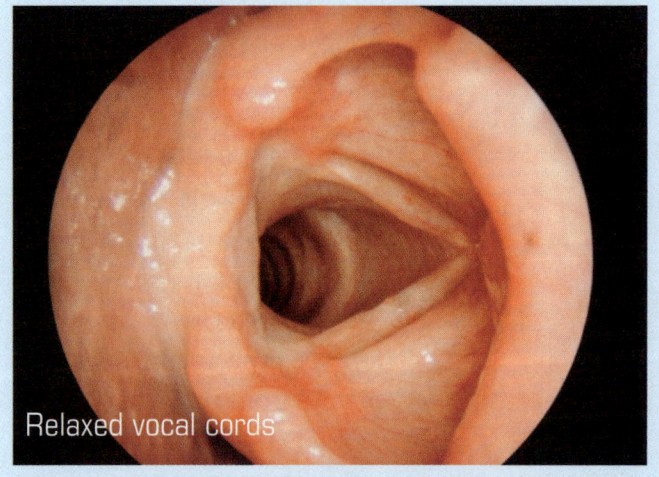

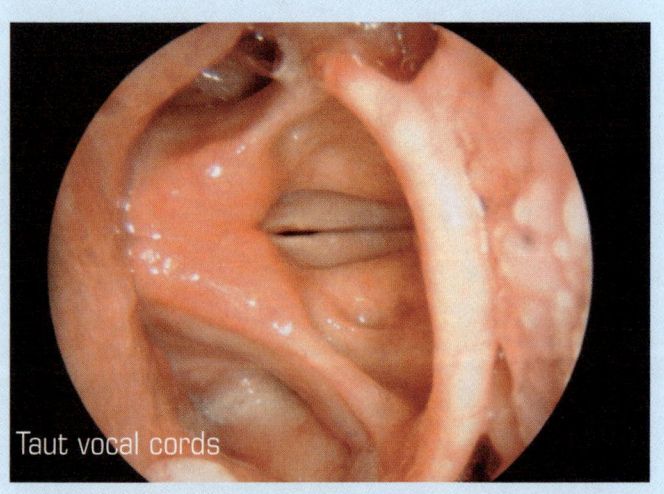

Relaxed vocal cords

Taut vocal cords

Vocal cords are located in the larynx, part of the neck. When taut or tight, they produce sound as air from the lungs is passed through them. This is used to form sounds such as singing and speech.

God's Wondrous Machine

Your body is wonderfully designed! If it weren't, even something simple like eating could become dangerous in terms of choking or food going into your lungs.

on the nose.

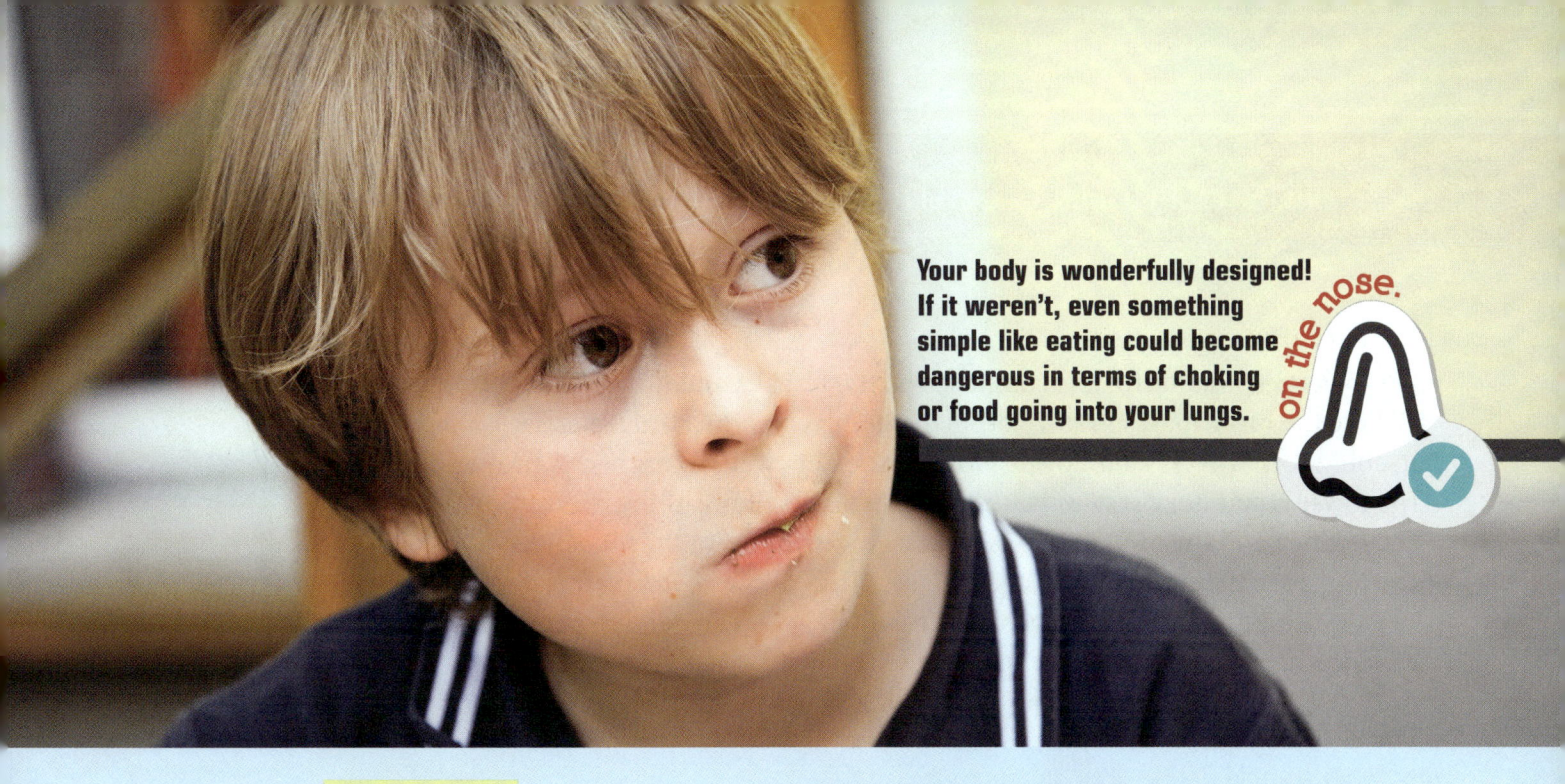

The Epiglottis

The larynx is the end of the line for the upper respiratory tract. It is at this point that you arrive at a fork in the road. The tunnel system splits. One part runs down to the lungs and the other part runs to the esophagus. The esophagus is the food tube that transports what you eat to your stomach. Your air and your food share the passage until arriving at this fork in the road. God has designed an ingenious and effective mechanism to prevent food from entering your lungs. He has designed the "lid." Well, it isn't really named the "lid." It is called the epiglottis. It is a little piece of cartilage that acts as a lid, covering the trachea and larynx when we eat and drink. It prevents us from choking when we swallow. Sometimes you can see the top of the epiglottis when you ask someone to stick out their tongue and say "ah."

You may have heard someone tell you, "Don't talk with your mouth full." Your body was not designed to breathe and swallow at the same time. In order to talk or laugh, air has to rush in and out of your lungs. The epiglottis remains open when you talk and laugh. When you swallow food, the epiglottis slams down like a lid to keep food stuff from entering your lungs. The epiglottis doesn't shut when you are eating and laughing at the same time. This may lead to food going down your "windpipe." This is called "aspiration" and leads to choking.

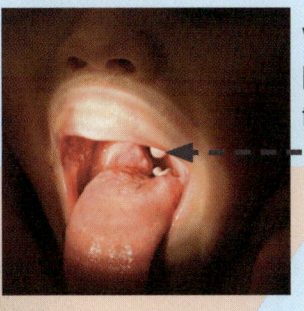

Visible epiglottis at the back of the throat on a two year old.

Epiglottis

97

Unit 2: The Breathtaking Respiratory System

4 The Structure of the Lower Respiratory Tract

The lower respiratory tract is composed of the trachea and lungs. The lungs include the bronchi, respiratory bronchioles, alveolar ducts, alveolar sacs, and alveoli. Wow! That is a mouthful. No worries. Let's walk by each, one by one. The lower respiratory system is where the business of breathing occurs. The trachea and the bronchi act as a passageway for air to the lungs. The lungs are the site for exchange of gases. They allow us to breathe. Just a quick point: the word alveolus is used when you are talking about a single one of these grape-like structures. The word alveoli is used when you are referring to many of these grape-like structures. It is the plural form.

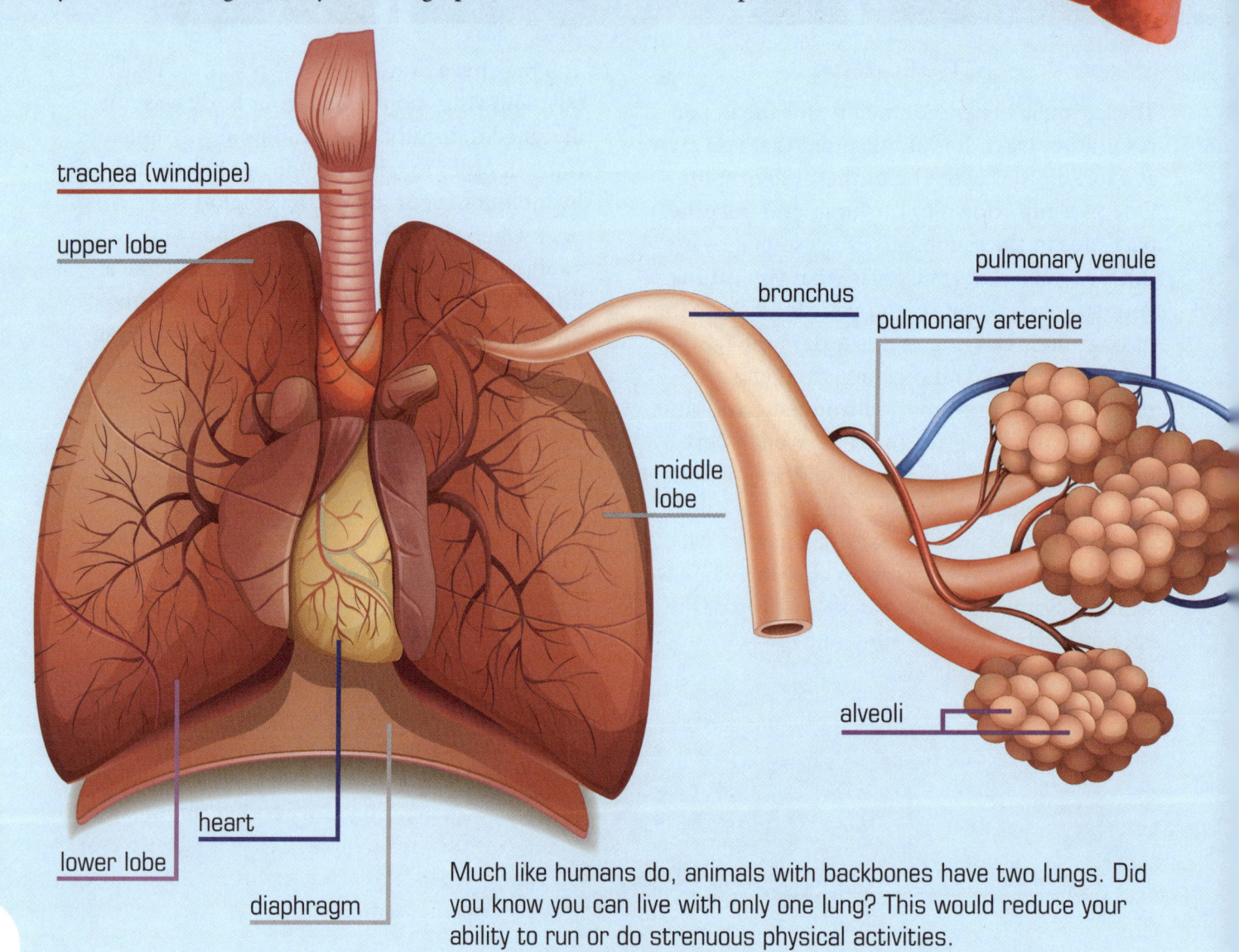

- trachea (windpipe)
- upper lobe
- bronchus
- pulmonary venule
- pulmonary arteriole
- middle lobe
- alveoli
- heart
- lower lobe
- diaphragm

Much like humans do, animals with backbones have two lungs. Did you know you can live with only one lung? This would reduce your ability to run or do strenuous physical activities.

98

God's Wondrous Machine

The Trachea

The trachea brings air into the lungs. It has many C-shaped flexible cartilage rings that run down its length. The structure of the trachea resembles the flexible aluminum or plastic tubing that is found on the back of your laundry dryer. These C-shaped cartilage rings help to keep the trachea from collapsing. The rings do not run completely around the trachea. Why do you think God designed it that way? Remember when we talked about that "fork in the road"? What structure runs directly behind the trachea? Bingo! The esophagus! If the trachea's rings ran completely around, when you swallowed food it would bounce through like a car on rumble strips on a highway.

Sometimes due to illness or a birth defect, a person may have problems maintaining an open airway in order to breathe. A tracheostomy may be used to help keep a person's airway open and make it easier to breathe. This procedure is indicated in cases where a person does not have a cough reflex. The cough reflex is normally triggered when something irritates the respiratory tract and causes one to cough. This reflex protects the airway. A tube is inserted below the vocal cords and allows them to breathe easier.

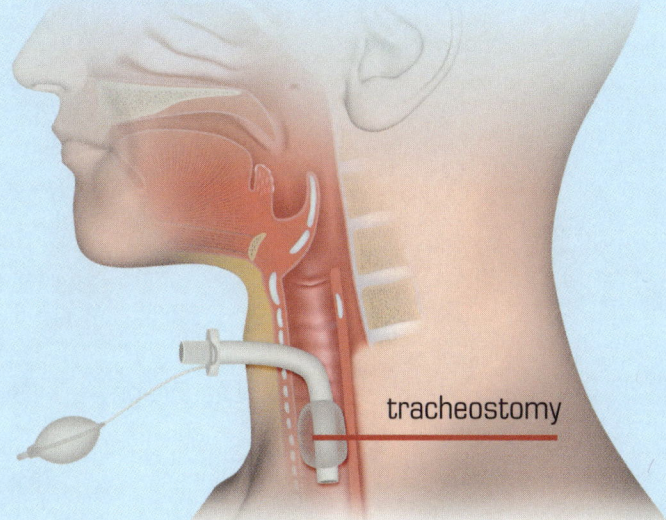

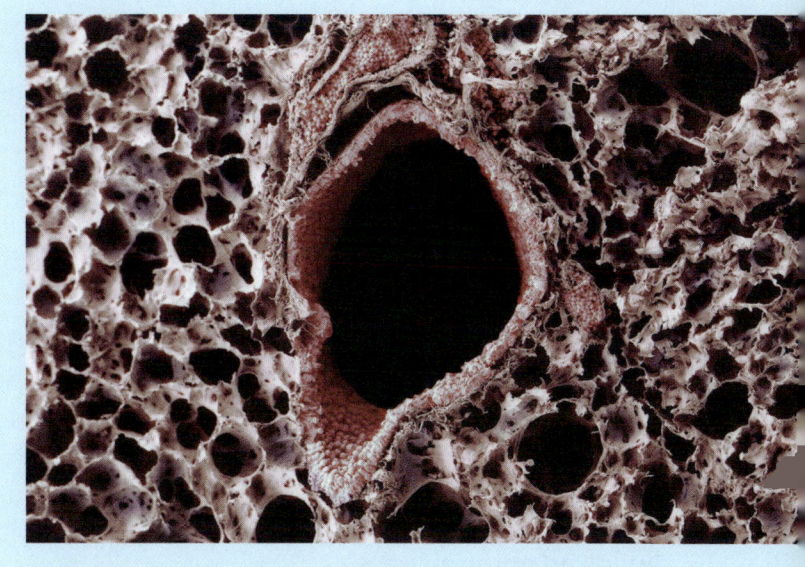

tracheostomy

Lung tissue

The Lungs

The lungs are spongy organs. They are composed of many passageways and microscopic air sacs. The lungs are encased in the pleura sac. This sac has two layers. It allows the lungs to expand and recoil without causing friction or rubbing on the ribs.

There are two lungs, the right and left. The right lung has three segments and the left lung has two segments. The left lung has one segment less due to the space that is occupied by the heart.

The trachea enters the lungs and divides into two tunnels, the right and left bronchus. The bronchus divides into smaller and smaller branches as the travel deeper into the lungs. The bronchi enter the lungs and branch into smaller secondary (second) and tertiary (third) bronchi, respectively. The tertiary bronchi divide into ever-smaller branches called the bronchioles. The tunnels become smaller and smaller. At the end of the bronchioles is a cluster of air sacs known as alveoli. These alveoli are grouped together like clusters of grapes. This is where carbon dioxide (CO_2) is traded for oxygen. Oxygen is needed for our body to perform all of its duties. We will look more at this momentarily.

Unit 2: The Breathtaking Respiratory System

Cilia

Cilia are hair-like projections that line the larger airways of the lungs. These hairs beat together in a coordinated motion that causes a current of mucus that is swept to the back of the throat to be coughed out or swallowed. The mucus in the lungs is produced by a special cell called the goblet cell. The mucus lies on the top layer over the cilia. Cigarette smoking is harmful to the cilia. If the cilia are unable to move, then mucus builds up in the airways.

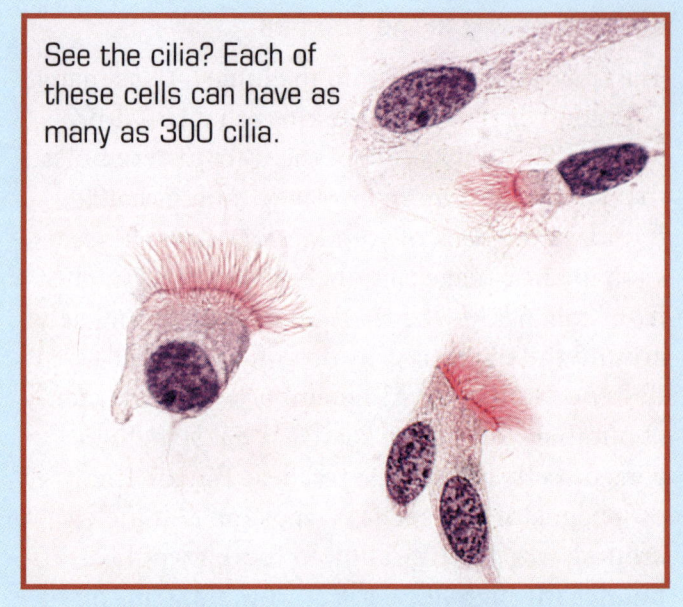

See the cilia? Each of these cells can have as many as 300 cilia.

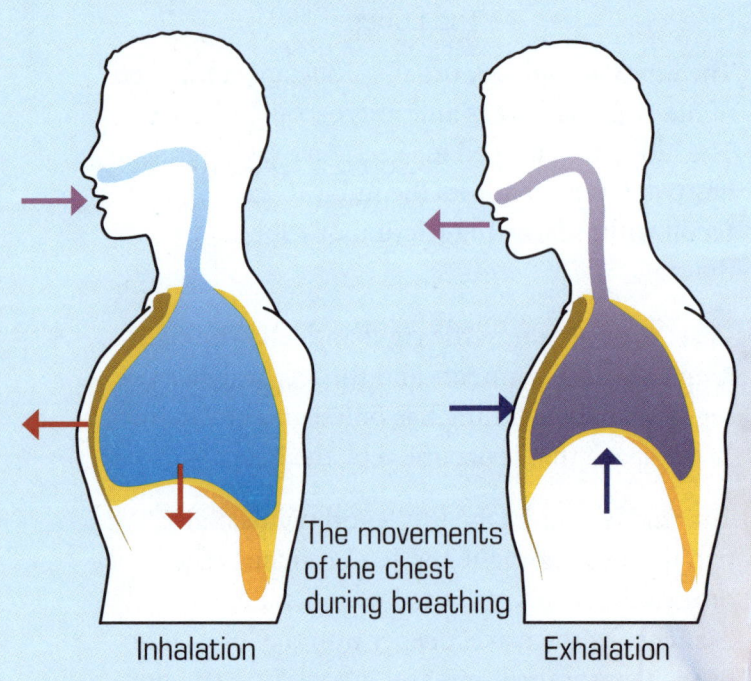

The movements of the chest during breathing

Inhalation   Exhalation

The diaphragm is a large sheet-like muscle that your lungs rest on. The diaphragm separates the thorax, the chest cavity, from the abdominal cavity. When you take a breath in, the diaphragm contracts and moves downward as your lungs expand. In exhalation, the diaphragm moves back up, expelling the air from your lungs.

Three other structures outside the lungs play an important role in breathing. Those three structures are the ribs, the intercostal muscles, and the diaphragm. The ribs surround your chest cavity. They attach in the back to your spine. In the front, most attach to the sternum, except for the last couple of ribs. The ribs function like the handle of a bucket. During inhalation your ribs are lifted up and out by the intercostal muscles, and during exhalation they move down and in.

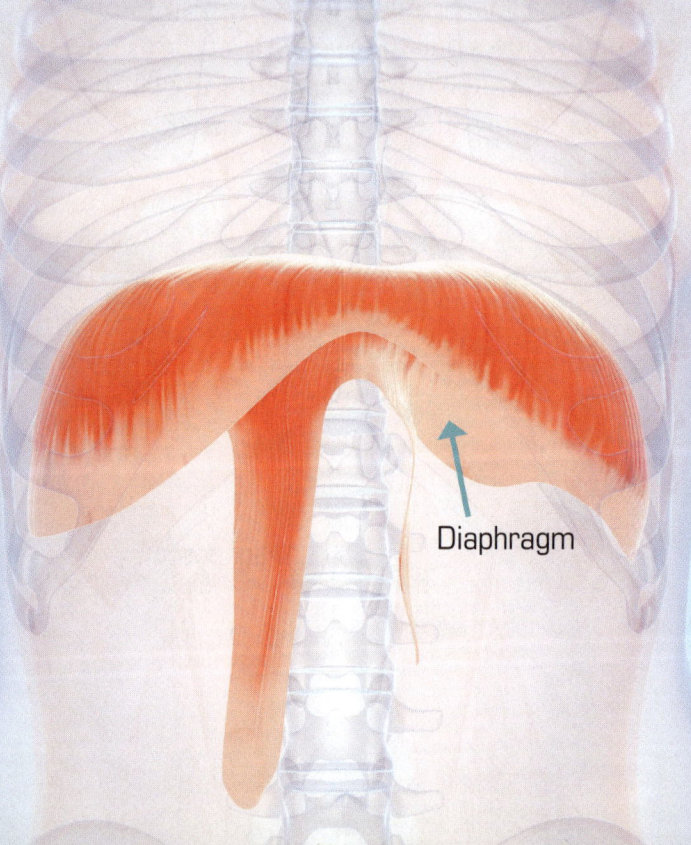

Diaphragm

Alveoli

Now, let's go back to the alveoli. Each alveolus has its own stem, called the alveolar duct. Alveoli are extremely small and have very thin walls. This allows for gases to diffuse across the membrane. The word diffusion is derived from the Latin word *diffundere*, which means "to spread out." Diffusion is movement of a substance from a region of high concentration to a region of low concentration. The gases that diffuse through the membrane are oxygen and carbon dioxide.

Carbon dioxide (CO_2) is waste or garbage made as a result of all the chemical processes that occur in our bodies. The CO_2 travels through the bloodstream and arrives in the lungs. We exhale this CO_2. God has designed everything so that none of this is wasted! Trees and plants use the CO_2. In a happy trade, the plants release oxygen to us. We happily inhale the oxygen. The red blood cells act like mini cargo trucks by picking up the oxygen atoms to deliver them to the rest of the body.

Gas		Inhaled Air	Exhaled Air
Oxygen	O_2	21%	17%
Carbon Dioxide	CO_2	0.04%	4%
Nitrogen	N	78%	78%

Remarkably, the concentration of the air that enters the lungs compared to the air that exits the lungs seems relatively similar. Don't let the numbers fool you! These precise concentrations provide enough of a diffusional difference that the carbon dioxide and oxygen travel in opposite directions. There is still oxygen in the air we breathe out.

When we inhale, air travels all the way down through the bronchioles to the alveolar duct to the alveolar sacs. A large network of blood vessels and capillaries surround the alveolar sacs. The red blood cells course by in almost single file, dumping carbon dioxide and loading up on oxygen.

A special cell in the alveoli produces a substance called surfactant. Surfactant helps to keep the alveoli open by decreasing the tug that water vapor has on the walls of these balloon-like sacs.

Your respiratory system does a wonderful job of putting moisture in the air you breathe. As a result, water molecules line the walls of the alveolus. Water molecules are strongly attracted to each other. This attraction creates a force called surface tension. The alveoli decrease in size when you exhale and the surface tension increases. This force could cause the alveoli to collapse and stick tightly together. The force to peel the air sac walls apart would be difficult. Hard to imagine? Surface tension can be seen with the circus-like performance of an insect called the water strider. If you look at the surface of a pond you might see a water strider walking across the surface of the water without falling in due to the surface tension.

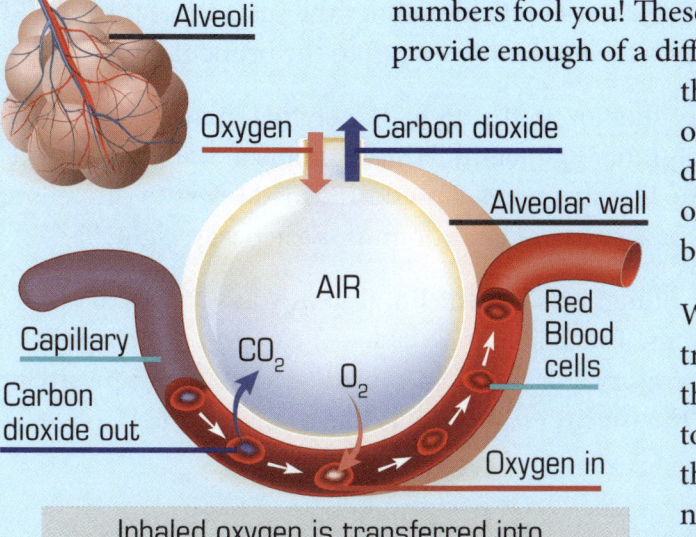

Inhaled oxygen is transferred into the blood while carbon dioxide is transferred to the alveoli to be exhaled.

Unit 2: The Breathtaking Respiratory System

The Respiratory Lining

The outside of your body is covered with skin, so are the passageways of your respiratory tract. The "skin" lining is called the epithelium. Epithelium lines the surfaces of the body. The lining is found on every aspect of the respiratory tract from the mouth to the bronchioles.

There are several types of epithelium in the body. The epithelium that lines the respiratory tract is called ciliated pseudostratified columnar epithelium. This is simply a descriptive name for the tissue. It is ciliated — covered with hair-like structures. Pseudostratified refers to the cells appearing to be lined up somewhat in layers. The cells are shaped like columns. Easy peasy, right?

The respiratory lining in the lungs acts like the lint trap in your clothes dryer. It traps all the unwanted particles that enter your lungs. The hair cells — cilia — lie on top of the epithelium and the mucus lies on top of the cilia. The respiratory cilia beat in a coordinated manner upward, and particles that enter get trapped in the mucus. The mucus escalator acts like a conveyor belt to send things up and out.

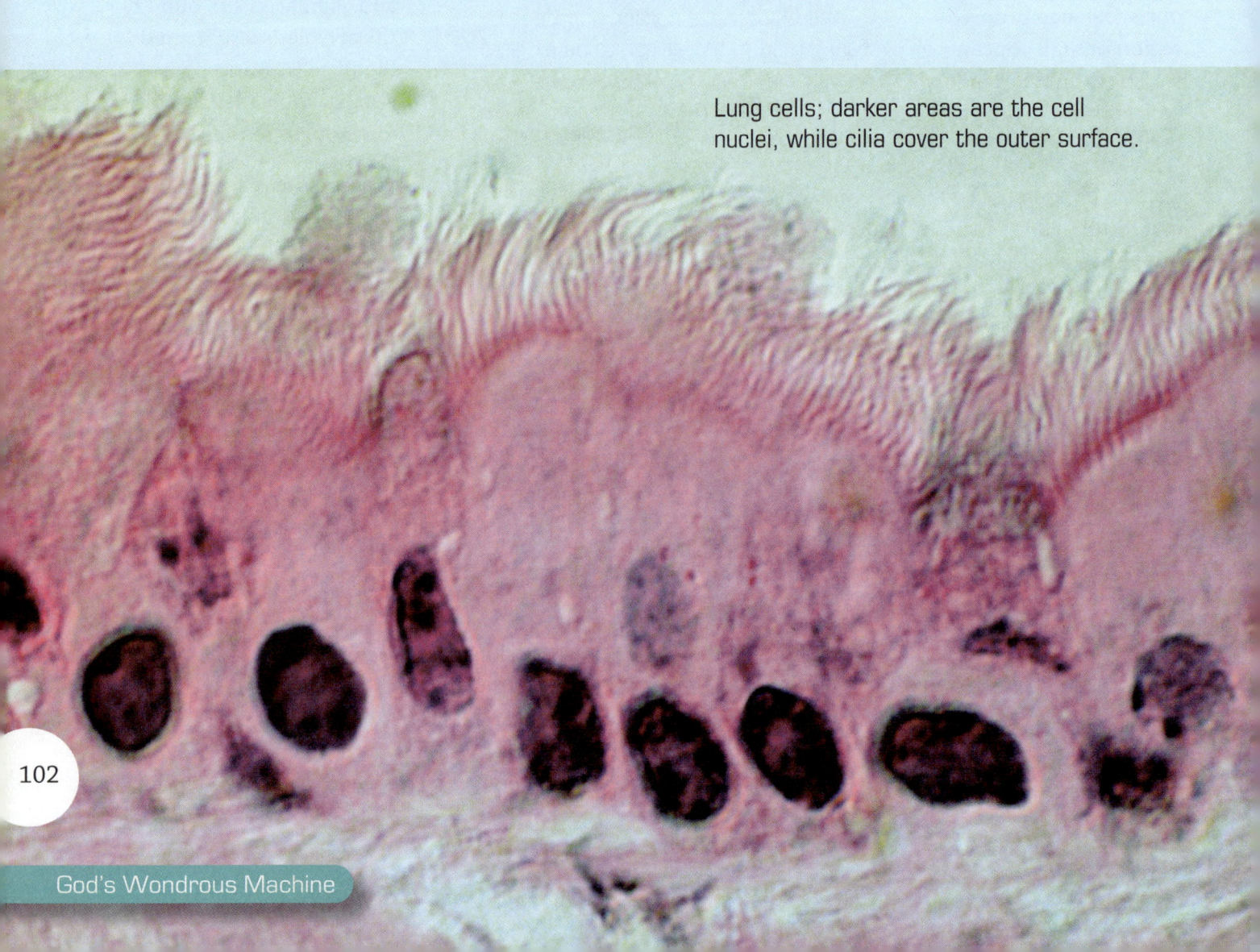

Lung cells; darker areas are the cell nuclei, while cilia cover the outer surface.

God's Wondrous Machine

Carbon Monoxide Poisoning

Gases other than carbon dioxide and oxygen can diffuse through the alveolar wall. As the weather becomes colder, there is a higher incidence of carbon monoxide poisoning. The furnaces in homes kick on for the first time as the weather becomes colder. If furnaces are not well maintained they can produce a colorless, tasteless, and odorless gas called carbon monoxide. Carbon monoxide is found in the fumes produced in things like cars, trucks, fires, small gasoline engines, stoves, and heating systems.

The chemical formula for carbon dioxide is CO_2. It has one carbon molecule and two oxygen molecules attached together. Carbon monoxide is CO. It has one carbon and one oxygen molecule attached. Carbon monoxide is less dense and lighter than carbon dioxide. When it is inhaled, it diffuses more readily across the alveoli to the red blood cells in the lungs. Carbon monoxide pushes oxygen off the red blood cell and takes its spot. The tissues and organs of the body are unable to get oxygen. The carbon monoxide binds to the red blood cells. The person will begin to experience headache, tiredness, vomiting, confusion, and dizziness, and will eventually lose consciousness. To overcome this oxygen starvation the body experiences, the treatment is to give 100 percent oxygen to remove the carbon monoxide from the red blood cells.

This is why carbon monoxide detectors in the home are important. It is also important to maintain equipment and appliances, and have yearly furnace checks. Never use gasoline-powered equipment in areas that do not have good air circulation.

MEDI+MOMENT

Deep sea diving provides a breathtaking opportunity to see incredible wonders that God has designed. Unlike the fish and other inhabitants of the deep, we were not designed to occupy such spaces. In order to go below the surface of the ocean, divers must breathe heavily pressurized gases to prevent their lungs from collapsing from the high pressures exerted on their bodies.

If divers ascend too quickly to the surface of the water after a deep dive, they can experience a potentially life-threatening condition called "the bends."

The bends or decompression sickness is caused by formation of bubbles of gas in the blood, like a carbonated soda. These bubbles of gas accumulate and travel in the bloodstream and form in the tissues. It is extremely painful. The gases can lodge in joints and in many places in the body, including the brain.

If the lungs were able to be filled with a liquid instead of a gas most of these problems could be avoided. In experimentation is the use of perfluorocarbon (PFC), a synthetic liquid that is clear and odorless. It has a high capacity to carry oxygen and carbon dioxide. It carries three times more oxygen and four times more carbon dioxide than air. The mixture actually sinks to the bottom of the lungs and opens up the alveoli. This liquid is being explored for utilization in life-threatening situations in the emergency room.

Unit 2: The Breathtaking Respiratory System

5 Respiration – Ventilation Getting Into the Act

Respiration and ventilation are sometimes used interchangeably but the two words do not mean exactly the same thing. Respiration is the actual exchange of oxygen and carbon dioxide at the surface of the alveoli and capillaries in the lungs. Ventilation actually means the movement and flow of air in and out of the lungs. There are many terms used to measure the lung volumes and the movement of air in the lungs at different phases in the breathing process. These volumes can be measured utilizing a special device called a spirometer. Pulmonary Function Tests (PFTs) are a group of measurements that can assess how well the lungs take in and release air. (*Pulmo-* comes from Latin, and it means lung.) It evaluates how much oxygen breathed into the lungs actually enters the blood circulation for the body to use.

Pulmonary Function Testing is conducted in an enclosed booth, much like an old-fashioned telephone booth. A person seals their mouth around a mouthpiece and a plastic nose clip is applied. This ensures no air will escape from the nose and only the air from the mouth is measured. The mouthpiece is connected to the spirometer. It measures the flow of air when you exhale and the rate of the flow of air. These tests can be used to diagnose diseases of the lungs and monitor any changes in existing lung diseases.

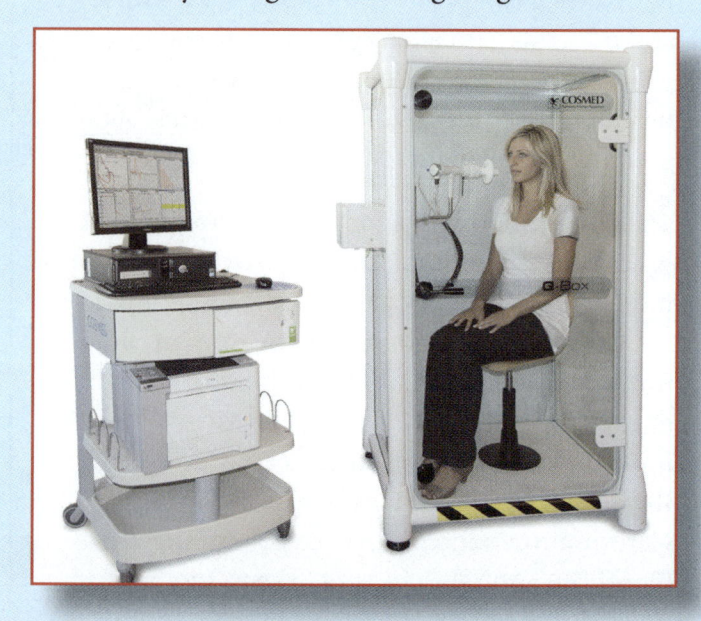

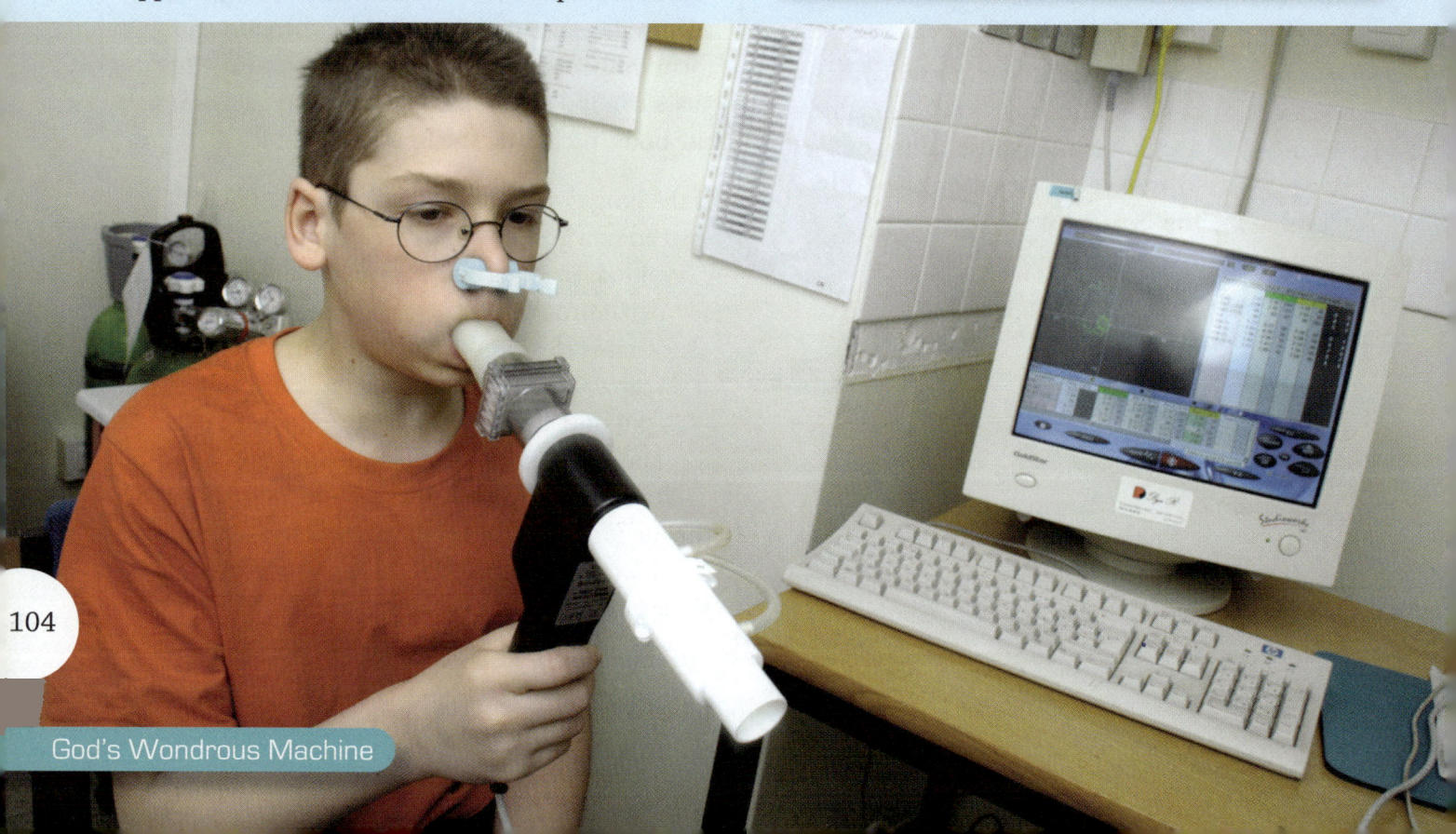

Averages In Men	
IRV	3.0
TV	.5
ERV	1.1
RV	1.2
TV + IRV + ERV = VC	
VC	4.6

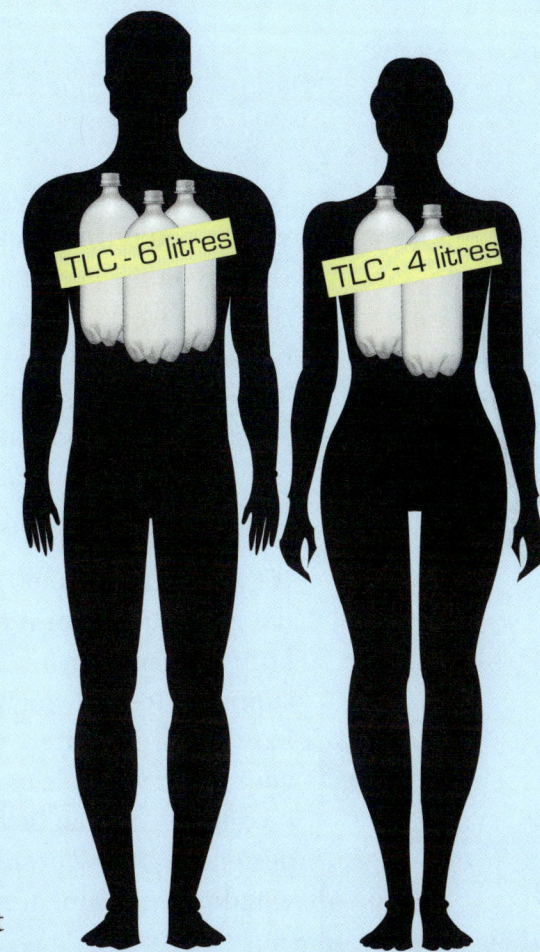

TLC - 6 litres

TLC - 4 litres

Averages in Women	
IRV	3.0
TV	.5
ERV	1.1
RV	1.2
TV + IRV + ERV = VC	
VC	3.1

Take a deep breath! Being tested on a spirometer as we see here is an important tool for doctors to find out how well your lungs are working. Doctors might order a test like this to find out if your lungs are working properly, if you have a disease like bronchitis, or why you might be short of breath. Whether you are tested in a closed booth or with a specific type of spirometer (there are several different kinds), both will give the doctor a very clear reading (as shown above) to help diagnose where the problem may be. See the following page for other devices that help doctors figure out how well your respiratory system is working!

Volume	Definition
Total Lung Capacity (TLC)	The maximum amount of air that a person is capable of holding in their lungs, 4 to 6 liters of air in an adult
Inspiratory Reserve Volume (IRV)	The amount of air that can be taken in forcibly over the tidal volume, approximately 2 to 3 liters
Tidal Volume (TV)	The amount of air we breathe in and out when resting, about 500 mL
Expiratory Reserve Volume (ERV)	The amount of air that can be forced out of your lungs after you exhale a normal breath at rest
Residual Volume (RV)	The amount of air that remains in your lungs after you exhale
Vital Capacity (VC)	The total amount of air in your lungs TV+IRV+ERV

Other factors can impact your lung volume:

Larger volumes	Smaller volumes
People who are taller	People who are shorter
Healthy weight	Overweight
Healthy lungs	Chronic lung-related diseases or conditions
Born and living in high altitudes like the mountains	Born and living in lower altitudes like along the ocean

Unit 2: The Breathtaking Respiratory System

Pulse Oximeter

Infant's Pulse Oximeter

Incentive spirometer

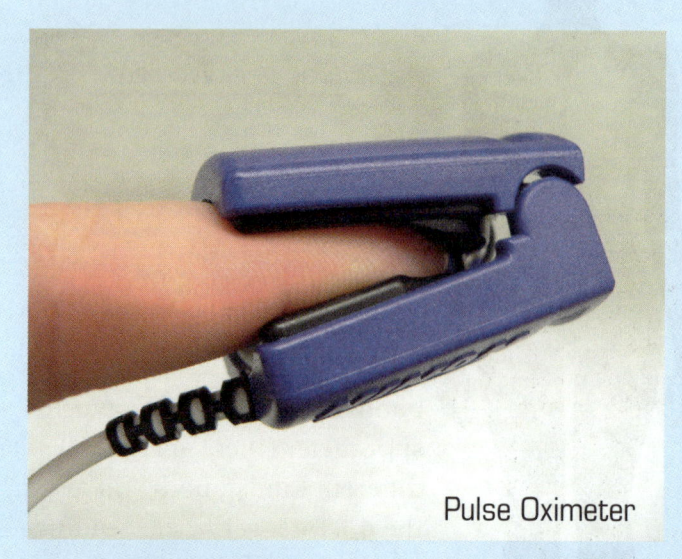

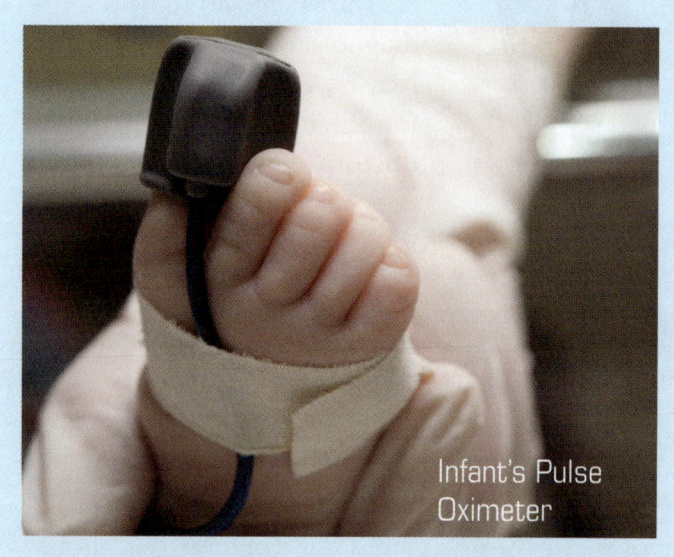

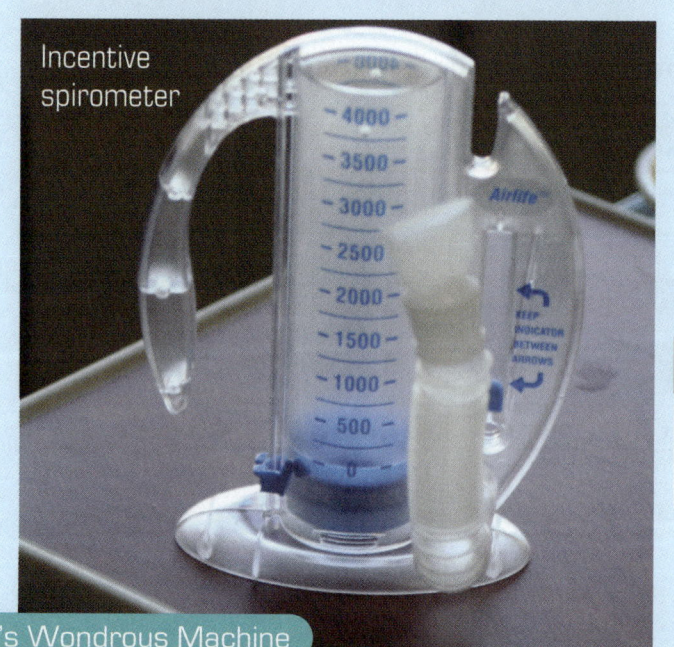

A quick and easy way to see how much oxygen is in your blood is to use a pulse oximeter. It is usually slipped on the end of a person's finger. The pulse oximeter works by determining the percentage of oxygen absorption in the blood. It uses a red light. The amount of light absorbed depends on how much oxygen is bound in the red blood cells. An oxygen saturation (absorption) of 95% or higher is normal.

If the level is below 90 percent, it is considered dangerously low, or if it falls below 80, then your body's organs may not be functioning like they are supposed to, and you may need to be given oxygen in order to get better. As with any other aspect of your body, too little or too much is not good when it comes to oxygen in your bloodstream. God designed us to be perfectly balanced in making our wondrous machine work the very best!

People who have lung disease or have just undergone some kind of surgery are often given an incentive spirometer. This is used to help your lungs function better. Even some musicians who use wind instruments use them to improve the flow of air from their lungs. When using this device, you breathe in from the machine as slowly and deeply as you can. Then you hold your breath for several seconds — as many as 5 or 6 seconds. This helps open the alveoli. An indicator on the incentive spirometer notes how your lungs are working, and when used a number of times a day, you can improve your lungs functions.

Word Wise!

"GESUNDHEIT" is another customary response when one hears a sneeze. It is a German word and means "good" health!

God's Wondrous Machine

Regulation of Breathing

Your rate of breathing changes depending on the needs of your body. Even your emotions can cause your respiratory rate to change. When you are fearful, you may hold your breath. During times of emotional distress, your rate of breathing may increase. When was the last time you had to remind yourself to breathe? You certainly can consciously decide to control when you breathe for periods of time.

Fortunately, God has designed our breathing under our voluntary and involuntary (occurs without you thinking) control. It would be incredibly distracting if you had to remember to breathe. There are two respiratory centers located specifically in the medulla oblongata of the brain. They are called the apneustic center and pneumotaxic center. The apneustic center controls the intensity of your breathing and its rate. The pneumotaxic center restricts the breathing in order to ensure that you don't overdistend your lungs with air. It also helps you maintain alternating between inspiration and expiration.

Chemoreceptors are additional respiratory regulators. They are located strategically in structures within the chest cavity. These sensors pick up on the chemistry of the blood. They take a chemical signal and send electrical impulses to the brain to adapt the respiratory rate as needed. Chemically, they detect the levels of carbon dioxide in the blood. If carbon dioxide increases in the blood the receptors will signal to the brain to increase the respiratory rate to get rid of more of this waste product from the body.

Unit 2: The Breathtaking Respiratory System

6 The Development of the Lungs

During the course of development in its mother's womb, a baby's lungs are not necessary for life. The lungs' ability to function upon leaving the womb is vital to life as the child greets the world. The organogenesis of the lungs begins at four weeks' gestation. Gestation is the period of development in the mother's womb from conception to birth. *Organ* refers to an organ and *genesis* refers to the origin or beginning of something. As the Bible states in Genesis in the Bible, God created the earth and its inhabitants in only six days. The organogenesis of the lungs takes place over the entire 40 weeks of gestation.

The production of amniotic fluid in the womb that surrounds the baby is important to the development of the lungs. Amniotic fluid is "inhaled" and "exhaled" by the baby. The baby does not actually breathe in this watery environment. This fluid, which goes in and out of the lungs, assists in lung development, protects the baby, and allows for freer movement in the womb. In addition to the amniotic fluid, surfactant is produced by the type 2 cells of the lungs. The type 2 cells do not begin manufacturing surfactant until 26 weeks' gestation.

This image has been put together from the scans of a 12-week-old fetus. In addition to the parts of the skeletal system seen (skull, spine, rib cage) in white, you can also identify the two lungs, shown in purple, above the kidneys highlighted in bright pink.

I AM wonderfully made!

Unlike other organs that develop in the womb, the lungs are organs that are not needed for breathing, yet they have to be ready to work at the moment of birth. Lungs develop throughout the entire period in the mother's womb and for some months after being born. What amazing planning has been built into God's design of our bodies to function when and how they should!

108

God's Wondrous Machine

The phases of lung development are depicted below.

Phrase	Development in the Womb	Illustration
Embryonic phase	4–5 weeks; first segments of the lungs appear at this time	
Pseudoglandular phase	Occurs between 5 and 16 weeks; the entire conducting tunnels of air are completed from the trachea all the way to the terminal bronchiole	
Canalicular Phase	Occurs between 16 and 26 weeks. The actual respiration parts develop: the lung tissue, alveolar sacs, and type 1 and 2 cells.	
Saccular Phase	This phase occurs from 26 weeks to birth. The grape-like clusters of the alveoli develop at the ends of the terminal bronchioles.	
Alveolar Phase	This occurs in the last couple of weeks of pregnancy. Only a third of the 300 million alveoli have grown to completion. The number of alveoli increases dramatically over the first 6 months after birth. This growth of alveoli continues for the first year and a half.	

In the alveolar phase the alveoli form like little buds on a tree at the end of the alveolar sacculi and grow larger in diameter as the baby matures.

Unit 2: The Breathtaking Respiratory System

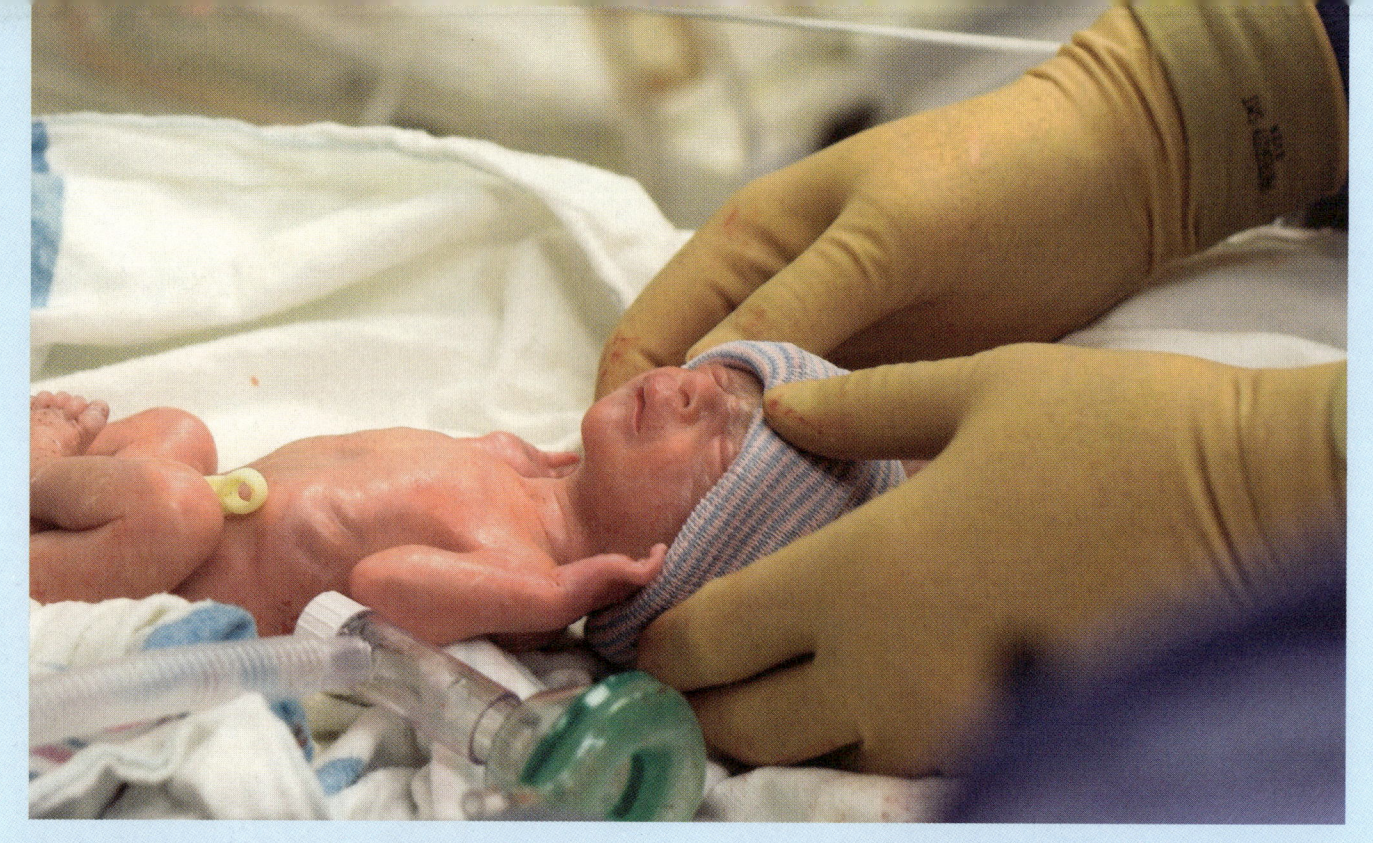

Sometimes babies are born early. The lungs of a baby may not be ready to fully function if born prior to 36 weeks of gestation. Their lungs may be immature and the baby's body has limited muscle strength and energy for effective breathing. Often they lack a substance that makes them unable to overcome the surface tension in their alveoli. If a mother goes into early labor during pregnancy, doctors may give the mother steroids, a medicine that can help the baby have better lung function on delivery.

Respiratory distress is a term used to describe someone who is having difficulty breathing. How a person attempts to overcome breathing difficulty can look and sound different, depending on the age of the person. For example, if you were to stand up and go for a run around the block as fast as you could, more than likely you would be out of breath. You would instinctively do maneuvers to help yourself grab a bigger breath of air. For example, you might bend over and put your hands on your knees. This allows you to lift up your ribs in an attempt to retrieve more air. Your nostrils would flare and your head might bob up and down with each breath. When someone is in respiratory distress, they may appear the same way.

A baby who is unable to sit up cannot do these types of maneuvers if he is having difficulty breathing. In order to force air into his lungs, a sick baby in respiratory distress may actually grunt. This is a worrisome sign. Take a quick moment and give it a try. Make the sound of a quick grunt. Try it again. What do your lungs feel like when you do a forceful grunt? The grunt increases the pressure in the alveoli in an attempt to fully open them to take in more oxygen. The grunt is a way that the baby increases his PEEP. Not a peep like a baby chick. PEEP stands for Positive End Expiratory Pressure. This is the positive pressure that is exerted in the alveoli at the end of exhalation.

> **Word Wise!**
> SACCULI is Latin for a small sac. This word was used in the 1600s to mean a small bag or sack of herbs applied to the body.

God's Wondrous Machine

MEDI+MOMENT

Enterovirus-D68 (EV-D68) sounds like the name of some science fiction space craft. This could not be further from the truth. It is actually a virus that can make you sick. There are many different types of enteroviruses — over 100 types.

Early in the fall of 2014, an outbreak of EV-D68 occurred in the United States, causing many children to become ill with respiratory symptoms. This virus was first identified in California in 1962. Of the very ill, many required care in the intensive care units of hospitals, a place for the sickest of patients. This enterovirus had some characteristics similar to the polio virus from long ago. Not only did children experience respiratory problems but in rare cases they were accompanied by weakness eerily similar to the polio outbreak of the 1950s.

Purdue University has used a special technique, X-ray crystallography, to discover the exact structure of EV-D68. They are currently studying the effects of binding it to an anti-viral compound in hopes of finding a treatment.

A vaccine has not yet been developed to prevent EV-D68, nor is there a specific medication to combat it. There are specialized tests to determine if the enterovirus is EV-D68, but it is not readily available in most places. And despite the success of current antibiotics on other illnesses, they do not work for EV-D68 or other viruses.

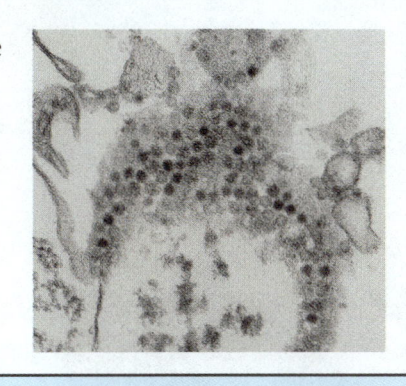

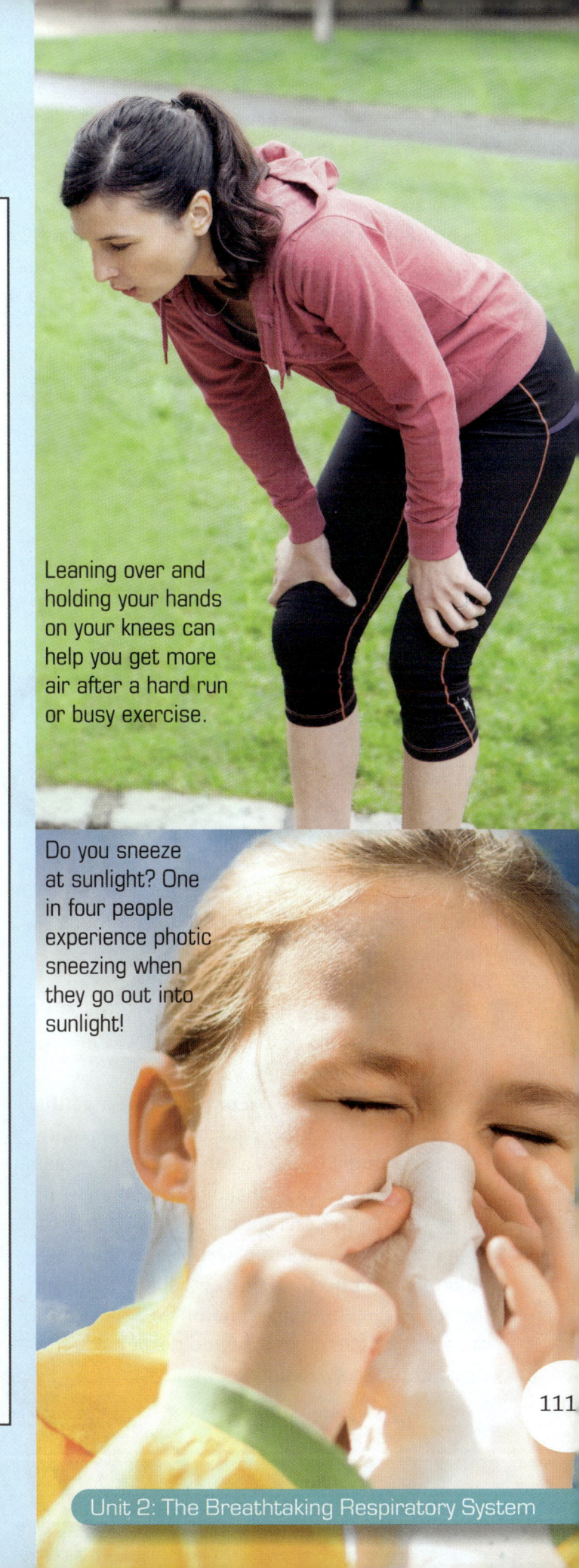

Leaning over and holding your hands on your knees can help you get more air after a hard run or busy exercise.

Do you sneeze at sunlight? One in four people experience photic sneezing when they go out into sunlight!

Unit 2: The Breathtaking Respiratory System

7 Technology

If you lived in the 18th century and had a cough, your mother might have reached for a "common" remedy. Steaming hot barley boiled in a pot mixed with water, snail slime, and a touch of brown sugar would fix you up in a jiffy. Not really? Well, you are probably right. Prior to the turn of the century, our technology and knowledge were limited when it came to effective ways to evaluate and treat the lungs. Today there are many ways that doctors can assess our lungs to see how they are working.

Breath sounds are either normal or abnormal. Fluid in the lungs, heart failure, asthma and even pneumonia will alter the normal sounds of the lungs

The Stethoscope

The stethoscope is a tried and faithful tool of the doctor. It is used to listen to the sounds of the body, from the beating heart to the air moving through the lungs to the rumbling of the stomach. It is the oldest of tools and was invented by physician Theophile René Laennec, who demonstrated the use of a tube for investigating the lungs and heart. He realized that one could listen to sounds through a tube. It was improper for a doctor to place his head on a woman's chest to listen to heart sounds, he rolled a piece of paper into a tube and placed it over the area of her heart to listen. He invented it in 1819. In 1855, George Phillip Cammann, an American doctor, took Laennec's idea and developed the stethoscope we know today.

God's Wondrous Machine

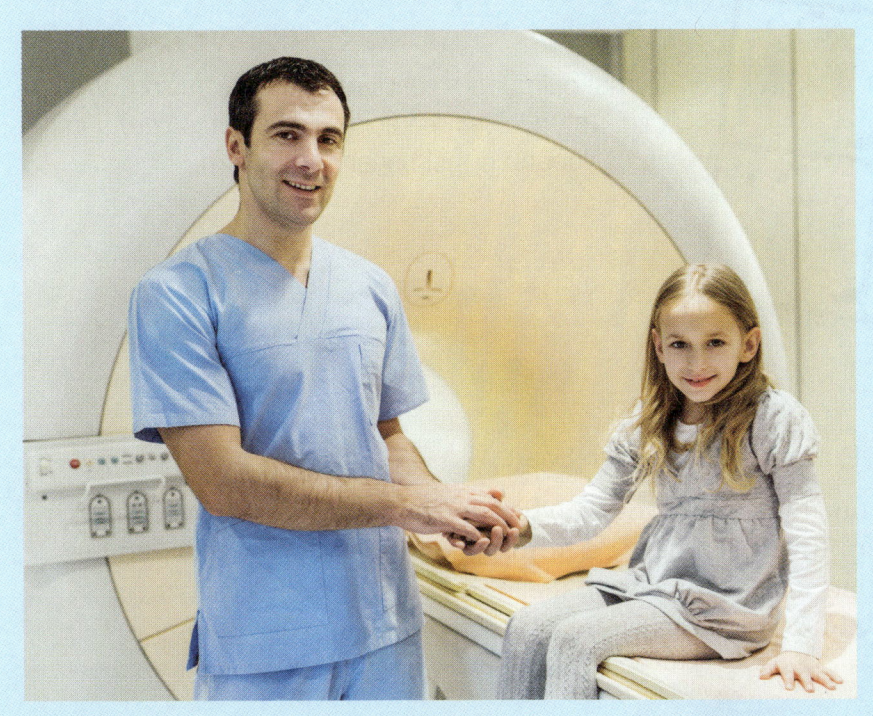

PET scan

PET or Positron Emission Tomography Scan is a type of imaging study. In order to perform the scan, a small amount of radioactive dye called a tracer is injected into a vein in the arm. The dye travels in the body and collects in areas of the lungs. The patient is placed on a table and slid into a large scanner. A computer takes the images of the lungs and generates 3-D pictures. This test can evaluate how well the lungs and the tissues are working.

Computed Tomography Scan (CT Scan)

The CT scan stands for computed tomography. CT scans are excellent tools to look at images of the lungs. Multiple images are taken in cross-sectional segments of the lungs. The slices are much like slicing a hard boiled egg. Placing a hard-boiled egg in an egg slicer and pressing down on the lever. The egg is perfectly evenly sliced. You are able to look at the inside of the yolk in various locations. This is similar to the images taken in a CT scan, but no actual physical cuts are made in the body. The computer generates these images. This scan is helpful in the diagnosis of diseases of the lungs, for example, to possibly assist in finding the causes of a persistent cough, shortness of breath, or chest pain.

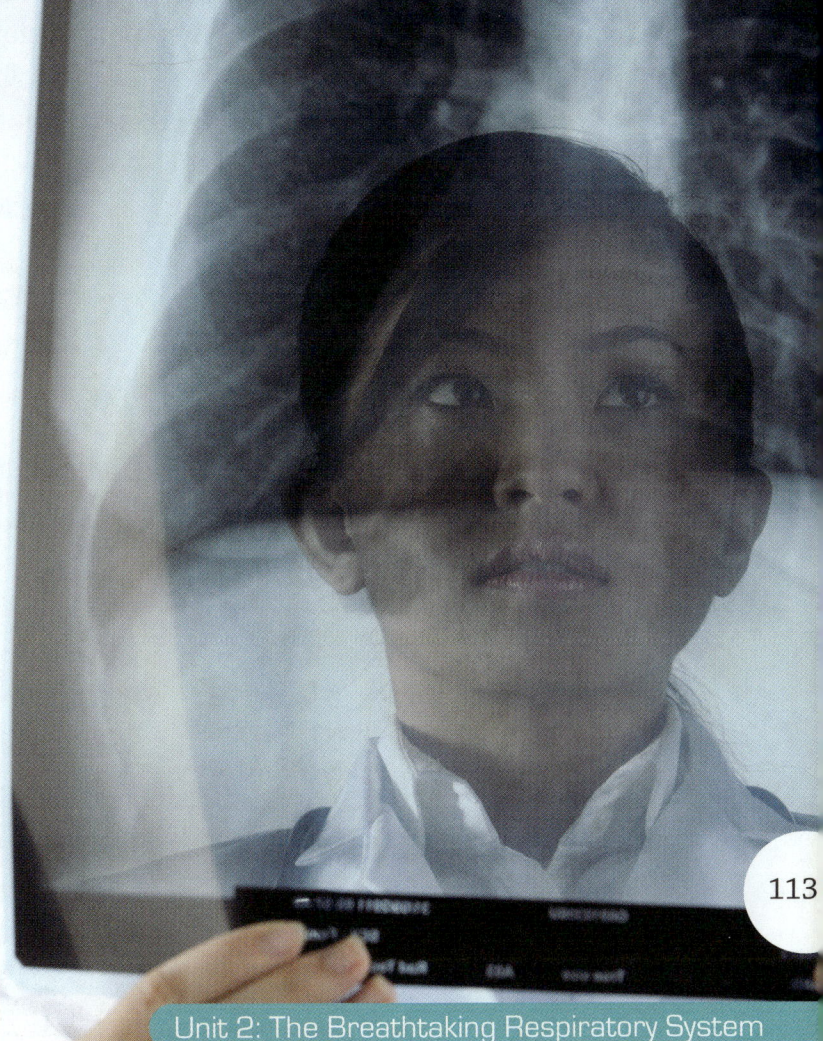

Unit 2: The Breathtaking Respiratory System

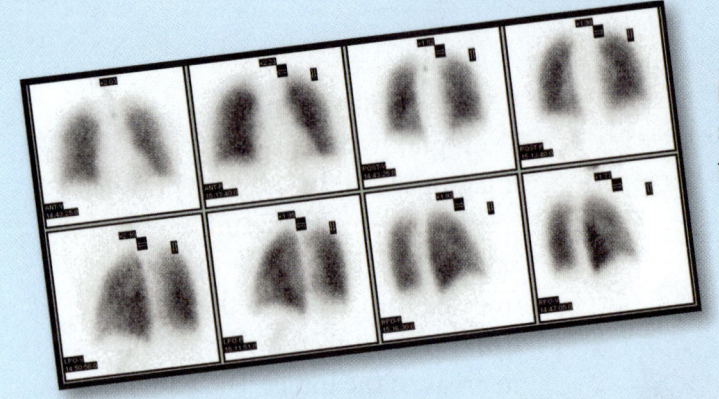

Normal pulmonary ventilation and perfusion (V/Q) scan. The nuclear medicine V/Q scan is useful in the evaluation of pulmonary embolism.

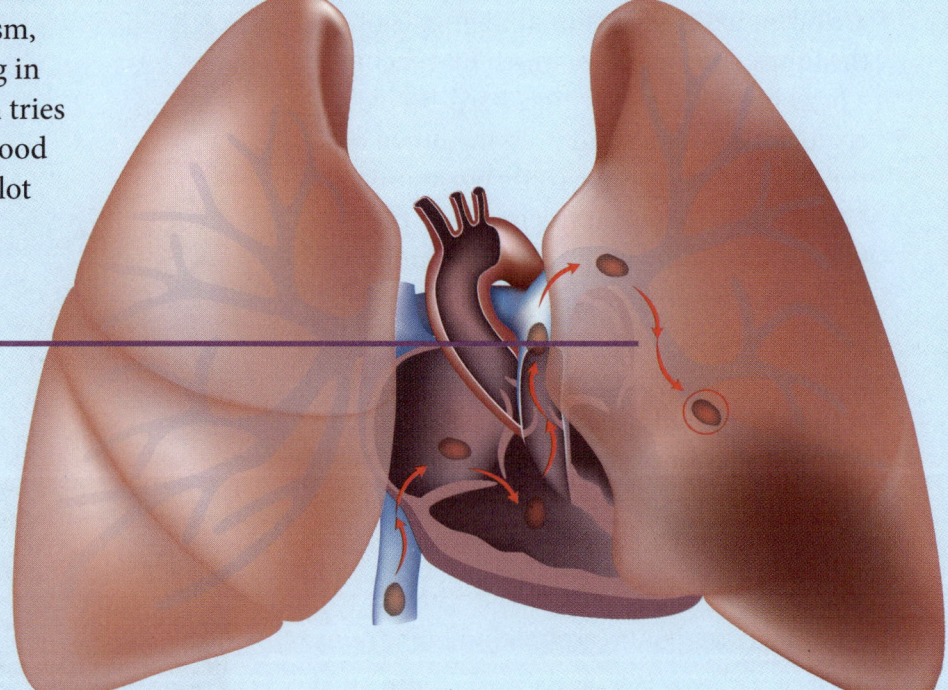

Pulmonary Perfusion Scan

Air flows in and out of the lungs. The function of the lungs can become limited if something blocks the flow of oxygen into the bloodstream. The Pulmonary Perfusion Scan measures air and blood flow in your lungs. It compares the ventilation (where air flows in the lungs) and the perfusion (where the blood flows in the lungs). This type of scan is very helpful in identifying a possible pulmonary embolism. Let's break that down a bit.

Pulmonary means anything pertaining to the lungs. Embolism originates from the Greek word *embolus* which means "plug" or "stopper." An embolism is a clot of blood that hardens in the blood stream and breaks off. It usually travels up from the vein of a leg and plugs up an artery in the lung. This blocks blood from flowing to that part of the lung.

This test compares the perfusion to the ventilation. In a pulmonary embolism, the ventilation is high (air is moving in the lung passageways) as the person tries to breathe, but the perfusion (the blood flow to that area) is low due to the clot blocking the flow.

Pulmonary Embolism

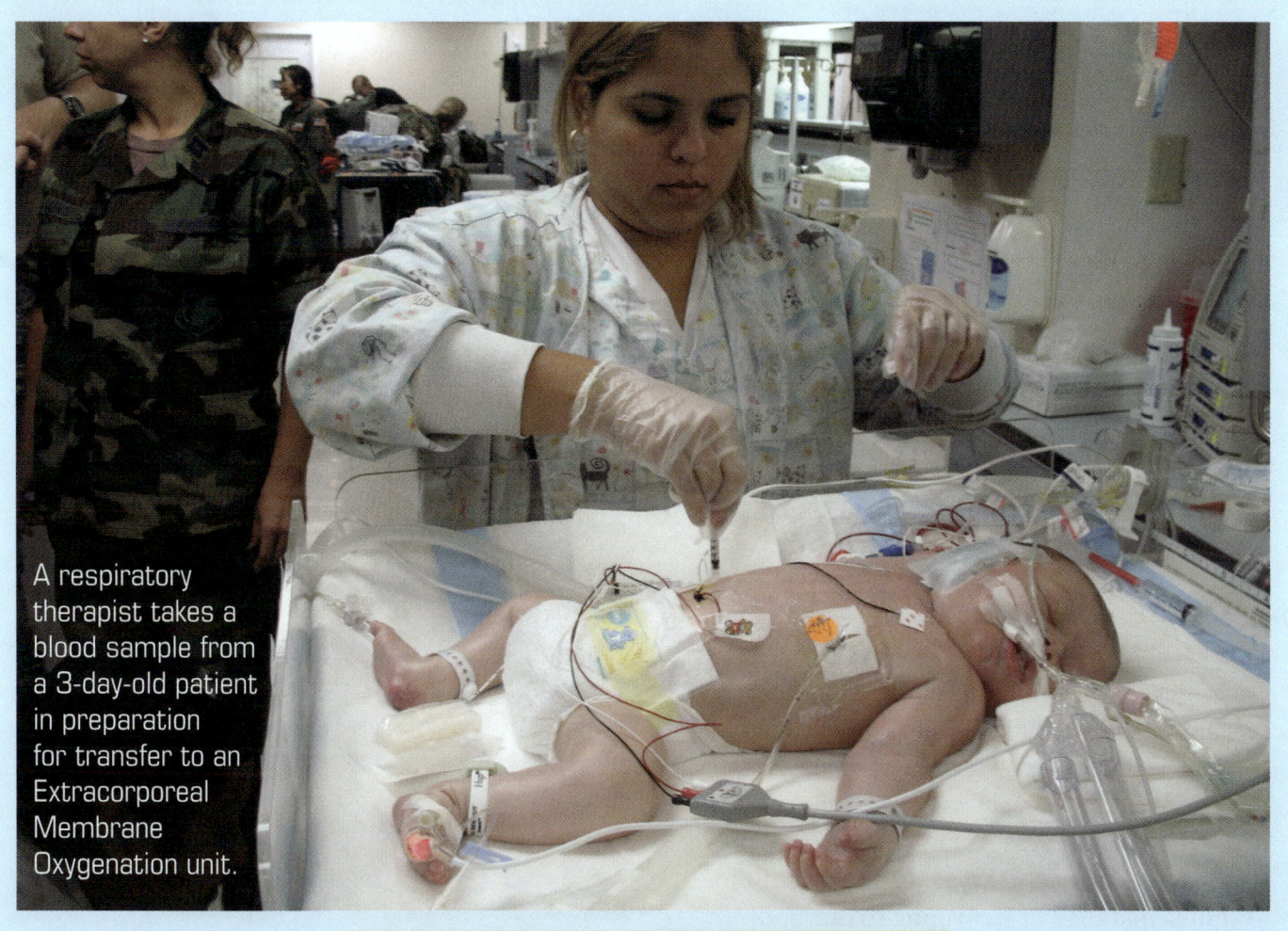

A respiratory therapist takes a blood sample from a 3-day-old patient in preparation for transfer to an Extracorporeal Membrane Oxygenation unit.

ECMO (Extracorporeal Membrane Oxygenation)

ECMO, or Extracorporeal Membrane Oxygenation, is a procedure that can be used in some of the smallest and sickest of patients whose heart and lungs cannot function normally on their own. The ECMO machine performs most of the work and allows for the heart and lungs to work more easily. Special tubes allow the blood from the patient to pass through the ECMO machine where the blood is oxygenated and carbon dioxide is removed like an artificial lung. The blood is returned to the patient. This type of invasive procedure can only be utilized for a few weeks. It allows time for the body to heal.

Unfortunately, there are people whose lungs are so damaged that their lungs will not recover. ECMO is a short-term solution to serious lung and heart problems. Individuals who are waiting for a lung transplant from a donor cannot use this technology. Dr. Robert Barlett, a surgeon at the University of Michigan Medical Center, is part of a research team trying to develop an artificial lung. It is called the BioLung.

The BioLung does not use a mechanical pump. The blood from the patient doesn't even leave their body. The heart of the patient continues to beat. The BioLung is packed with special hollow plastic fibers with teeny tiny holes that allow only gas to pass through. Similar to real lungs, these fibers allow carbon dioxide to leave the blood, and oxygen is allowed to enter. This oxygenated blood is in the heart and can then be pumped to all the organs of the body. The BioLung is still in development. It holds great promise for those whose lungs no longer work well.

Unit 2: The Breathtaking Respiratory System

8 Health and Illness

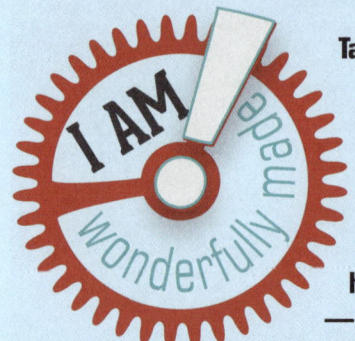

I AM wonderfully made!

Take Good Care

Therefore, I urge you, brothers and sisters, in view of God's mercy, to offer your bodies as a living sacrifice, holy and pleasing to God — this is your true and proper worship (Romans 12:1).

We are told here by Paul to surrender our all to God. As believers in Christ, we are to be a "living" sacrifice. No longer, as we were commanded in the Old Testament, do we offer animal sacrifices to God. We offer ourselves. We are tempted by many things and pleasures in life. We have the ability to desire many things in excess, from food to things that may be damaging to our bodies. These things hold promises of short-term enjoyment with lifetime damage. In order to serve God effectively, we have to be good stewards of what He has given us, including our bodies.

God has given us a wonderful gift. We are to care for our bodies. Here are three helpful tips for keeping your lungs healthy:

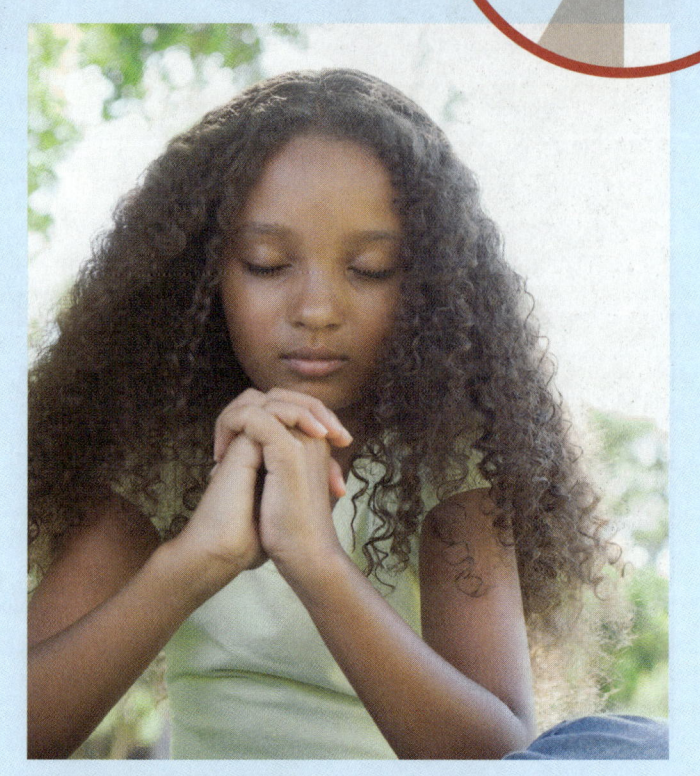

It was once believed the breath was the soul. It was once thought that your soul escaped your body during a sneeze, and saying "God bless you" would keep the devil from taking your soul before it could get back safely.

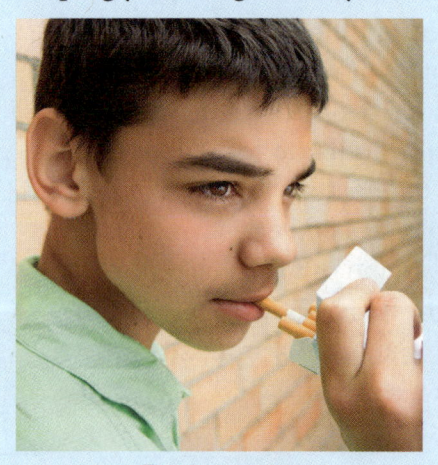

on the nose.

Don't smoke

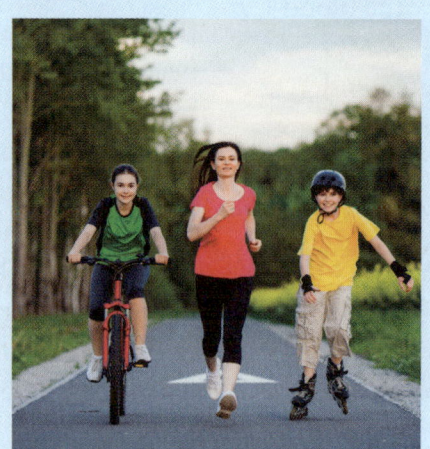

Get plenty of exercise

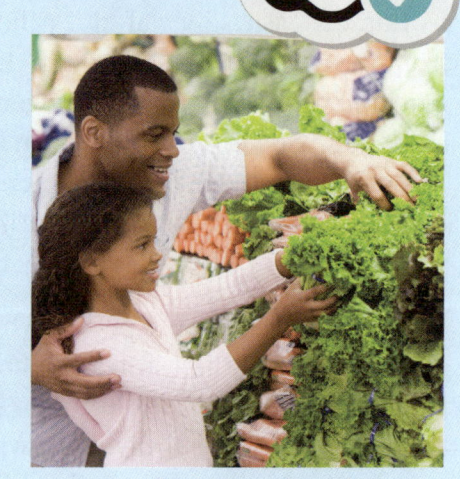

Eat a healthy diet

God's Wondrous Machine

Smoking and Your Lungs

We continue to expand our knowledge of what God has created around us and in us. Smoking has proven to be very damaging to the lungs. Smoking has gone in and out of favor in public circles through the years. Today, smoking is prohibited in most public areas. Today, we understand the damage that smoking causes to the lungs.

In the late 1600s, King James II of England despised smoking. He hated it so much that anyone who was caught smoking was treated as a criminal. The offender would be thrown in jail if caught committing this horrible crime.

Smoking is a very difficult habit to break once you get started. Many people who practiced this habit were addicted. (An addiction occurs when one becomes enslaved to a habit or practice despite the negative consequences.) People began to find new ways to satisfy their addiction in order not to be found guilty of a crime. They began chewing tobacco. One of the unsavory products of chewing tobacco is that much tobacco "juice" is produced. If one swallows this "juice," they experience a great deal of intestinal unrest and spew their stomach contents.

Enter stage right — upper right — the spittoon or cuspidor. A spittoon or cuspidor is a container used for spitting into. In years past, you could find a spittoon just about any place: stores, saloons, banks, hotels, and even at churches. Spittoons were considered the polite way to practice spitting in public. It was far more hygienic to spit in a spittoon than on the floor.

It is known that President Andrew Jackson (1767–1845) wanted to care for guests, and he had 20 spittoons placed in various places throughout the White House.

Today, we know that smoking causes 90 percent of the cases of lung cancer. We also know that the nicotine in cigarettes is incredibly addicting. In times past, it was commonplace to see advertisements for cigarettes on TV. In April 1970, Congress passed the Public Health Cigarette Smoking Act, banning the advertisement of cigarettes on TV.

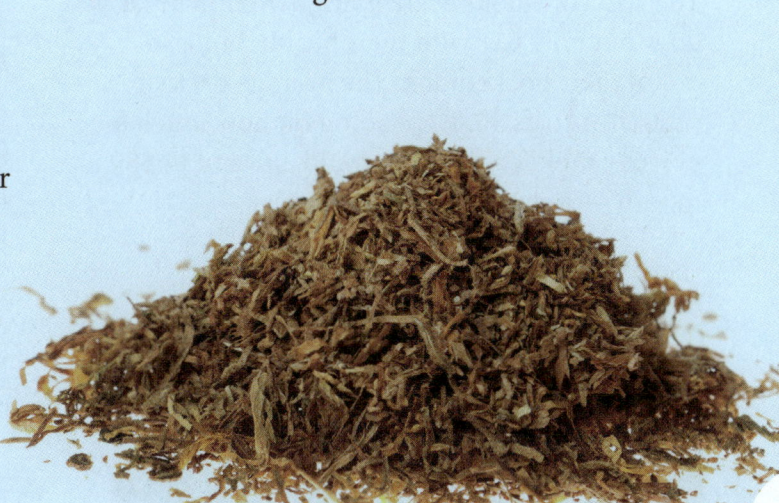

Unit 2: The Breathtaking Respiratory System

What do cigarettes do to the lungs?

1. The lungs lose their ability to be elastic and stretchy. Normally, as you breathe, your lungs expand and decrease in size to accommodate the volume of air. Smoking damages the tissue by depositing a sticky substance called tar. It becomes very difficult to exhale (breathe out).

2. Smoking causes a great deal of mucus to be manufactured. This mucus clogs the airways. It is common for smokers to experience the "smoker's cough." This is their body's attempt to dislodge the sticky mucus to clear the air passages.

3. The cilia, (hair cells), of the lungs cannot clear dirt and chemicals that become caught in the airways. The air sacs in the lungs are unable to function, and many will actually break open due to excessive pressure.

4. It causes cancer in the lungs as well as other lung diseases like emphysema, asthma, and chronic obstructive pulmonary disease (COPD). All of these diseases prevent the lungs from working properly. Smoking also causes heart disease and bladder cancer.

The costs of smoking are many. An individual does not only pay with their health, but also out of their pocketbook. The average pack of cigarettes costs $6. Depending on how much a person smokes a day, this could amount to $89 a month — a staggering $1,068 a year.

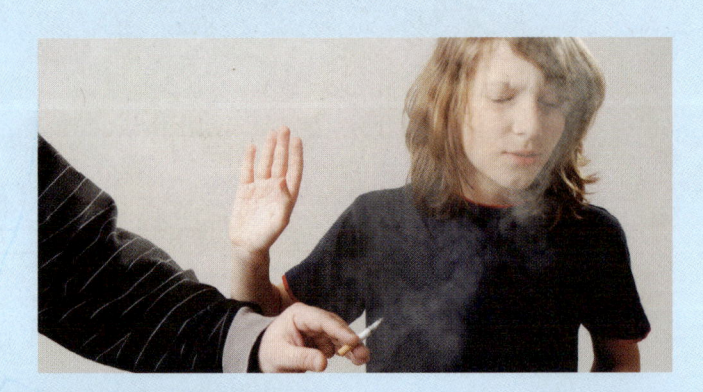

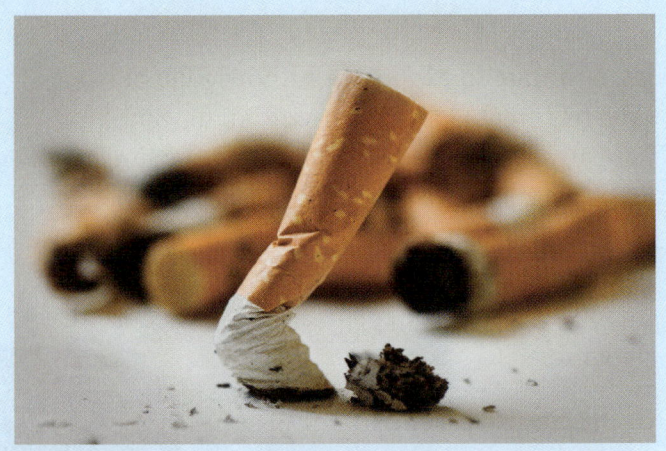

In April of 1994, according to the United States Department of Health and Human Services, five major American cigarette companies submitted a list of ingredients in cigarettes. The master list reveals that 599 ingredients are added to cigarettes. Many of these additives are carcinogens. (A carcinogen is a substance that is known to cause cancer in humans or animals.) Take a look at the list below of some of the known additives that are found in cigarettes. See if you recognize any that you would want to put into your body.

Additive	Where it is typical found
Arsenic	poison, used in rat poisons
Formaldehyde	used to preserve dead specimens and for embalming
Naphthalene	moth balls
Ammonia	household cleaner
Cadmium	used in batteries
DDT	a banned insecticide
Polonium-20	a cancer-causing, nuclear waste radioactive element
Acetylene	fuel used in torches
Benzene	gasoline additive
Carbon Monoxide	car exhaust
Hexamine	explosive ingredient
Methanol	rocket fuel

God's Wondrous Machine

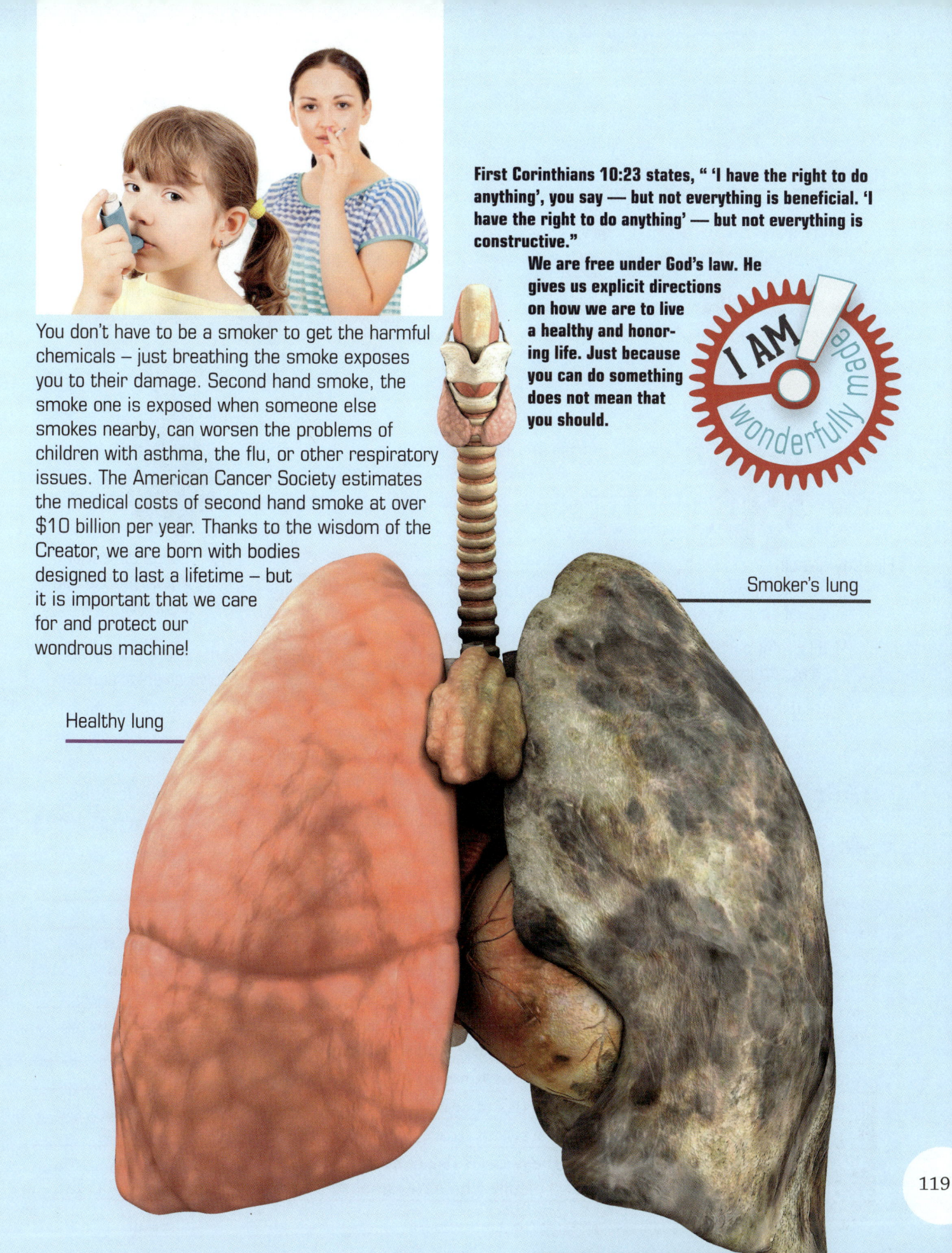

You don't have to be a smoker to get the harmful chemicals – just breathing the smoke exposes you to their damage. Second hand smoke, the smoke one is exposed when someone else smokes nearby, can worsen the problems of children with asthma, the flu, or other respiratory issues. The American Cancer Society estimates the medical costs of second hand smoke at over $10 billion per year. Thanks to the wisdom of the Creator, we are born with bodies designed to last a lifetime – but it is important that we care for and protect our wondrous machine!

First Corinthians 10:23 states, " 'I have the right to do anything', you say — but not everything is beneficial. 'I have the right to do anything' — but not everything is constructive."

We are free under God's law. He gives us explicit directions on how we are to live a healthy and honoring life. Just because you can do something does not mean that you should.

I AM wonderfully made

Smoker's lung

Healthy lung

119

Unit 2: The Breathtaking Respiratory System

Healthy lungs   Lung Damage   Emphysema

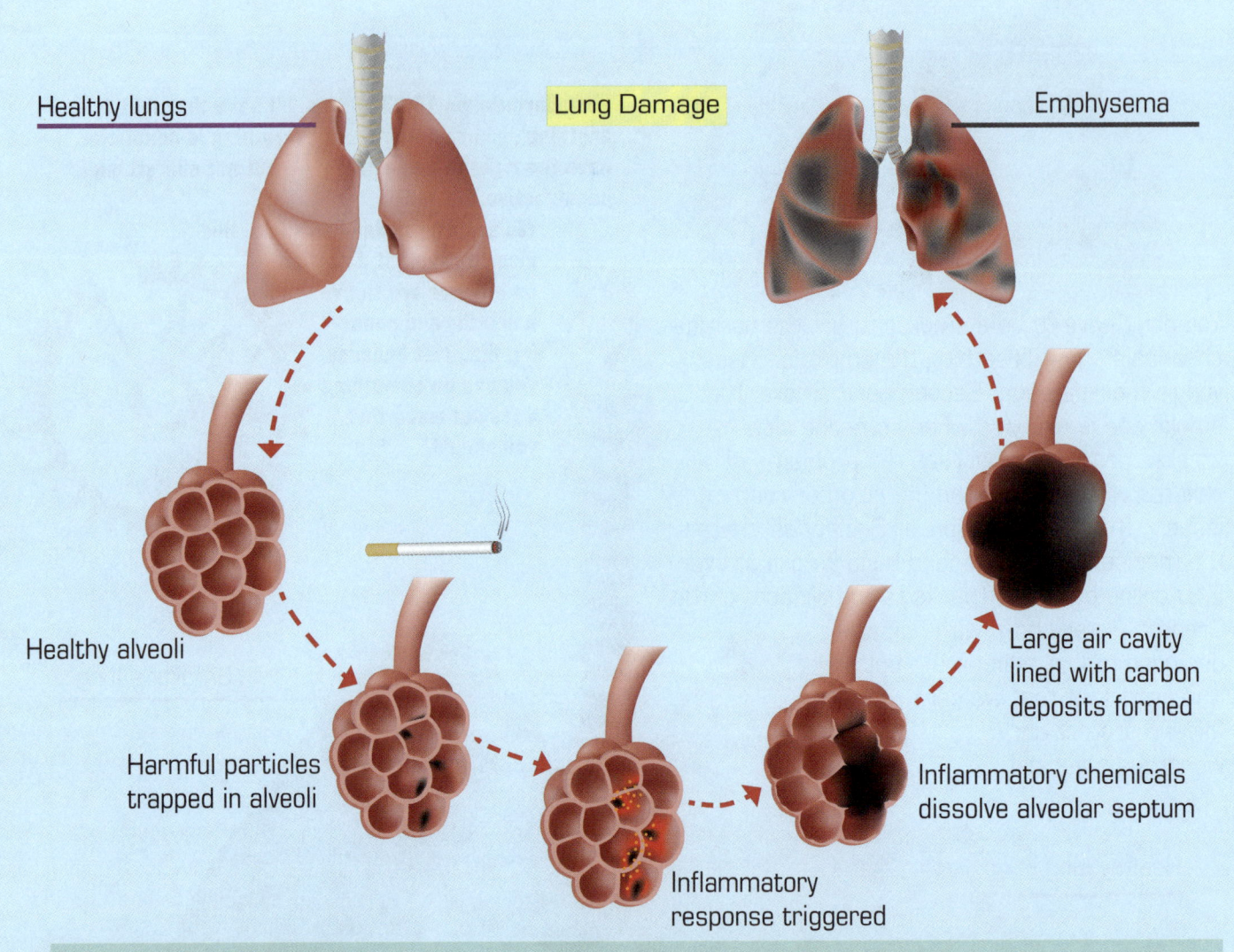

Healthy alveoli

Harmful particles trapped in alveoli

Inflammatory response triggered

Large air cavity lined with carbon deposits formed

Inflammatory chemicals dissolve alveolar septum

Quitting Smoking: Now that we have seen some of the bad news about smoking, it's time for some good news. Once the hard and challenging decision to quit smoking occurs, the ex-smoker will begin to experience the positive effects of stopping.

20 minutes after one's last cigarette	The blood pressure and pulse decrease.
	The temperature in the hands and feet increases.
8 hours after one's last cigarette	The blood in the body begins to recover and the levels of carbon monoxide decreases. The oxygen levels return to normal.
48 hours after one's last cigarette	The nerve endings in the mouth and nose begin to regenerate sense of taste, and smell improves.
A few weeks after one's last cigarette	The lung function improves.
1 year after one's last cigarette	The risk of heart disease has been cut in half.
5 years after one's last cigarette	The risk of stroke, bleeding in the brain, is decreased.
15 years after one's last cigarette	The person's risk of heart disease is now comparable to someone who never smoked a single cigarette in his or her life.

God's Wondrous Machine

Illnesses of the Lungs

Germs That Make You Squirm

There are things that we put in our bodies that can cause damage to them. However, there are other infectious agents, germy critters like bacteria and viruses, that can cause illness to the body. God has equipped our bodies with defenses to fight against uninvited guests. He has made special cells, proteins, tissues, and organs in our bodies to fight against germs. The major cells that help fight against disease are white blood cells. They are the military intelligence and soldiers that go to battle. As our soldiers are battling within our bodies, we can experience symptoms while the war rages. Viruses and bacteria can produce similar symptoms like vomiting, diarrhea, fever, rashes, and cough. These symptoms are ways that our bodies attempt to show these infectious agents the door.

Viruses and bacteria have some basic differences. Viruses are 100 times smaller than a single bacteria. A bacteria is 10 times smaller than a single human cell. Viruses are not alive by themselves and cannot survive long outside the body. Viruses and bacteria enter the body via the mouth, nose, or open wounds. A virus enters the body and hijacks the cells. It causes the cell to use its machinery to produce more viruses. The viruses are mass produced and fill the cell until it ruptures open. The newly formed viruses try to take over other cells. Bacteria, on the other hand, can survive outside the body for a longer period of time and are more complex than viruses. Most of the earth's biomass is made up of bacteria — it is believed to be about 5 nonillion (5×10 to the 30th power by USA measurement!). Some bacteria are very helpful and even aid in our digestion. Only about 1 percent of all bacteria cause disease.

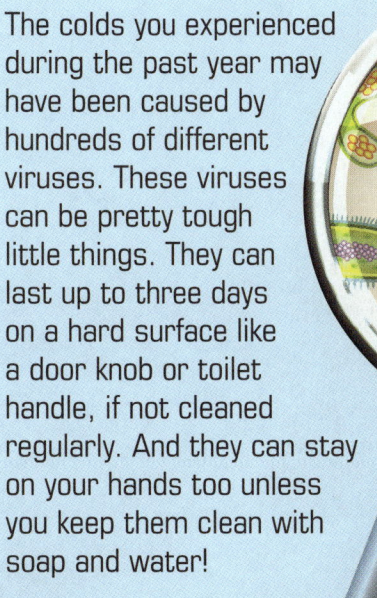

The colds you experienced during the past year may have been caused by hundreds of different viruses. These viruses can be pretty tough little things. They can last up to three days on a hard surface like a door knob or toilet handle, if not cleaned regularly. And they can stay on your hands too unless you keep them clean with soap and water!

Unit 2: The Breathtaking Respiratory System

Epidemic vs Pandemic

We have seen great outbreaks of disease and illness over the ages that affect the lungs. The word, epidemic, is used to refer to increased outbreaks of disease that affect a particular region or area. A pandemic occurs when there is an outbreak of a disease that expands over large geographic areas and continents.

Every winter there is always an increase in respiratory illnesses. One of the biggest factors that contributes to this increased occurrence of illness is that many people stay indoors and are in close confines with one another. Good hand washing, covering your mouth or nose when you cough or sneeze, and staying home from school/work when you are sick is important in decreasing other's exposures to illness.

The Flu Can Make You Blue

Major outbreaks of Influenza have occurred over the years. Influenza is the same thing we call the "flu." It is caused by a virus. People who suffer from influenza experience fever, cough, sore throat, runny nose, body aches, headaches, and tiredness. At the end of World War I in 1918, influenza was a wartime killer that claimed the lives of 40 million people. Nearly half the world's population was infected. This was indeed a pandemic.

Word Wise!

"STERNUTATION" means to sneeze.

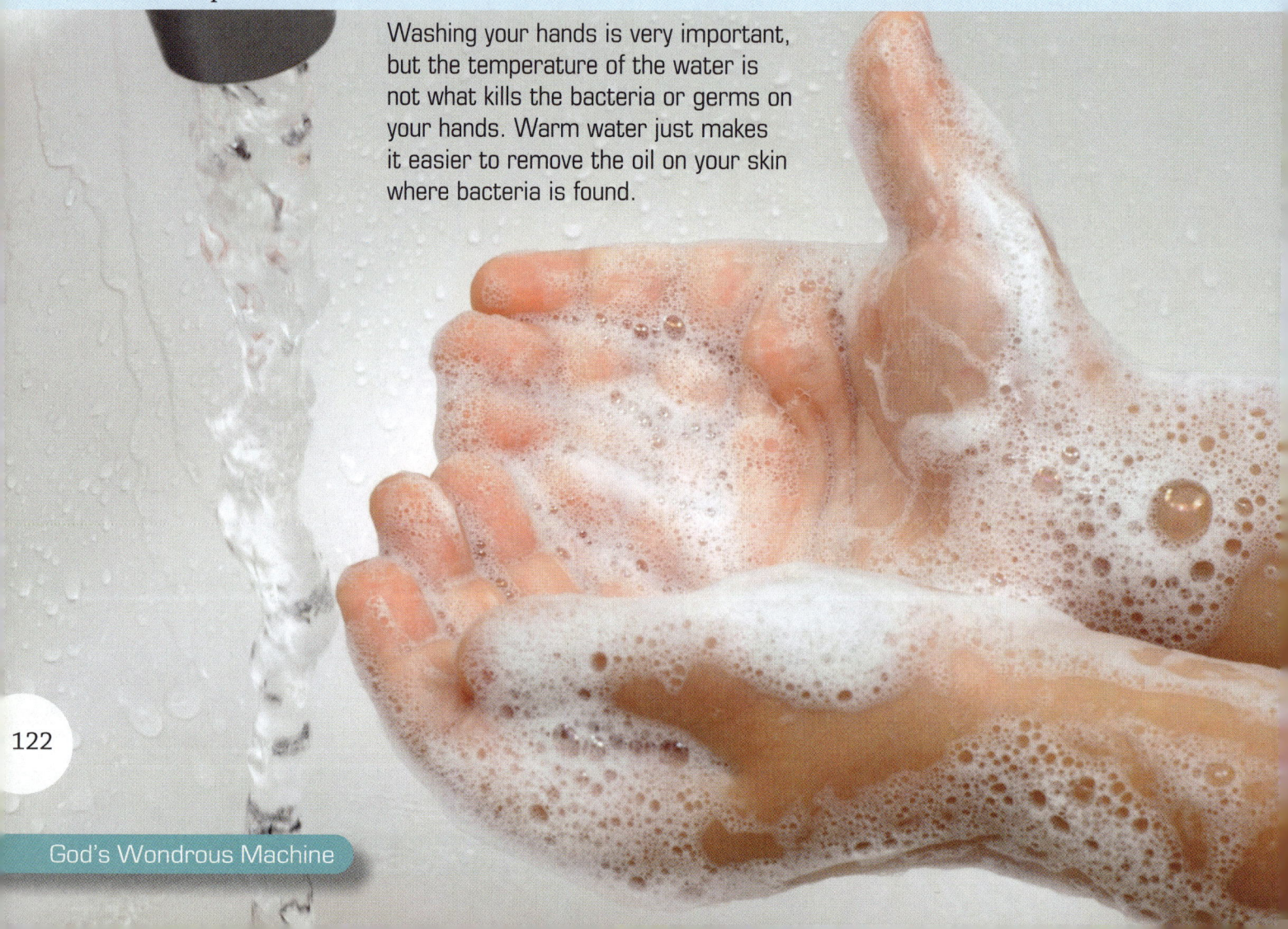

Washing your hands is very important, but the temperature of the water is not what kills the bacteria or germs on your hands. Warm water just makes it easier to remove the oil on your skin where bacteria is found.

Tuberculosis

Tuberculosis (TB) is a disease caused by a bacterium called *Mycobacterium tuberculosis.* It is a highly contagious disease. ("Contagious" refers to something that is easily spread from one person to another.) TB is spread by droplets from coughing, sneezing, talking, or spit. It typically affects the lungs, but can also infect other parts of the body like the spine, brain, or kidney. It was the leading cause of death in the United States in the early 1900s. Due to the highly infectious nature of TB, sanitariums were erected in the United States. Sanitariums are places where individuals who suffer from contagious diseases are isolated from society in long-term medical facilities. These facilities were referred to as "waiting rooms for death."

In 1904, The National Association for the Study and Prevention of Tuberculosis was founded to lead the fight against tuberculosis. They began the Christmas Seal campaign in 1907 to raise money for a small TB sanitarium in Delaware. This organization's name was later changed to the one many know it by today, the American Lung Association. The tagline for its campaigns to promote good lung health was "It's a matter of life and breath." Today, its tagline is "Fighting for Air."

This is a far cry from the image that TB had in the 1700 and 1800s. Back then TB was called "consumption" because as the disease ravaged the body, the individual lost a great deal of weight and the disease consumed them. During those times, to have TB was considered to be very fashionable. It tended to kill many famous, wealthy, and incredibly talented people. There were romantic painters who depicted TB as an elegant disease. The person would appear pale and gaunt with rosy cheeks.

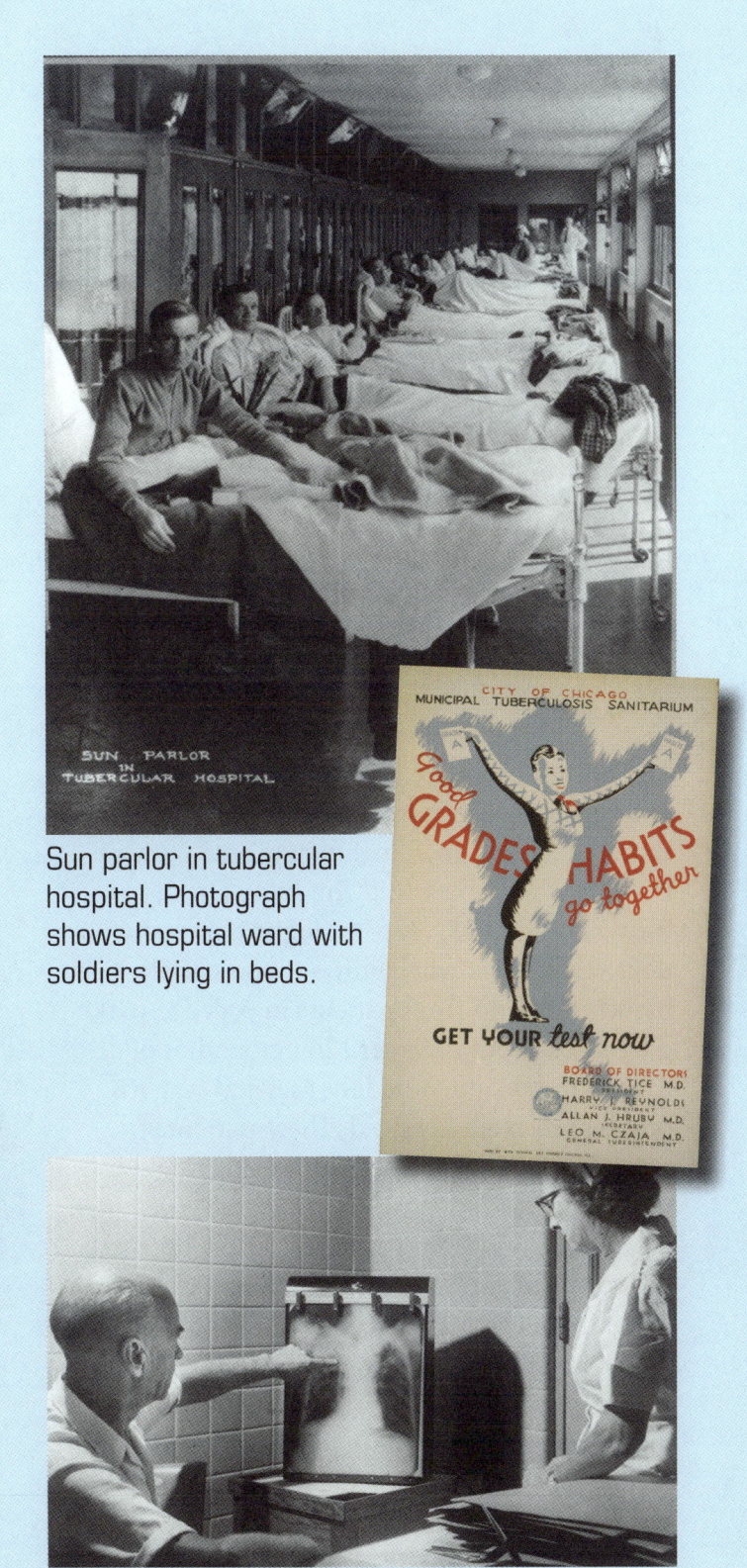

Sun parlor in tubercular hospital. Photograph shows hospital ward with soldiers lying in beds.

If a skin or blood test reveals TB bacteria, a chest x-ray or sputum sample may show TB disease.

Unit 2: The Breathtaking Respiratory System

Cystic Fibrosis

Cystic fibrosis is an inherited disease. It is a disease passed from parent to child in their genetic instructions. The complexity and precision with which God designed the body blows our minds. A small addition, change, or deletion in the genetic instructions in the body can cause huge malfunctions. Cystic fibrosis is a result of a specific genetic defect that interferes with the body's ability to carry salt and water to and from the cells. Due to this defect, many organ systems in the body are impaired. Thick, gummy mucus builds up and clogs the lungs and the digestive tracts. It affects the lungs, pancreas, liver, intestines, sinuses, and reproductive organs, the areas that are high producers of mucus in the body.

The host of problems that cystic fibrosis patients suffer from was observed by Dr. Dorothy Andersen, a pathologist at Columbia-Presbyterian Babies and Children's Hospital in New York in 1938. (A pathologist is a medical doctor specialist who studies tissue samples, blood, and fluid from patients in order to make diagnoses about illnesses.) In her studies of these patients, she noted that several systems of the body were involved. These patients experienced thick, sticky mucus clogging their lung passageways. They became sick more often and were extremely susceptible to infections of the lungs. The mucus blocked the ducts in their pancreas, which prevented the pancreatic enzymes from exiting the pancreas. These enzymes are important in helping in the digestion of food, in particular fats, proteins, and carbohydrates. The patients' appetites were great, but they suffered from malnutrition. The sweat glands in their skin did not work well, and they had a salty taste to their skin. This was noted when parents kissed their child.

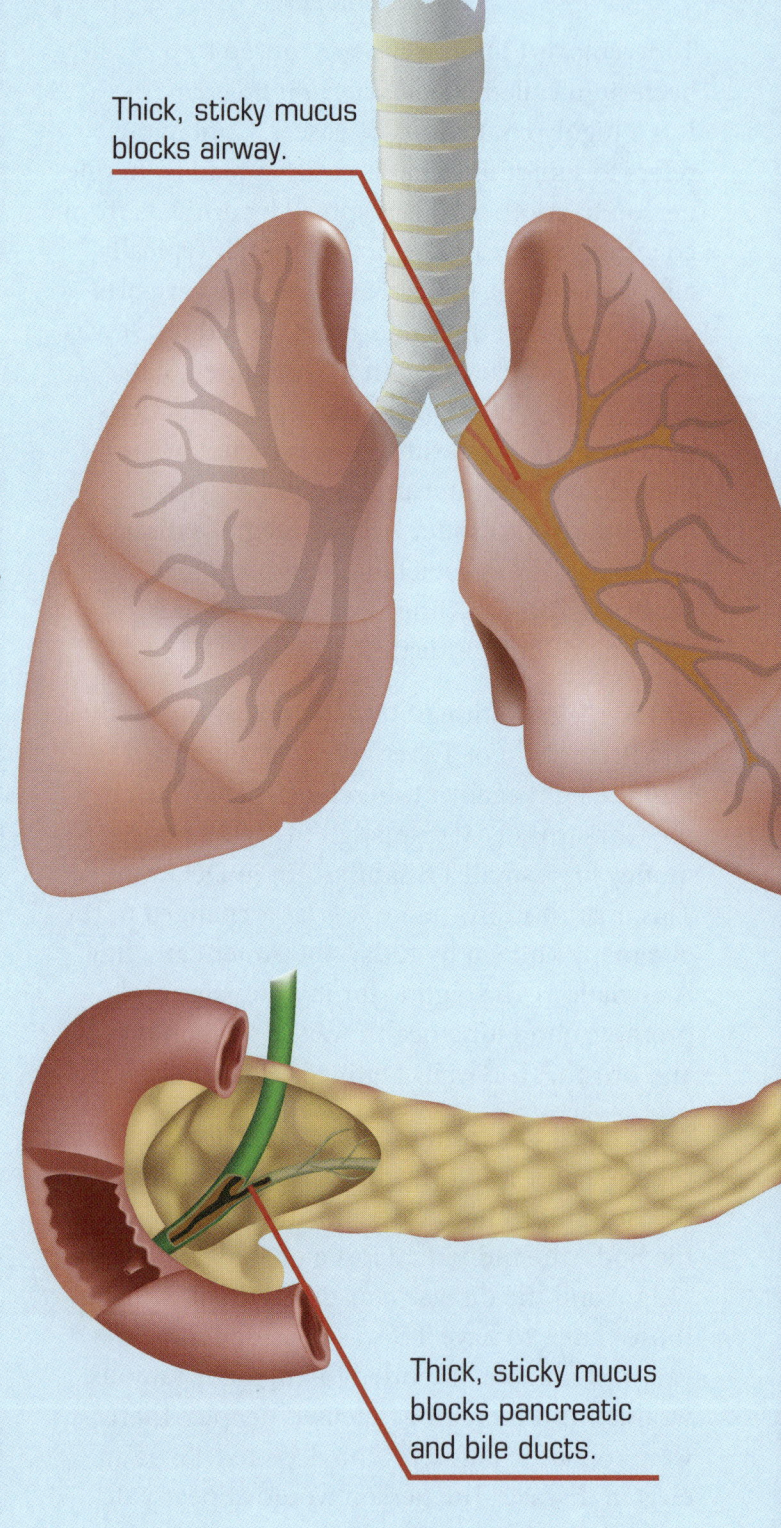

Thick, sticky mucus blocks airway.

Thick, sticky mucus blocks pancreatic and bile ducts.

God's Wondrous Machine

The specific gene, cystic fibrosis transmembrane conductance regulator, or CFTR, that causes cystic fibrosis was discovered in 1989. The disease occurs primarily in those of northern European descent — 1 out of 3,500 white children. The disease is much less common in non-white children with 1 out of 12,000 affected. Some diseases may continue to occur because they have some protective qualities against other ailments. Diarrhea was a common cause of death in early times, but still remains a threat in Third World countries. Those who carry the defect in the CFTR gene are less affected by deadly diarrheal illnesses but tormented by the effects of the genetic disorder.

Dr. Paul di Sant'Agnese developed an effective technique of diagnosing cystic fibrosis in 1953. He developed the "gold standard" for diagnosis called the "sweat test." The sweat test measures the concentration of chloride in the sweat. It is a painless test. There are two parts to it. First, a chemical that has no odor or color is placed on a small area of the skin, usually the arm or leg. An electrode with a very weak electrical charge is placed on top of the area. The combination of the chemical and the electrode causes the area to sweat. This step lasts for about five minutes. Second, the area is cleaned and the sweat is collected. The sweat is sent to a specialty lab to measure the amount of chloride found in the sample.

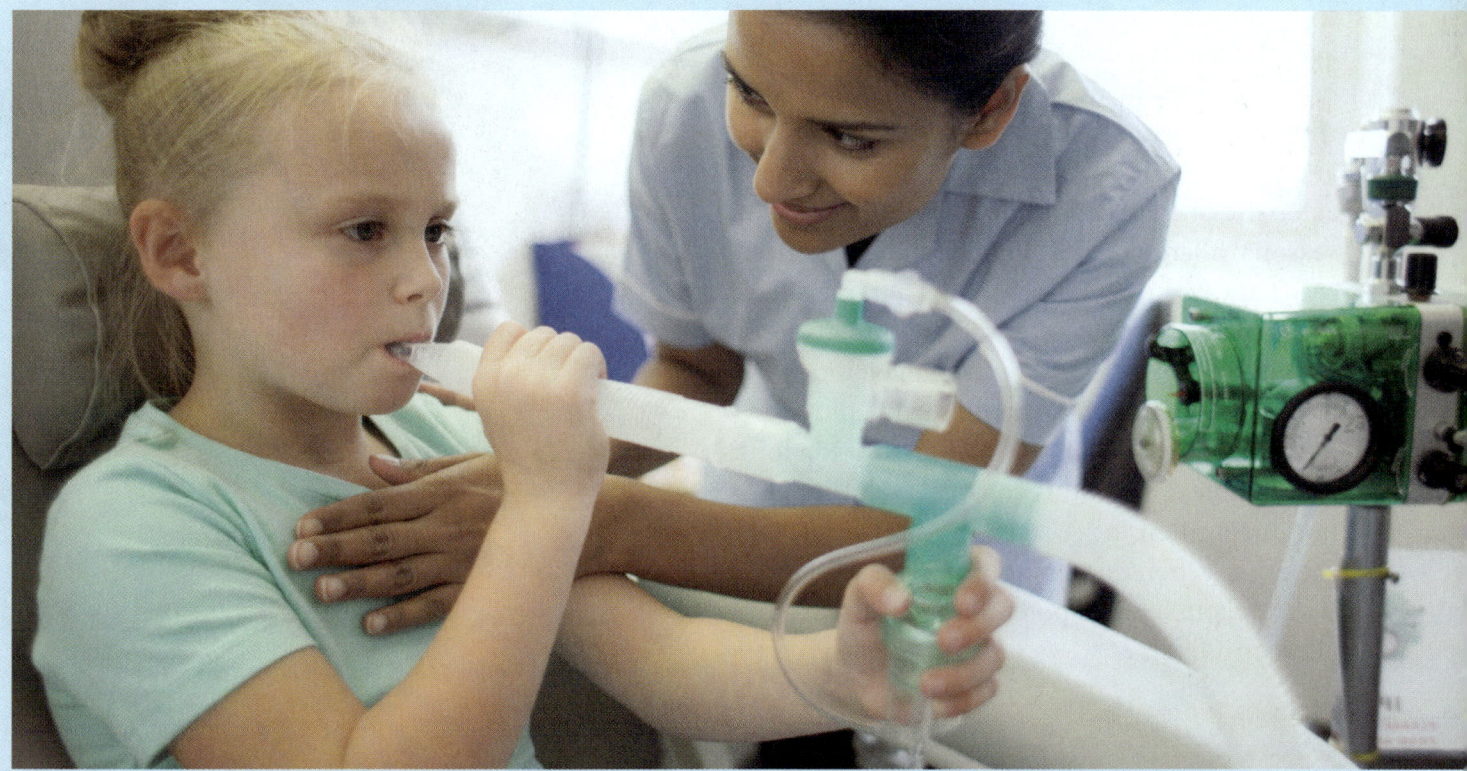

CFTR Gene Chromosome 7

IPPB (Intermittent Positive Pressure Breathing) therapy for Cystic Fibrosis is a therapy utilized in patients who have difficulty with their lungs. It delivers a controlled pressure of a gas to help in air movement and expansion of the lungs. Aerosol medications can be given with the treatment.

Unit 2: The Breathtaking Respiratory System

Allergic Rhinitis or Hay Fever

Achoo! Sniff! The warm sun beats down. The flowers are in full bloom. *Sniff!* It is a glorious time of the year. *Achoo!* Yep, allergy season is in full bloom also. (An allergy is an exaggerated reaction of the immune system to a foreign body.)

Allergic rhinitis, or, as it is "affectionately" called, hay fever, tends to hit people who suffer from it in the spring. It is an allergic response to the stuff that floats through the air causing inflammation of the nasal airways. The stuff that causes such a reaction is called allergens. An allergen can be anything such as dust mites (little critters that can live between the sheets of bedding), tree and grass pollens, fungi, molds, dust, or animal dander (the particles of hair and skin shed by an animal). The immune system kicks into high gear and becomes overreactive to these irritants.

Symptoms can consist of increased mucus production in the nasal passages accompanied by rhinorrhea (runny nose), sneezing, watery eyes, and pressure in the sinus cavities. A unique characteristic of children suffering from this type of seasonal allergy is the "allergic salute." Children aren't always known for grabbing a tissue when their noses are runny. Frankly, anything will do to wipe the nose . . . a shirt or even the hand. Habitually, the palm of the hand is rubbed upward at the opening of the nose, and the motion looks like a salute. Due to this constant "saluting," it is not uncommon to see a crease near the bridge of the nose. When doctors spot this crease they see it as a helpful clue in potentially identifying an allergy sufferer.

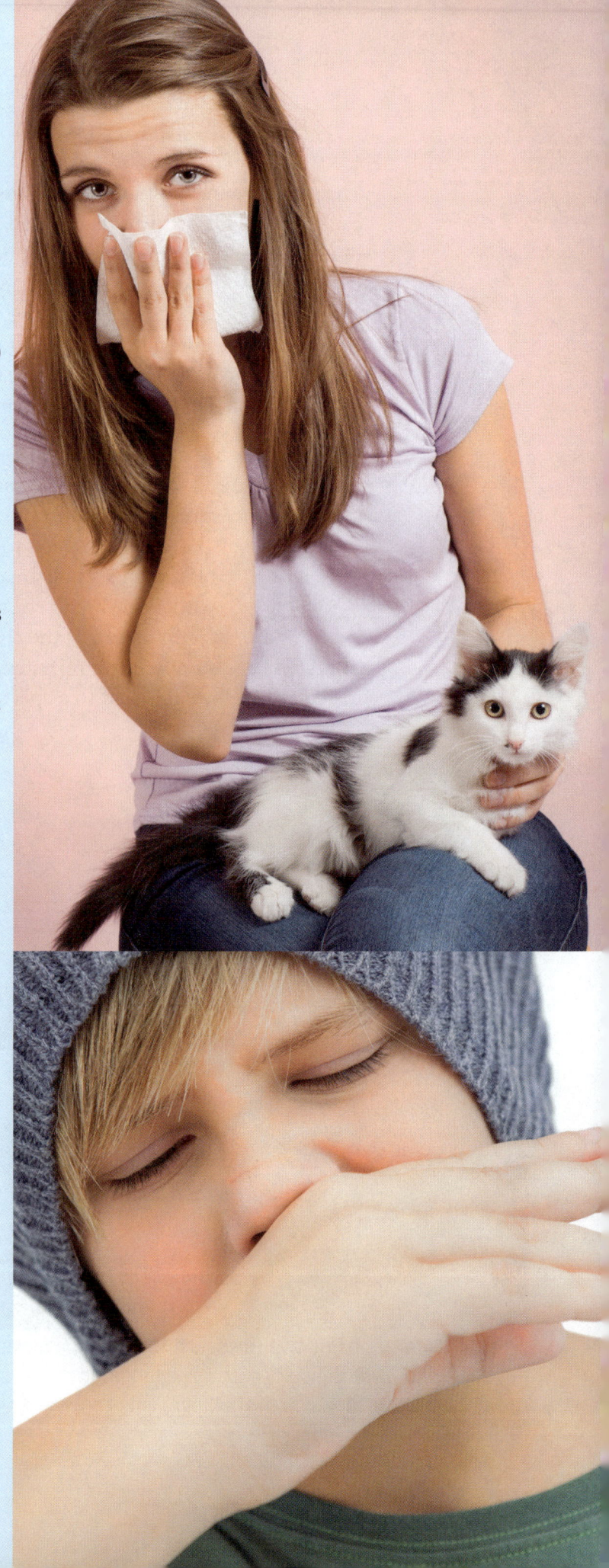

God's Wondrous Machine

Air trapped in alveoli

Relaxed smooth muscles

Wall inflamed & thickened

Normal airway

Asthmatic airway

Asthmatic airway during attack

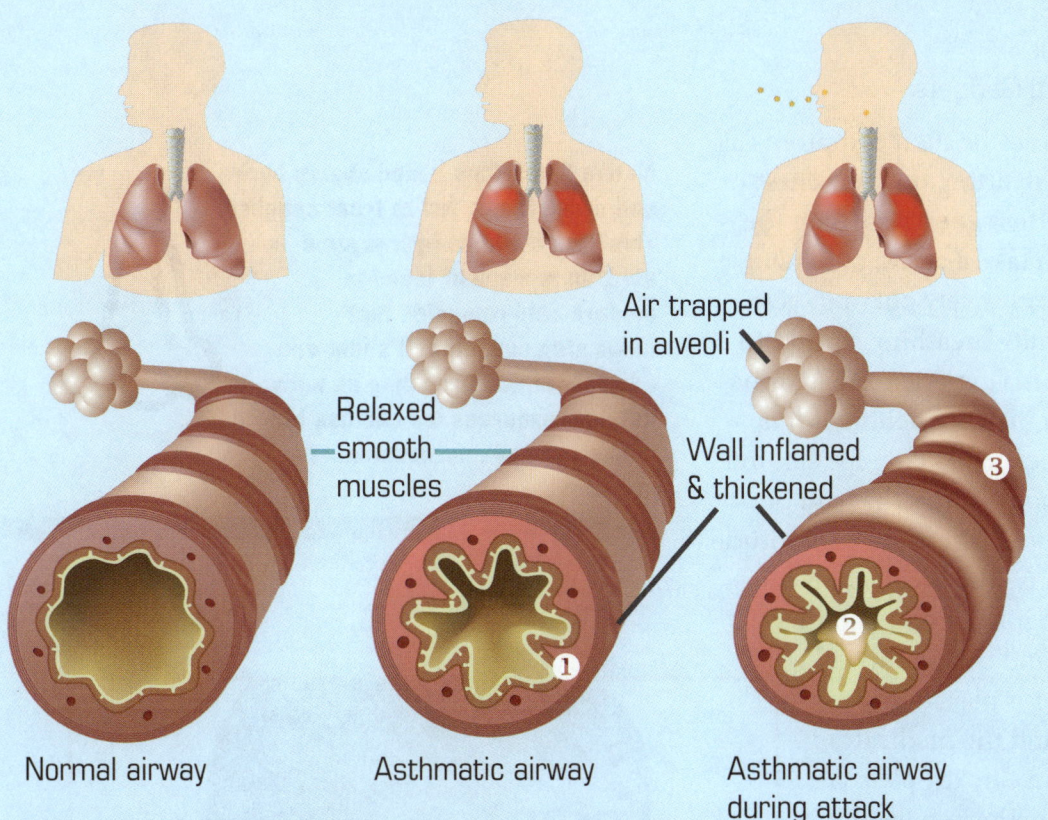

In an asthma attack, three things occur to the lung passageways.

1. The lining of the airways becomes inflamed and swollen. This swelling narrows the passageway.

2. The lungs increase production of mucus. This mucus clogs the airways, further narrowing the area.

3. The tiny straps of smooth muscle that encircle the bronchioles spasm and tighten around the tubes.

Asthma

Asthma is a chronic lung disease that is in the same family of illnesses as allergic rhinitis. In fact, many people who suffer from asthma also suffer from allergic rhinitis. What is asthma anyway? Asthma is a reversible, recurring inflammation of the lung passageways. It tends to run in families. An asthma "attack" can occur in response to environmental things, allergies, exercise, or infections. During an asthma "attack," a person becomes acutely short of breath and experiences chest tightness and wheezing. Wheezing is a high-pitched sound made as the person breathes. Coughing occurs due to the mucus that accumulates in the narrowed airways. Do you have asthma or know someone who does? According to the National Heart, Lung, and Blood Institute, approximately 25 million people in the United States suffer from asthma; 7 million of those are children.

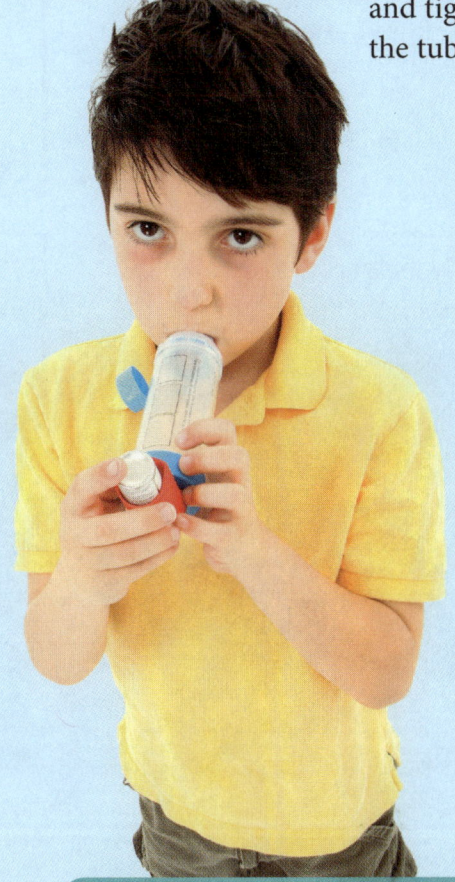

Unit 2: The Breathtaking Respiratory System

Asthma Gadgets

Many asthmatics will describe their symptoms as feeling like an elephant is sitting on their chest or that a vise is squeezing their chest, trapping the air inside. If you were to take a straw, pinch it a bit, and try to breathe exclusively out of it, you would experience difficulty breathing similar to what a person with asthma experiences. Asthma can be serious and even life-threatening if it is not properly treated. There is no cure for asthma. Fortunately, there are many things that can be used to treat the symptoms. There are a multitude of inhalation medications. The medication can be delivered through an inhaler or a nebulizer. The inhaler is portable and can be carried anywhere. The nebulizer is placed in a mouthpiece container and the medication is suspended in the air in tiny droplets via an electrical compressor. The nebulizer is great for small children or people who are having great difficulty taking a good breath.

on the nose.

Native Americans boiled cherry bark and drank it as a tea to treat coughs. This bark contains hydrocyanic acid, an ingredient found in modern cold remedies that helps stop coughing. It's just one example of God providing us with natural resources we can use for medicines and improvements in our lives!

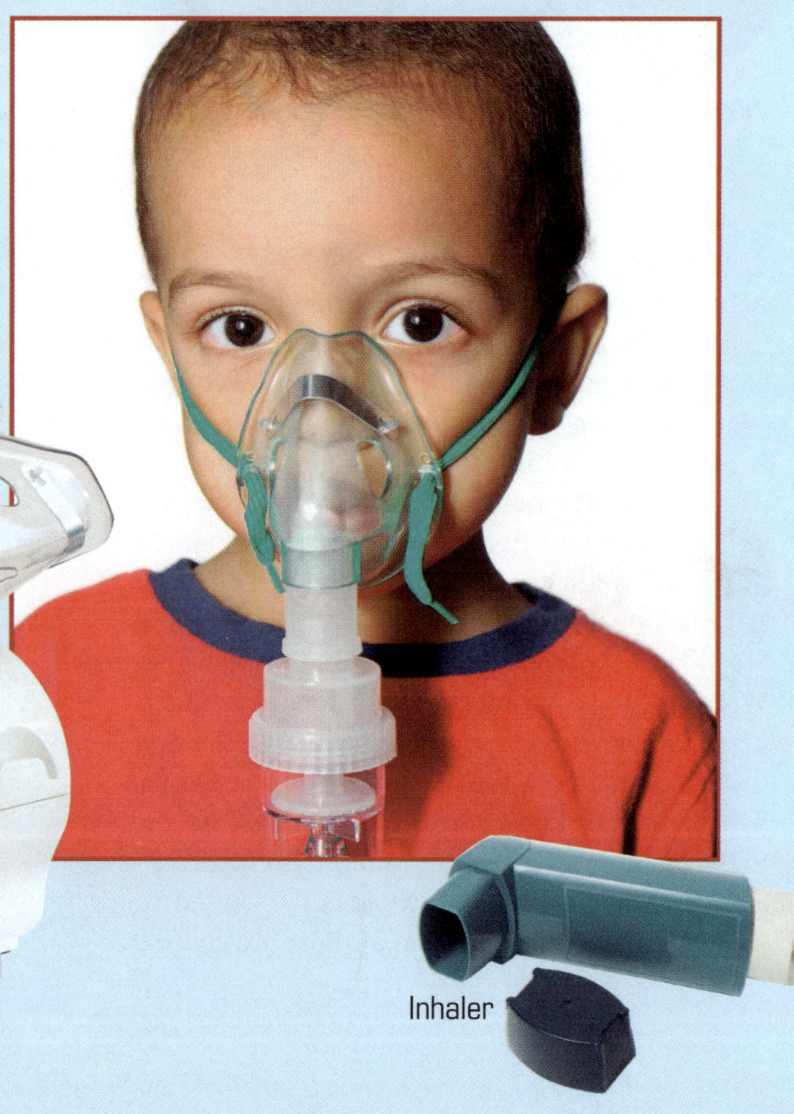

Nebulizer

Inhaler

God's Wondrous Machine

Laryngitis

Laryngitis is inflammation of the larynx. Swelling occurs in the area of the vocal cords. It is caused by viral and bacterial infections. In addition, singers, coaches, and enthusiastic sports fans can experience overuse of their vocal cords, causing pain and inflammation. The throat feels "scratchy" and the voice is hoarse. One illness you may have heard of is laryngotracheobronchitis. Whew, let's break that down in common layman's terms. Laryngotracheobronchitis is also known as "the croup." Typically, this illness occurs in the winter months in young children. The child's cough sounds like a seal barking. Most cases of croup are caused by viruses. Treatment is aimed at comforting the sufferer and allowing the body to heal itself. Air humidifiers, hot showers, and drinking plenty of fluids are helpful.

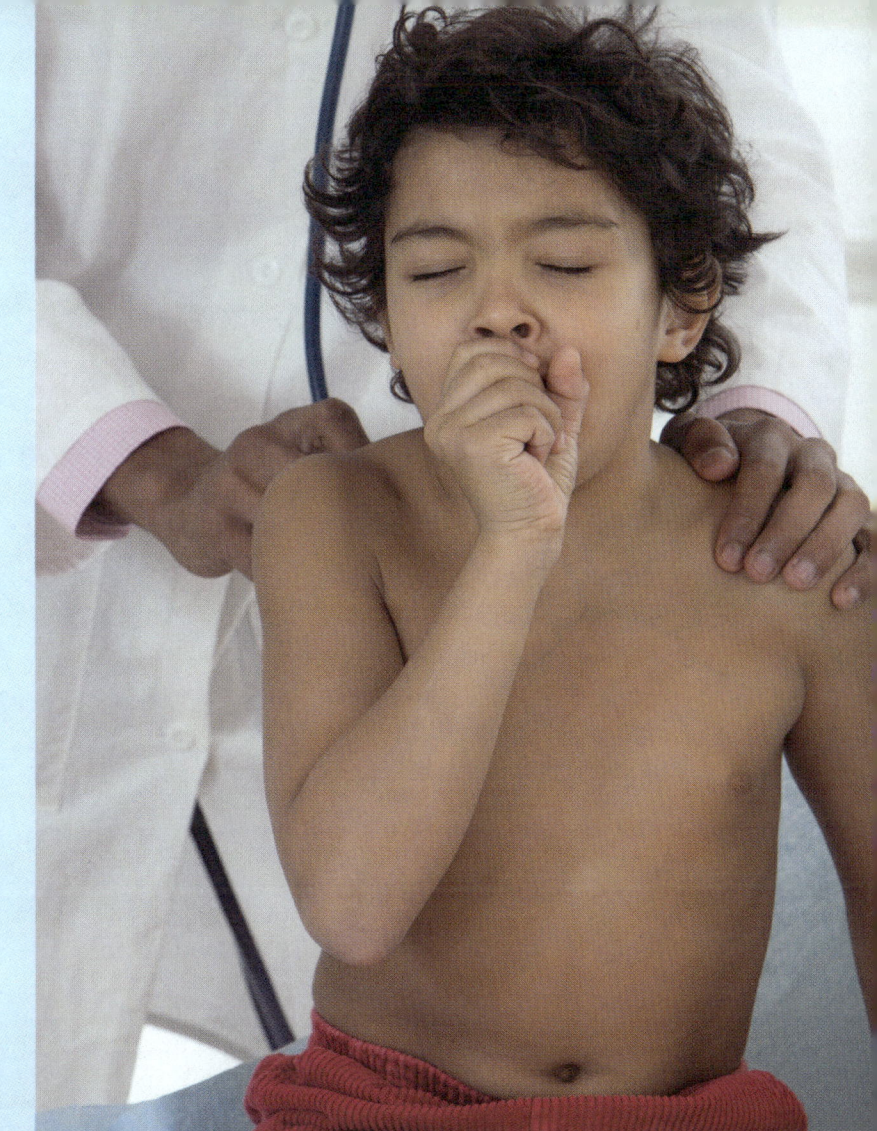

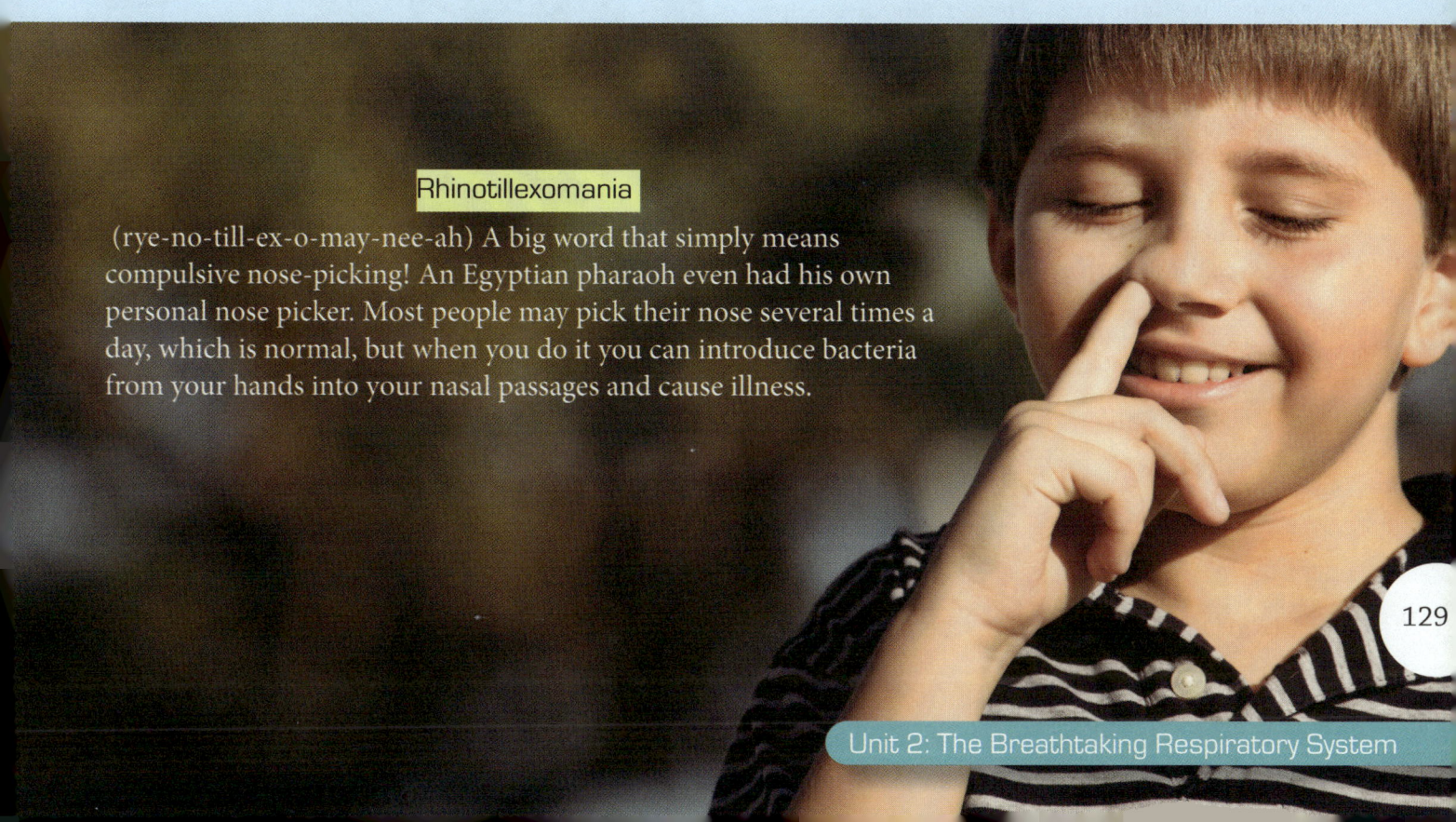

Rhinotillexomania

(rye-no-till-ex-o-may-nee-ah) A big word that simply means compulsive nose-picking! An Egyptian pharaoh even had his own personal nose picker. Most people may pick their nose several times a day, which is normal, but when you do it you can introduce bacteria from your hands into your nasal passages and cause illness.

Unit 2: The Breathtaking Respiratory System

9 The Story of Polio

Poliomyelitis, also called polio, is a disease that affects not only the lungs but many other organ systems as well. It can lead to debilitating deformities of the legs, impairing the ability of walk. Polio is caused by a virus that invades the spinal cord and can lead to paralysis (the inability to move) of legs and the diaphragm, breathing problems, and death. A devastating epidemic occurred in the United States in 1952, over 57,000 people were afflicted with the disease.

Dr. Jonas Salk and Dr. Albert Sabin are credited with bringing this horrible crippling disease under control. In 1955, Dr. Jonas Salk developed a polio vaccine. It is called the Inactivated Polio Vaccine (IPV). The inactivated polio virus is injected into a person and the body's immune system mounts a response to the virus by producing protective antibodies. These antibodies help to protect a person from contracting the disease. In 1957, Dr. Albert Sabin developed a vaccine that used a live weakened version of the polio virus that was taken by mouth. It was called the oral polio vaccine (OPV). The OPV vaccine was discontinued in the United States in 2000 because of its association with a rare serious reaction.

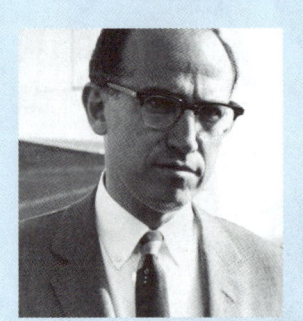

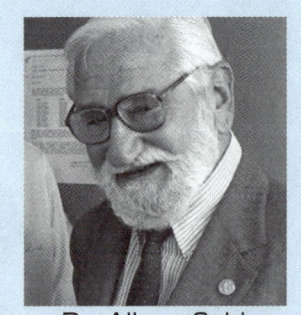

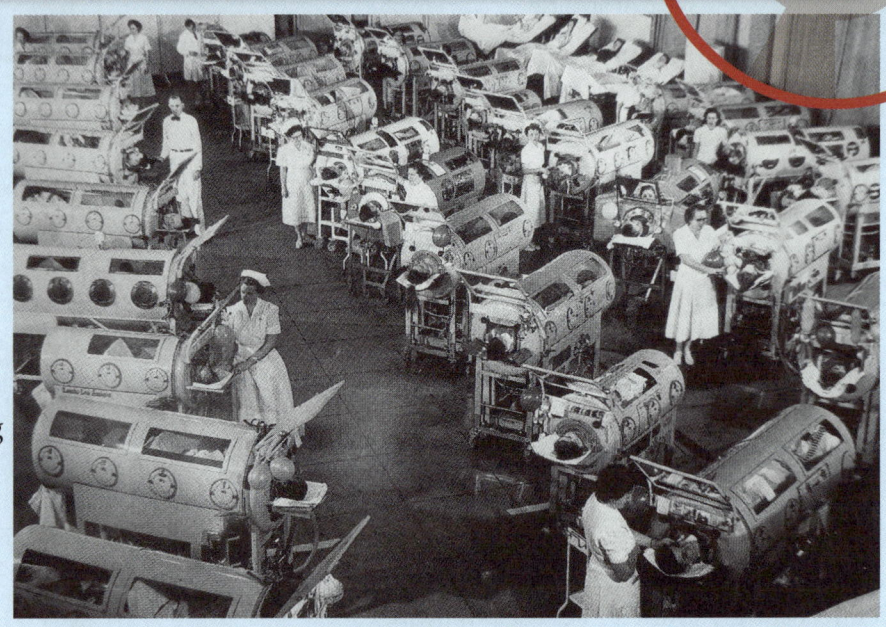

Iron lung ward filled with polio patients, Rancho Los Amigos Hospital, California (1953)

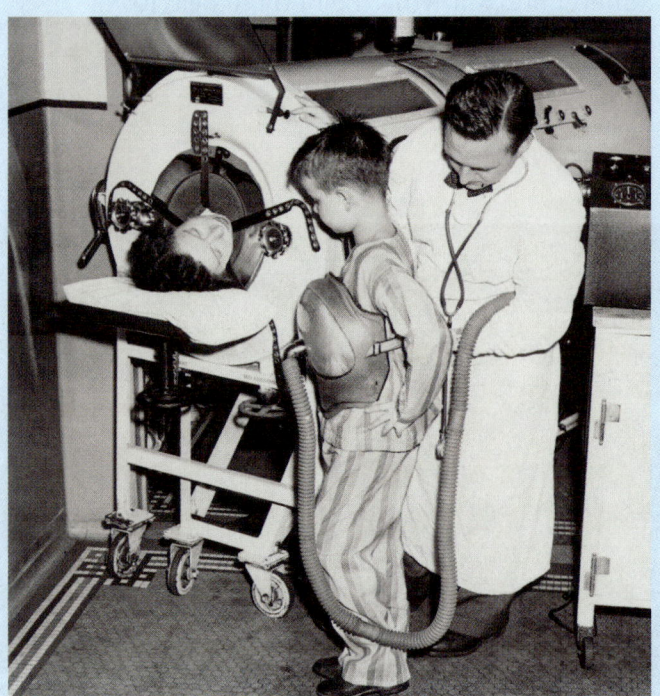

Dr. Jonas Salk   Dr. Albert Sabin

At the height of a polio epidemic, Dr. Harry Seanor, fastens the one-pound lung on an eight-year-old boy to show the difference in size to that of the 700-pound lung at left. Iron lungs were respirators to assist patients with breathing, (1949).

God's Wondrous Machine

Paralytic Poliomyelitis

1	The poliovirus enters the body through the mouth, usually from hands contaminated with the stools of an infected person or by ingestion of contaminated food or water.
2	The poliovirus travels to the digestive tract and attaches to receptors on the intestinal walls and replicates. The poliovirus can spread from the intestinal walls into the bloodstream.
3	In 99% of cases the poliovirus causes only mild flu-like symptoms or no symptoms at all. But in 1% of cases the poliovirus spreads from the bloodstream to the central nervous system.
4	The poliovirus attacks the central nervous system, destroying nerve cells in the spinal cord.
5	The virus may destroy the nerve cells governing the muscles necessary for breathing, and the muscles in the limbs, causing paralysis, most often in the legs.
6	The poliovirus is highly contagious. Even in mild cases the poliovirus is excreted in feces that can contaminate hands, food, and water.

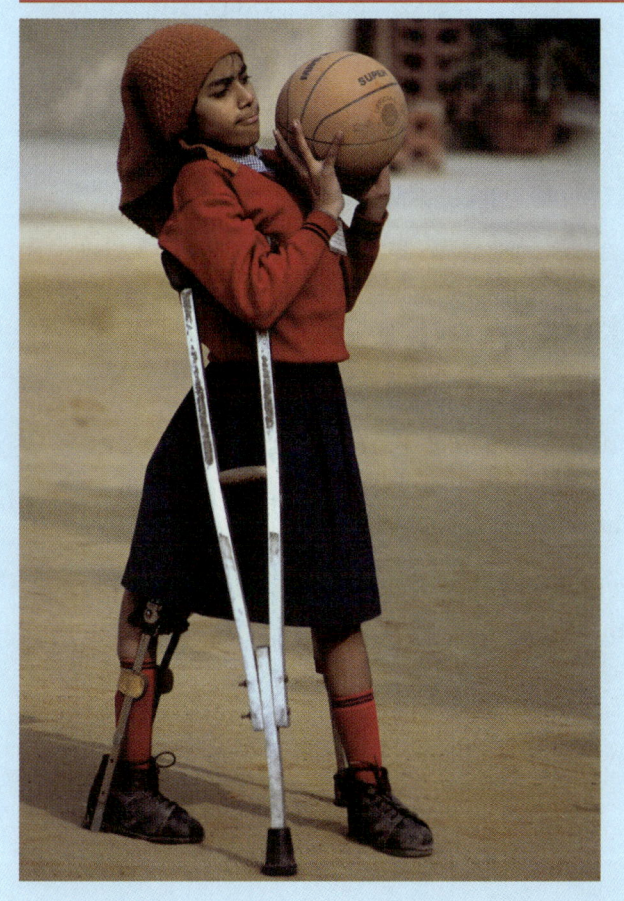

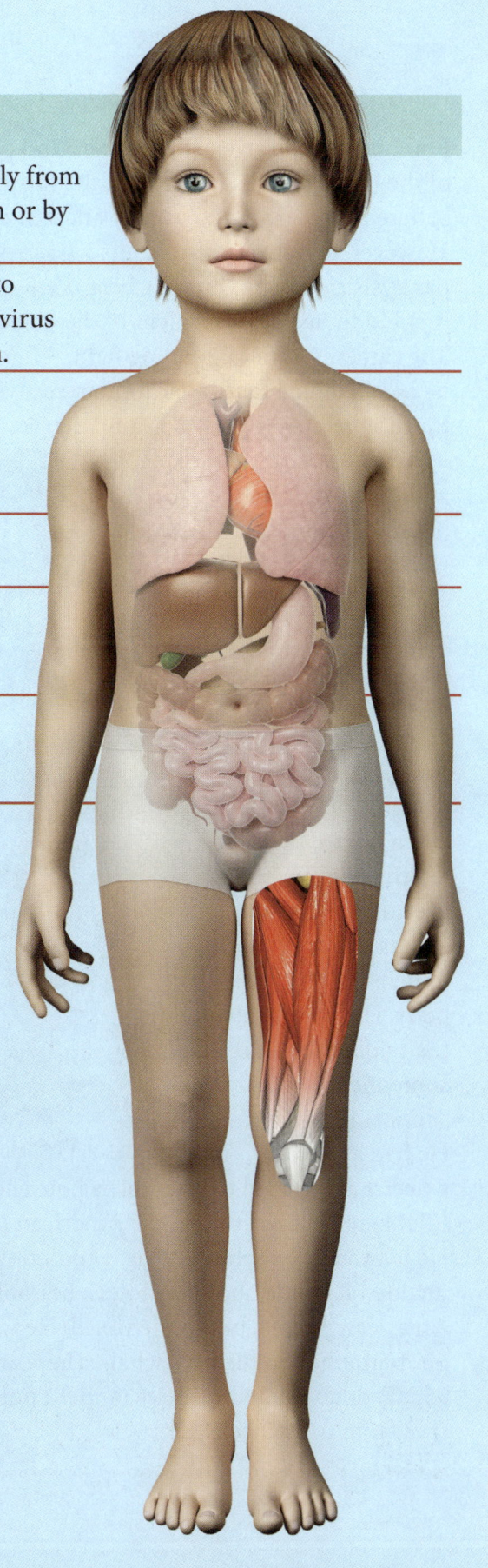

Unit 2: The Breathtaking Respiratory System

Franklin D. Roosevelt (FDR) and the March of Dimes

Franklin D. Roosevelt (FDR), the 32nd president of the United States, was one of the most famous sufferers of polio. Polio usually affected children. However, there were also adults who experienced paralysis from this virus. In 1921, FDR lost his first bid to become president of the United States. The campaign was a grueling fight. After his loss, he escaped on a family vacation to recover from the fatigue of being on the campaign trail. He was 39 years old, married with five children. He became ill while on vacation for a period of time. He recovered but never regained the full use of his legs. His legs were paralyzed. He was unable to walk. FDR kept his disability a secret when he decided on another run for the presidency. He wore braces under his pants to help support his body. He leaned into the podium or held someone's arm to support his weight. He had a special wheelchair created to resemble a household chair. FDR kept his secret from the American people. He felt that if people knew he could not walk unaided it would show weakness, not only to the American people, but to the world. He was rarely photographed in his wheelchair. There are over 35,000 documented pictures of FDR; only two show him in a wheelchair.

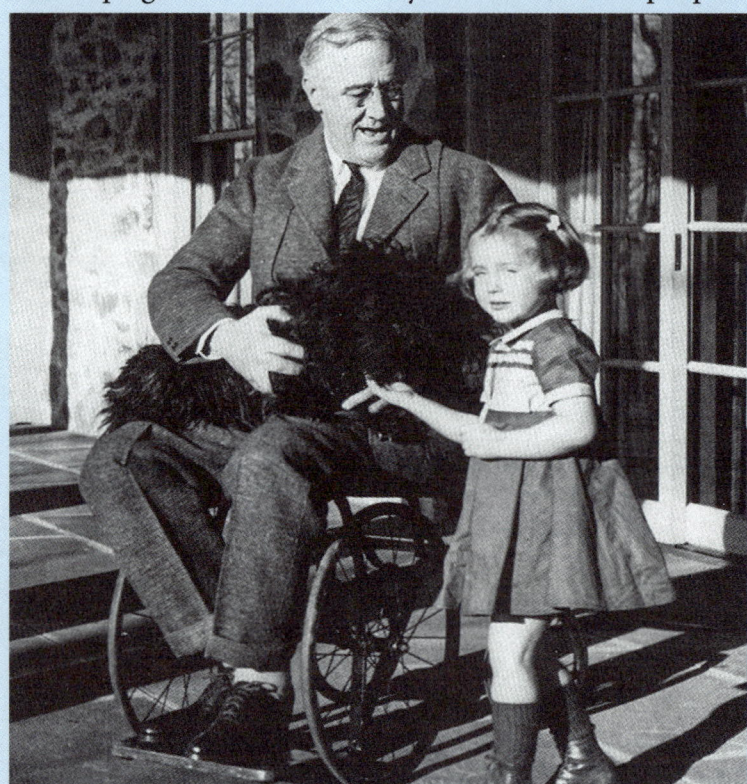

President Franklin D. Roosevelt

An old proverb states that "necessity is the mother of invention." This means that only through great need are we inspired to create new things and solutions to problems. In 1938, Roosevelt, on the wings of the polio epidemic, established the National Foundation for Infantile Paralysis. Infantile paralysis was another name for polio, since children were the most affected by this disease. The purpose of the organization was to connect scientists and volunteers to assist the victims of polio as well as provide financial support for research. The National Foundation for Infantile Paralysis stills exists today. The name was changed to the March of Dimes. This name change was instituted after a nationwide campaign to raise money to fund the organization. FDR called on everyone to give whatever money they could spare. He emphasized that even amounts as small as a dime would be of great service.

"Franklin's illness... gave him strength and courage he had not had before. He had to think out the fundamentals of living and learn the greatest of all lessons — infinite patience and never ending persistence." —Eleanor Roosevelt, wife of FDR

132

God's Wondrous Machine

Life in the Iron Lung

The whirling rush of air sounds rhythmic throughout the room. Lying face up, your arms pinned to your sides and only your head peeking out of an 800-pound steel can, you try to relax as the next wave of pressure pushes the air out of your lungs.

This is a small glimpse of life in an iron lung. Though the iron lung is no longer produced, it made the difference between life and death for thousands of people during the polio epidemic in the 1950s. Today, only about 10 people worldwide still live life in the iron lung. Phillip Drinker, an engineer, and his colleagues at the Harvard School of Public Health invented a respirator that enabled paralytic polio patients to breathe. It was called the Drinker Respirator and was first introduced in 1927. It became commonly known as the "iron lung" due to its appearance.

The Drinker Respirator was very large and heavy. The magnificent thing about this life-saving technology was, it could accommodate a great range of different-sized patients. A small child to a man as large as 6 feet 4 inches and weighing up to 225 pounds could use the apparatus. Many people who required the aid of the iron lung would use it for only a few weeks until their bodies recovered from the paralysis of polio. There were others who never regained the use of their muscles or their diaphragms to assist in breathing. They were confined to the metal case for the rest of their lives.

How does it work? Great question. A person is laid on a padded cot and slid into the apparatus. The metal enclosure is snapped shut. The only thing that lies outside the container is the person's head. A soft flexible rubber collar seals the opening around their neck and the machine. There are windows along the body of the tube to allow health providers access to the patient. A mirror is suspended over the person's head, allowing the patient a limited view of the room. A mechanical arm connected to a bellow at the foot of the chamber and was powered by an electrical motor.

Air is not actually pushed into the person's lungs. It is the pressure differences in the airtight container that allow the person to breathe. As the arm of the machine works like a piston with the bellow, it creates positive and negative pressures. When the pressure in the tube is more negative than the pressure inside the lungs, the patient's diaphragm draws down. The person inhales. When the pressure becomes more positive, higher than the pressures within the lungs, it causes the person to exhale.

Up to 100 iron lungs would run at the same time in hospital units at the peak of the polio epidemic. According to the Smithsonian Institution, the cost of an iron lung was extremely high. In the 1930s, an iron lung would cost a family a whopping $1,500. That was the going price of a house at that time. To put this in perspective, a dollar in the 1930s is equivalent to $14.25 today.

So doing the math, $1,500 in the 1930s would be over $21,000 today.

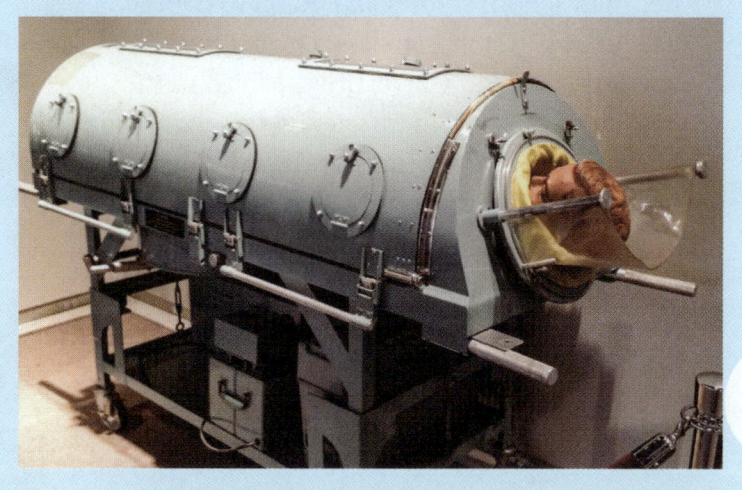

Unit 2: The Breathtaking Respiratory System

The Woman with the Iron Will: Martha Mason

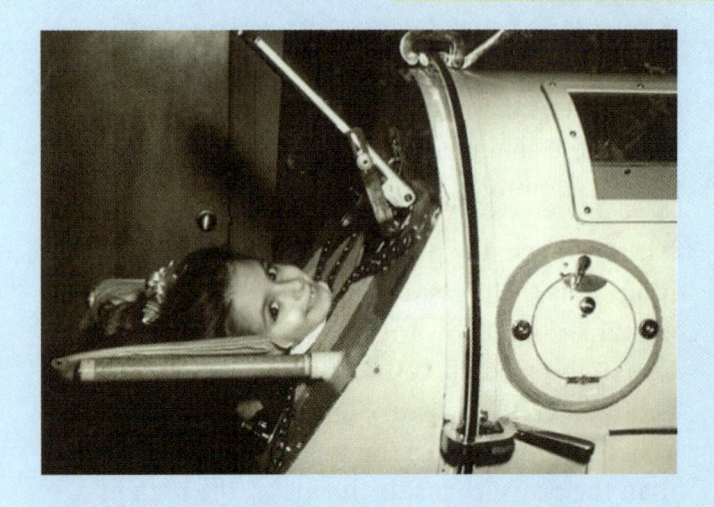

The year was 1948. On the 13th day of September, three days after her brother died from polio, 11-year-old Martha Mason began to feel ill. She became stricken with the same grave illness as her brother. Martha stayed in the hospital for a year. Finally, her parents were able to bring her home in an iron lung with assistance from the March of Dimes Foundation. It was in the iron lung that she would live the remainder of her life. Martha lived in her metallic cocoon, unable to breathe on her own, for 61 additional years.

But Martha's spirit was never paralyzed. She spread her wings and soared. With the help of multiple friends, her loving parents, and the town in which she lived. Martha was able to complete her high school studies and go on to college, graduating first in her class. During her time at Gardner Webb University she lived in the basement and communicated via intercom with her classmates and professors. She wrote for the local paper after graduation with the help of other's hands and a voice-activated computer.

As technology advanced, Martha's living situation remained the same. She stated, "By the time [alternative ways of respiration] were readily available, I had already established a lifestyle in an iron lung. After investigation and observation, I've learned that these people have [tracheotomies]; they have infections that have a lot more problems. I don't know of any one of them who has used that equipment for 60 years and had a good life with it." Mason felt her iron lung allowed her to be independent because the operation of it required no monitoring by medical professionals and allowed her to stay in her own home.

The iron lung that she lived in had a backup generator. This generator was crucial to her survival in the event of a power outage. Everyone in her town knew her. If the power went out, the fire department would immediately dispatch a crew over to her house to make sure her iron lung was functioning properly. In 2010, Martha published her memoir, *Breathe: A Lifetime in the Rhythm of an Iron Lung*. She never saw herself as a victim. Martha indeed lived a full life. She demonstrated resolve and an iron will.

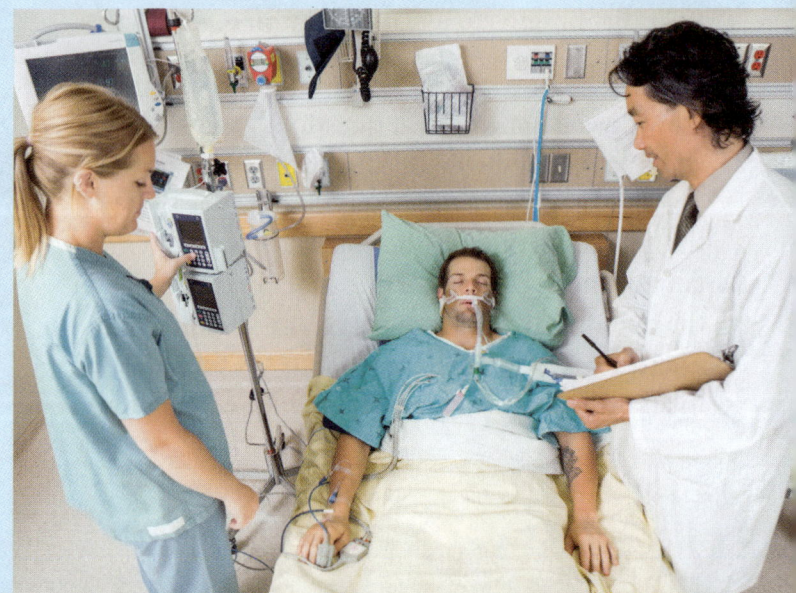

Today the "iron lung" is no longer used. A special machine called a ventilator is now used to support the breathing of patients who are too sick to breathe on their own.

God's Wondrous Machine

The Woman Who Could Fly: Wilma Rudolph

Her life got off to a rocky start. She entered this world on June 23, 1940, a sickly-premature baby, born the 20th child in a family of 22 children. At the tender age of four, this small African-American girl lost the use of her right leg due to polio. Her name was Wilma Rudolph.

Wilma's parents were told that she would never be able to walk normally. With dogged determination, they refused to accept the doctor's verdict. The Rudolphs who did their best to make a living to support their large family, knew their daughter would walk one day.

Refusing to accept no for an answer, Wilma's mother began to take Wilma for intensive therapy sessions at Meharry Hospital. It was the only facility at that time in history that would treat African Americans. Meharry was over 50 miles away from their home. Wilma went twice a week. She endured painful and grueling exercises. On Wilma's sixth birthday, she was able to walk with the assistance of leg braces, special shoes, and crutches. But her recovery did not stop there. Her mother refused to treat Wilma any differently than her siblings. By 12 years old, she was able to walk on her own. She even began to learn to run and jump.

Wilma loved to watch her siblings play and always joined in. Upon entering junior high, Wilma decided to try out for the basketball and track team. She made it! She didn't play very much, but with each passing practice she grew stronger and stronger. Her nickname became "Skeeter" because she was like a buzzing mosquito eager to get in the games. She started to excel in athletics. At a track meet at the Tuskegee Institute, Wilma ran. She lost every race she ran.

Nevertheless, Ed Temple, a coach from Tennessee State University, took notice of young Wilma. He recognized Wilma's potential and invited her to train with his collegiate track team. Wilma ran so fast it was as if she could fly. She competed in two Olympic games, the first one at 16. In two games, she returned home with a bronze medal (third place) and three gold medals.

Franklin Delano Roosevelt, Martha Mason and Wilma Rudolph all overcame great odds to live life to the fullest. God gives us all varying talents. We all encounter varying degrees of difficulty in life. It is not what we lack but what we do with what is gifted to us.

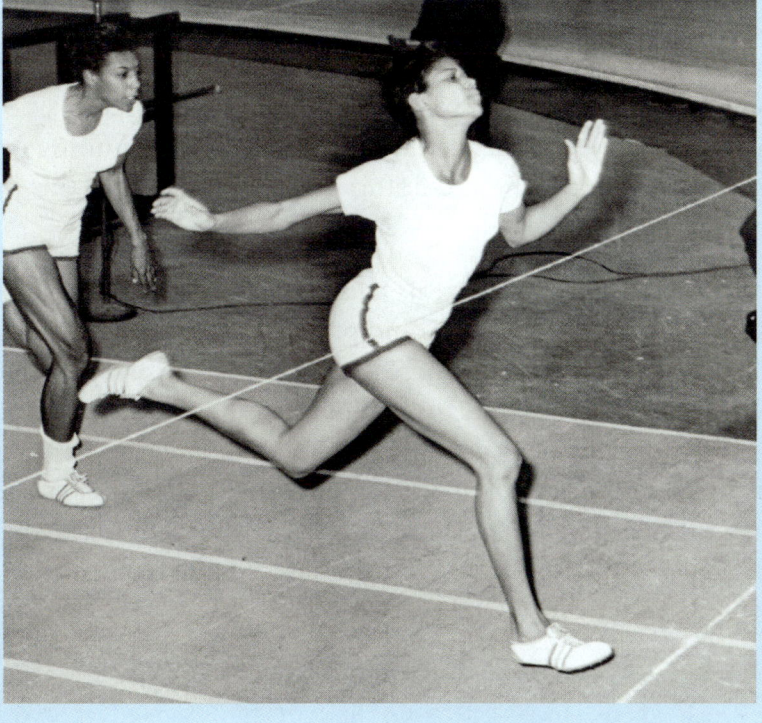

Unit 2: The Breathtaking Respiratory System

10 Ponder This

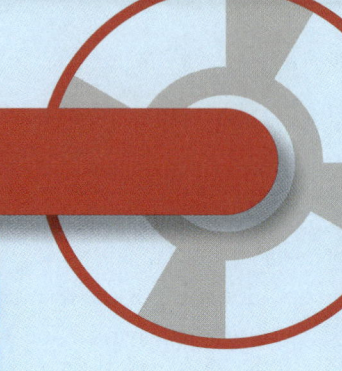

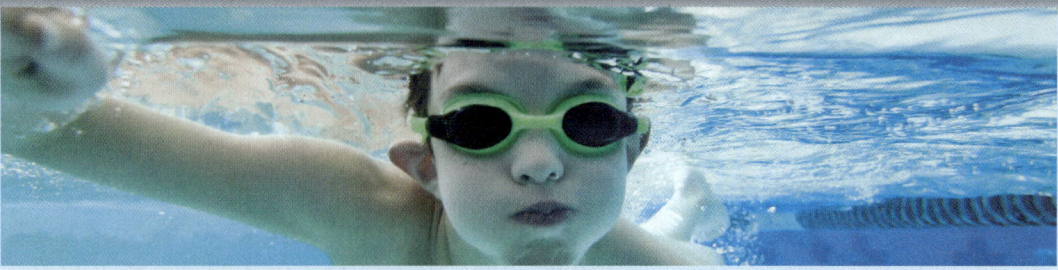

Why does my side sometimes hurt when I run and breathe hard?

Ouch! Some people call this sharp pain you experience with heavy exercise a "side stitch." The medical term for this is called exercise-related transient abdominal pain. Don't you love it when medicine can come up with terms to describe a common phenomenon and make it sound quite complicated? This pain can be experienced when you have been running or walking vigorously. Don't worry — the pain is temporary and nothing serious. Normally, this pain is felt on the right side, not far from your belly button.

There are many theories on the origin of this pain. Some think the exuberant movement of the legs increases the pressure in the abdomen and presses the diaphragm upward. Your respiratory rate is increased to satisfy your muscles' increased demand for oxygen, causing the lungs to press the diaphragm down. The diaphragm is then trapped in the middle, and these opposing forces give it a squeeze. The squeezing decreases the flow of blood and oxygen to the area, which leads to a sharp stabbing pain and/or cramping. Another theory is that the ligaments, special connective tissues that keep things in place, in the area of the diaphragm may experience stretching with the pounding and breathing action. To be honest, no one really knows. To be sure, the pain is real. But be assured, it won't hurt you.

Why do I hiccup?

The original term for such a reaction was "hiccough" in the early 1500s in England. The word evolved to what we now refer to as hiccups. We have onomatopoeia to thank for the name change. Onomatopoeia is simply a term for a word that is spelled and pronounced just like the sound it describes. A hiccup is produced when the diaphragm is irritated. It jerks down in a spastic manner. Air rushes into your lungs. As the air passes by your vocal cords they close suddenly and you make the well-known sound.

This irritation can be caused by eating fast, a stomach or throat annoyance, and even becoming frightened. Typically, they only last a few minutes. The world record for hiccups is held by Charles Osborne. He had the hiccups for 69 years! Not a record that you would be interested in breaking for sure. It was said that his hiccups began in 1922 after he tried to weigh a 350-pound pig that was to be slaughtered. They did not stop until 1990. It is estimated that he hiccupped over 430 million times. At the peak of his marathon, he would hiccup up to 40 times a minute.

God's Wondrous Machine

What causes me to sneeze when I leave a movie theater?

Achoo! I believe I've hit a snafu.

Achoo! This is no virtue.

Achoo! I can't stop, boohoo.

Cough. Sniff. I think I made a swap, yahoo.

We have all experienced that little tickle in the nose, and without any control you launch a snot rocket. This propulsion can occur due to many reasons aside from irritation. Believe it or not, some people sneeze when entering bright light after being in the dark; for example, after leaving a movie theater. This is called a photic sneeze, or a photic sneeze reflex. A reflex doesn't involve a conscious decision by the brain. You don't think about it, but your body just does it. Nearly 20 to 30 percent of all people may experience photic sneezes. So appropriately, it is also known as the ACHOO syndrome (Autosomal Dominant Compelling Helio-Ophthalmic Outburst Syndrome). It is believed to be a trait that runs in families.

The optic nerve is the nerve that connects your eyeballs to your brain. It carries signals that originate at the eye, and the brain interprets what you see. In a dark environment, your pupils dilate (become larger) to allow more light to enter your eye in the darkness. Upon exiting the theater, your optic nerve tells your pupils to constrict. This protects your eyes from the extra light. Enter another brain nerve, the trigeminal nerve. It is stimulated when your nose is irritated by something. The optic and trigeminal nerves are neighbors. They lie very close to each other. It is believed that some of the electrical impulse that runs down the optic nerve seeps over to the trigeminal nerve. This activates the trigeminal and triggers a sneeze.

Why does my nose run when I cry?

Crying produces a great deal of fluid runoff down your face. Did you know you actually have a drainage area near your eye? At the corner of your eye, you will find the lacrimal sac.

Tears flow into the sac and drain out near the tubinates in the nasal cavity. The more you cry, the more your nose runs.

Why does my nose run when it is cold?

One of the functions of your nose is to warm the air that enters it. The vessels that lie close to the nasal lining dilate (become wider) during colder conditions. This allows extra blood to flow by in order to provide additional heating power. The extra blood flow also produces extra mucus to stream out your nose.

Unit 2: The Breathtaking Respiratory System

Why is snot green?

Doctors like to ask gross questions when you are sick. They may even ask you to describe the color of your snot! This certainly isn't a common topic of casual conversations. No, doctors do not have some strange interest with your body fluids. They ask this question because it may provide a clue about your illness. When you are sick, your immune system (remember when we talked about your soldiers) sends out white blood cells to fight the battle. There are several different types of white blood cells. The white blood cells that are the foot soldiers at the site of the attack are called neutrophils. The neutrophils are armed inside with special enzymes that aid in the defense. The enzyme of interest is myeloperoxidase. This enzyme contains a great deal of iron. As the fight wages, the white blood cells sacrifice themselves and spill their innards out into the mucus. Then more bacteria to fight the more brave white blood cells are called into action. The myeloperoxidase released has the characteristic green color. This spilling enzyme helps to kill the unwanted invaders. This "sick" snot is composed of dead white blood cells, discharged enzymes, and half-eaten bacteria. The longer it sits around in your sinuses, the greener it gets.

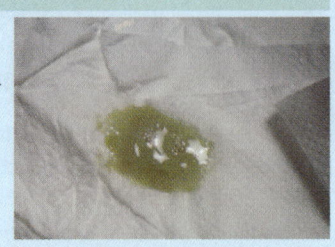

Why can fish breathe underwater and we can't?

All living animals require oxygen. Just like you, fish need oxygen. However, they satisfy their oxygen needs in a different way. The water that surrounds them is a compound of two hydrogens and one oxygen atom. Water is referred to as H_2O. This is the chemical shorthand for water's composition.

We cannot breathe the oxygen in the water because of its tight bond with hydrogen atoms. Fish "breathe" the oxygen that is dissolved in the water. (You can see an example of dissolved gases when you drink a soda pop. It fizzes when you pour it, tickling your nose. This is due to the dissolved carbon dioxide gas in it. When the gas is no longer present in the drink it becomes "flat" tasting.) Fish do not have lungs; they have gills. As they swim about, water is pushed through their gills. Interestingly, fish are cold blooded. We are warm blooded. One reason God has designed fish to be cold blooded is that it reduces their oxygen demands. The warmer you are, the more oxygen is required. Fish force water into their gills and the dissolved oxygen seeps into the walls of their blood vessels. Carbon dioxide seeps out of the vessels and is released out of the gills.

How do insects breathe?

God has created us uniquely different from the insect world. Like us, insects have the same need for oxygen in order to live. They do not have lungs like us but instead they have spiracles along the side of their exoskeletons. Spiracles are holes that allow air to enter the insect's body. The air travels down a series of tubes, and the oxygen actually dissolves into the liquid of their bodies. So insects do not technically "breathe" the way we breathe.

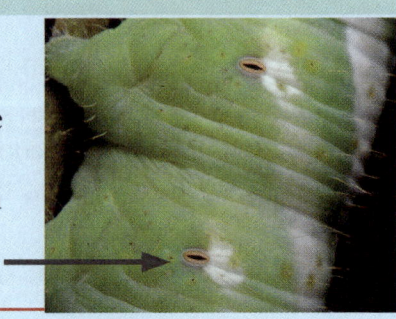

God's Wondrous Machine

What causes nosebleeds?

Remember when we were talking about the large network of blood vessels that line your nasal cavity? Because of their proximity to the surface, these vessels are particularly vulnerable. If you put your finger in your nostril, you increase your chances of producing an epistaxis (ep-i-STAK-sis). That is the smart word for nosebleed. There are other things that can cause nosebleeds. For example, a drying of the nasal passages is more common in the winter when the humidity in the air is low. Infections and allergies can also produce a nosebleed.

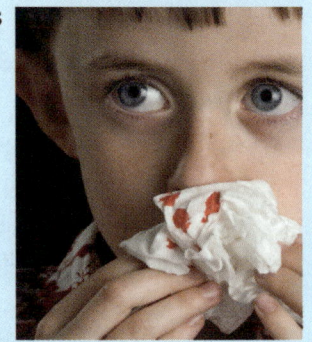

Why is it hard to breathe at high altitudes?

The higher you travel above sea level, the less oxygen concentration there is in the air. The oxygen concentration at sea level is much more dense. Another way of thinking about this is that the air molecules stack upon each other and exert a greater pressure the closer you move to sea level. Physical exertion at high altitudes requires more breaths of air to obtain the normal amount of oxygen your body demands. No worries. If you stay at higher elevation for a period of time, after a few days, your body gets used to these demands by increasing the production of red blood cells. With the addition, it allows for more oxygen-carrying capabilities.

Conclusion

Psalm 139 states that we are fearfully and wonderfully made. We are part of God's creation, and with the breath that He gives let us praise Him and marvel at His creation.

Praise the LORD.
Praise God in his sanctuary;
praise him in his mighty heavens.
Praise him for his acts of power;
praise him for his surpassing greatness.
Praise him with the sounding of the trumpet,
praise him with the harp and lyre,
praise him with timbrel and dancing,
praise him with the strings and pipe,
praise him with the clash of cymbals,
praise him with resounding cymbals.
Let everything that has breath praise the LORD.
Praise the LORD!

Unit 2: The Breathtaking Respiratory System

11 Fun Stuff

Facts: Bizarre and Gross

The desire of humans to compete in just about anything is unmatched. In Langenbruck, Germany, a competition for the longest nose in the world was held. I have no idea what type of training was required. Josef Dewold surpassed all contestants, proudly displaying his schnoz, winning the men's division with a nose measuring 4.8 inches. Margot Sikora, not to be left behind, won the women's with a 4.1-inch nose.

Medical treatments have improved over the years as our knowledge and understanding of the workings of the human body has grown. In ancient times, there were some unusual ideas of cures for diseases. Yikes!

- To cure whooping cough, ride a donkey seven times in a circle or crawl under the donkey seven times.

- To cure tuberculosis, breathe into a freshly dug hole in the ground or swallow live snails.

During the middle ages, people had no concept about the origin of infectious illnesses. They believed diseases were caused by evil vapors that permeated the skin. Bathing was not a normal practice. They thought a thick layer of sweat and dirt would keep them healthy. So they stopped bathing. In the 1500s, England's Queen Elizabeth I tried to get people to bathe more often. She felt it was a better, healthier practice. She encouraged people to take up her practice of bathing at least once a month whether they needed it or not. This was shocking and controversial. People of the time only bathed a couple of times a year.

Great or common mullein (Verbascum thapsus) has been used for almost 2,000 years as an herbal treatment for lung and skin ailments, ranging from asthma to burns. It is one of several natural herbs used for respiratory issues.

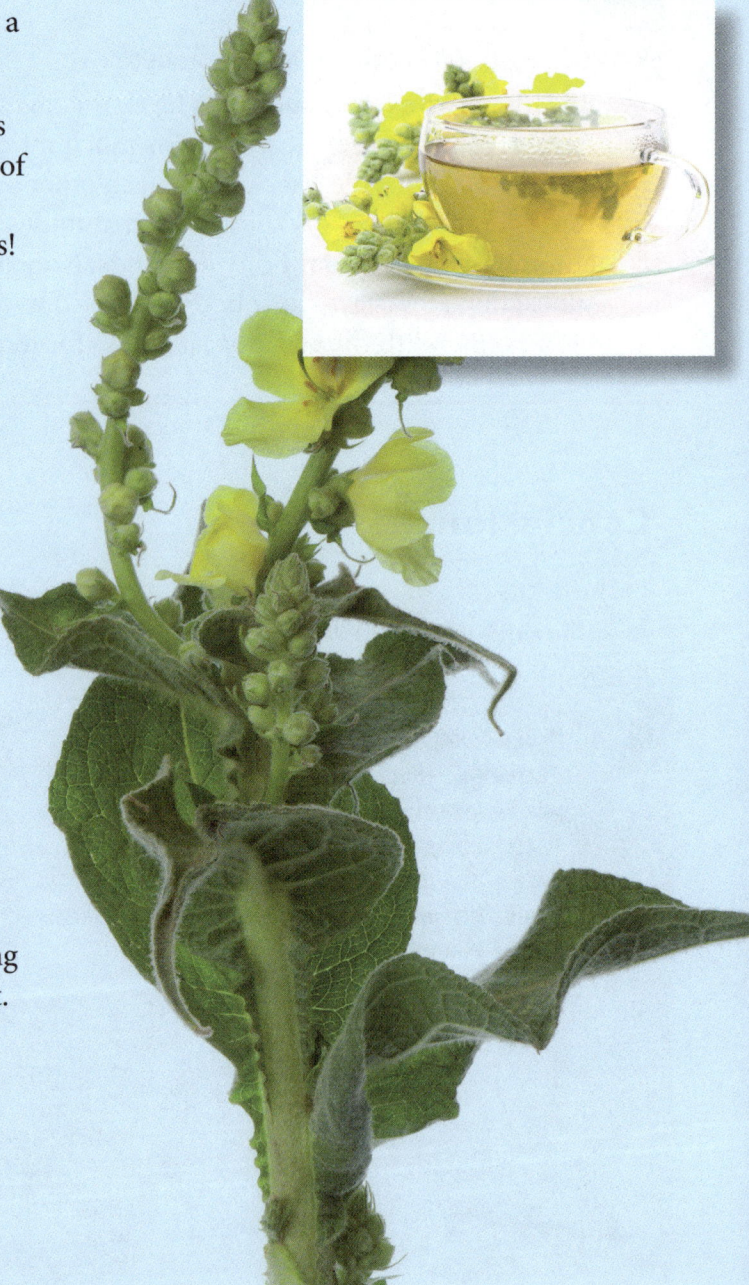

140

God's Wondrous Machine

You've Got to Be Kidding

What were the little snots afraid of when they went to bed?	The Booger Man.
What is brown and sticky?	A stick.
How do you make a tissue dance?	You put a little boogie on it.
Why did the boogie cross the road?	He was getting picked on.
Knock, Knock. Who's there? Snot. Snot who?	Your joke is snot funny.
What can you keep even if you give it away?	A cold.
Why was the nose so tired?	Because he had been running all day.
When you're out with your honey, And your nose is runny, You may think it's funny,	But IT'S NOT!!! (IT SNOT)
What does a booger in love tell his girlfriend?	I am stuck on you. Or I pick you.
What do you call a skinny booger?	Slim pickings.
What is the difference between boogers and broccoli?	Kids don't eat broccoli.
Why can't your nose be 12 inches long?	Because then it would be a foot!
Doctor, how do I stop my nose from running?	Stick out your foot and trip it.
How do you prevent a summer cold?	Catch it in the winter.
Doctor: Your cough sounds better today.	Patient: It should — I practiced all night.
What did the French man say after getting caught in the rain?	Eiffel a cold coming on.
Why did the hacker give his computer a box of tissues?	Because it had a nasty virus!
What do you give a cowboy with a cold?	Cough stirrup.
You can pick your nose and you can pick your friends…	…but you can't pick your friend's nose.
Did you just pick your nose?	No, I've had it since the day I was born.
What can you catch, but not throw?	A cold.
What did the nut say when it sneezed?	Cashew!
If we breathe oxygen in the daytime, what do we breathe at night?	Nitrogen!
What do you call a dinosaur that keeps you awake at night?	A Bronto-snore-us

Word Wise!

"BOOGER" A popular term for a small mass of congealed nasal mucus.

Unit 2: The Breathtaking Respiratory System

Breathtaking Quotes!

"Coughing in the theater is not a respiratory ailment. It is a criticism." *Alan Jay Lerner*

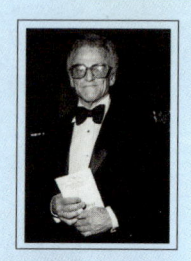

"When a man has lost all happiness, he's not alive. Call him a breathing corpse." *Sophocles*

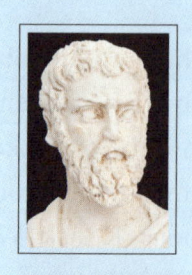

"To be a Christian without prayer is no more possible than to be alive without breathing." *Martin Luther*

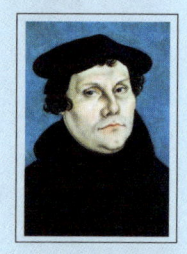

"What light is to the eyes — what air is to the lungs — what love is to the heart, liberty is to the soul of man." *Robert Green Ingersoll*

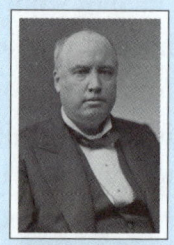

"Whenever I feel blue, I start breathing again." *L. Frank Baum*

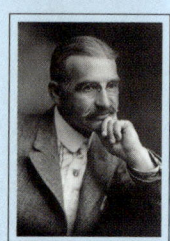

"The longest sword, the strongest lungs, the most voices, are false measures of truth." *Benjamin Whichcote*

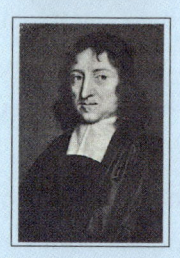

MED+MOMENT

Careers There are a lot of different kinds of medical careers, including many focused on the respiratory system. Here are just a few:

Respiratory Therapist	Manages the airway of patients; helps in establishing an airway after a trauma, for patients in intensive care units and for sedation; gives breathing treatments; sets up and manages ventilators
Pulmonologist	A doctor who specializes in the treatment of lung conditions and disease. Education: college 4 years, medical school 4 years, internal medicine residency 3 years, pulmonary fellowship 2 to 3 years. Total training after high school is 14 to 15 years.
Cardiopulmonary Lab Specialist	Helps patient understand and manage health problems, works with patients with diseases such as emphysema, heart attack, asthma, and Chronic Obstructive Pulmonary Disease (COPD)
Pulmonary Lab Tech	Conducts pulmonary function testing
Pulmonology	Medical specialty that deals with the study and treatment of diseases involving the respiratory tract

God's Wondrous Machine

"A large nose is the mark of a witty, courteous, affable, generous, and liberal man." *Cyrano de Bergerac*

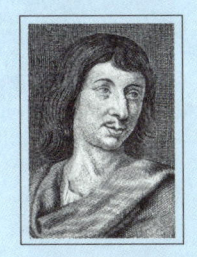

"The air is the only place free from prejudice." *Bessie Coleman*

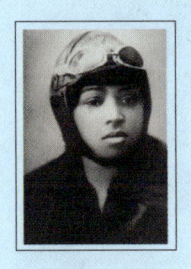

"A nation that destroys its soils destroys itself. Forests are the lungs of our land, purifying the air and giving fresh strength to our people." *Franklin D. Roosevelt*

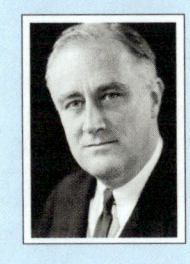

"The highlight of my childhood was making my brother laugh so hard that food came out of his nose." *Garrison Keillor*

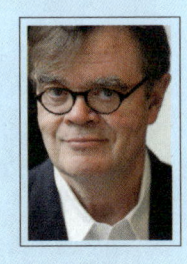

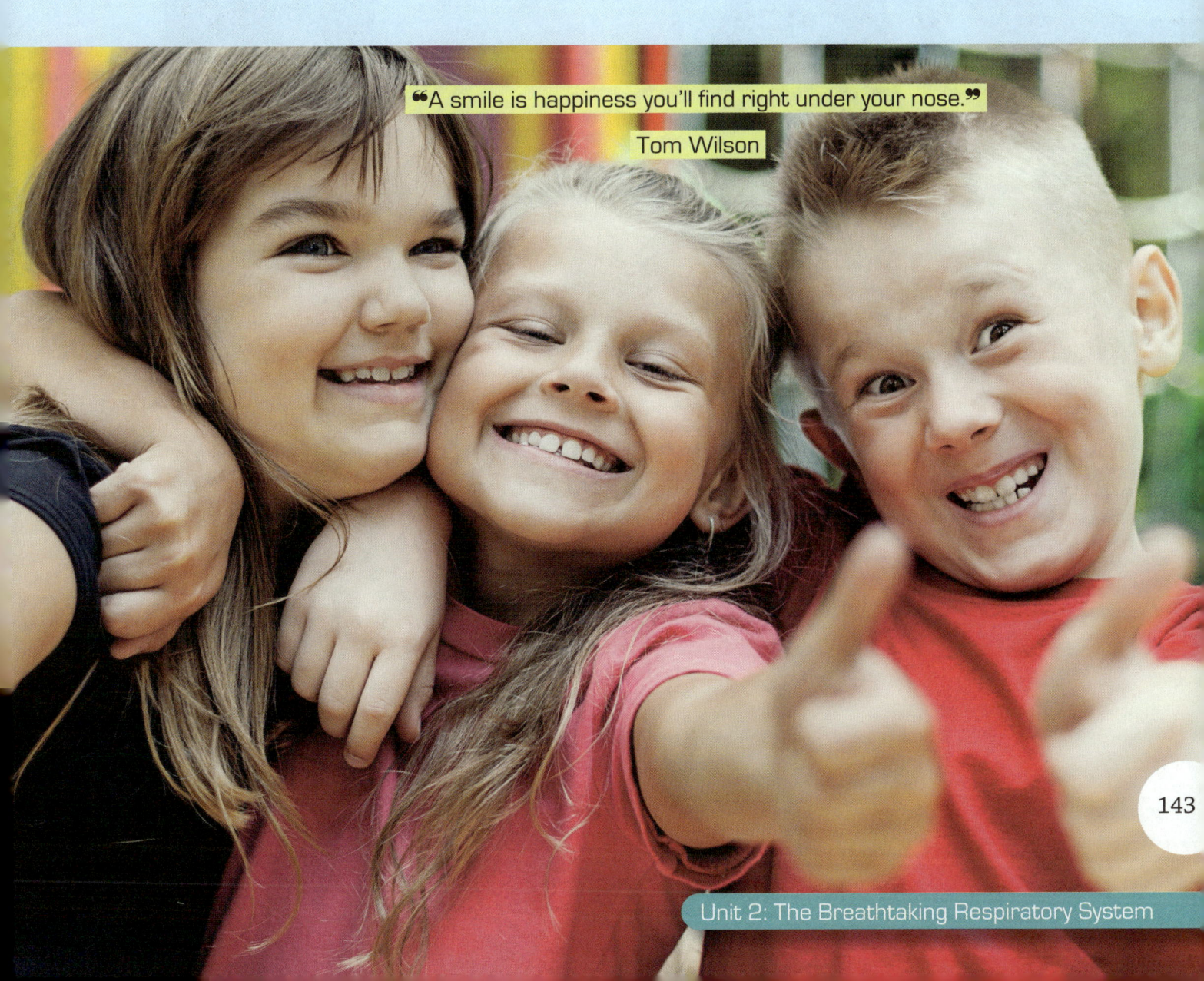

"A smile is happiness you'll find right under your nose."
Tom Wilson

Unit 2: The Breathtaking Respiratory System

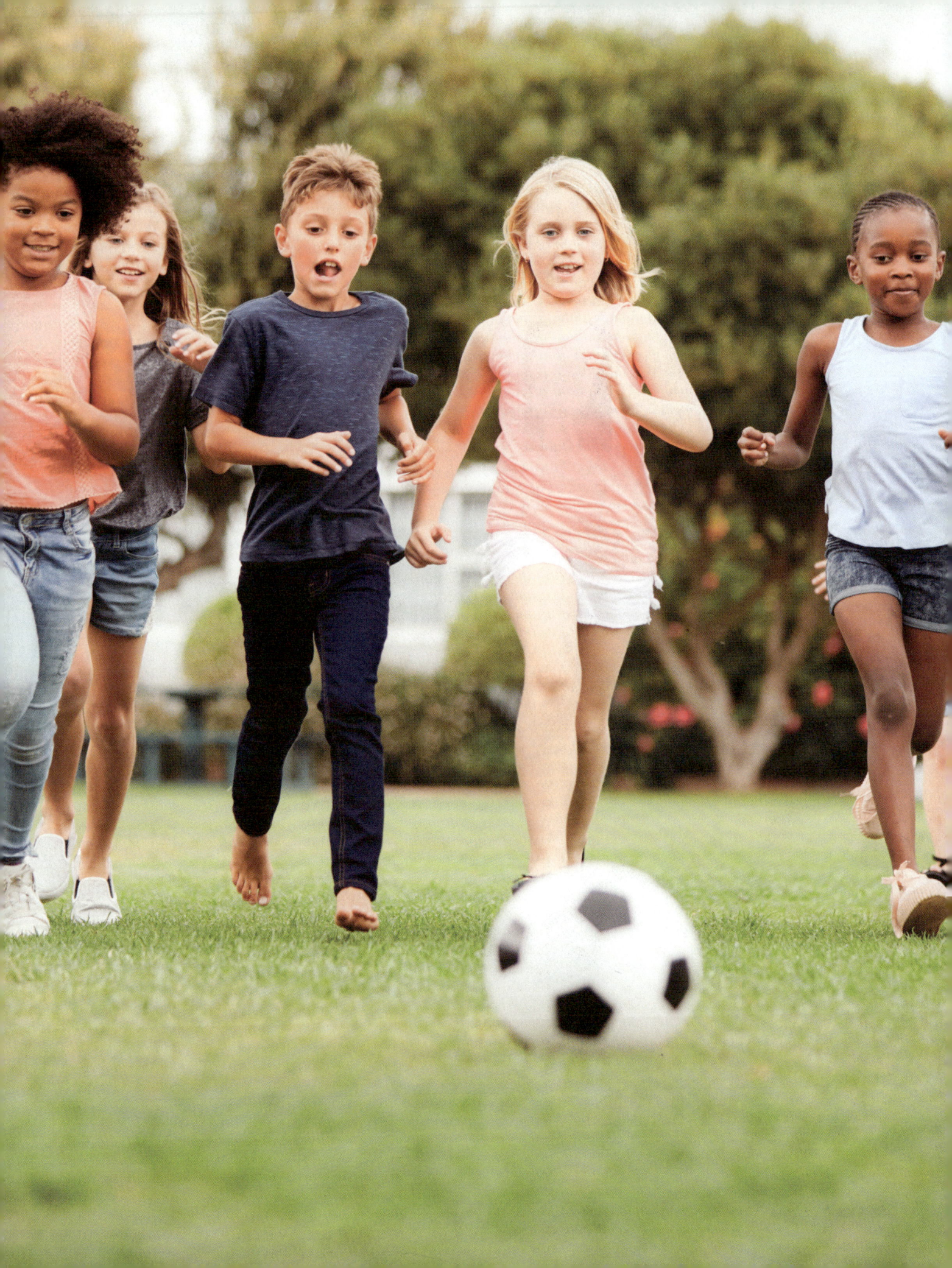

GOD'S WONDROUS MACHINE

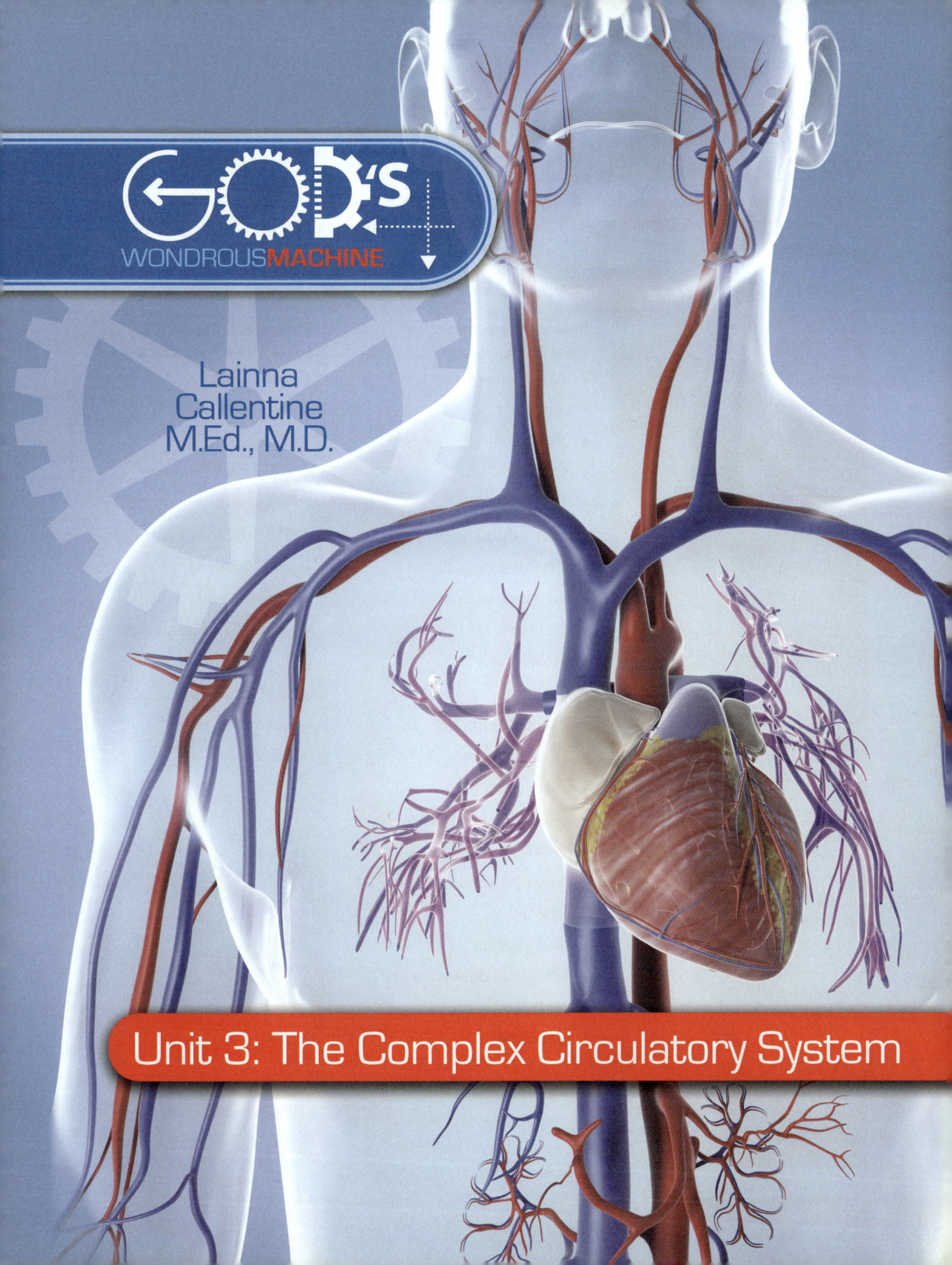

Lainna Callentine M.Ed., M.D.

Unit 3: The Complex Circulatory System

VOCABULARY LEVELS

Choose the word list based on your skill level. Every student should be able to master Level 1 words. Add words from Levels 2 and 3 as needed. More proficient students should be able to learn all three levels.

Level 1 Vocabulary

- Anemia
- Aorta
- Arteries
- Arterioles
- Atrium
- Bone marrow
- Closed circulatory system
- Fetus
- Hemoglobin
- Open circulatory system
- Prothrombin
- Red Blood Cells
- Stethoscope
- Valves
- Veins
- White blood cells

Level 2 Vocabulary

Review and Know Level 1 Vocabulary

- Antibodies
- Antigens
- Buffy coat
- Capillary
- Coronary
- Epicardium
- Erythrocytes
- Hematophagic
- Hemophilia
- Hemostasis
- Malaria
- Myocardium
- Pericardial sac
- Platelets
- Sickle cell anemia
- Stem cell
- Syncope
- Systole
- Tachycardia
- Universal donor
- Universal receiver
- Ventricles

Level 3 Vocabulary

Review and Know Level 1 and 2 Vocabulary

- Auscultate
- Bradycardia
- Centrifuge
- Chordae tendineae
- Diastole
- Electrocardiogram
- Endocardium
- Hematopoiesis
- Myocardial infarction
- Prothrombin
- Sinoatrial node
- Tricuspid valve
- Venules

God's Wondrous Machine

See It, Say It, Know It!

- 🟥 Level 1 Vocabulary
- ⬜ Level 2 Vocabulary
- 🟦 Level 3 Vocabulary

Word [Pronunciation]	Definition
Anemia [ah-ne´me-ah]	A problem with the blood in which oxygen delivered to the organs and tissues is decreased. It can be a symptom of many different diseases.
Antibodies [an-ti-bod-eez]	Blood proteins that are made to attack a specific invader, like bacteria or viruses. They set off a cascade of events to assist the body in a stronger defense.
Antigens [an´tĭ-jenz]	A foreign substance, like bacteria or virus, that triggers an immune response and causes antibodies to spring into action.
Aorta [a-or´tah]	The largest artery in the body that originates from the left ventricle and sends oxygenated blood to the body.
Arteries [ahr´ter-ez]	Vessels that carry oxygenated blood from the heart to the body.
Arterioles [ahr-te´re-ōlz]	Small vessels that carry oxygenated blood that connects to capillaries.
Atrium [a´tre-um]	The upper chambers of the heart in which blood enters the heart. There are two atrium, the right and left atriums.
Auscultate [ô´skəl-tāt´]	To listen; to listen to the sounds of the body.
Bradycardia [brady-car-dia]	A slow heartbeat that is typically less than 60 beats a minute for an adult.
Bone marrow [bohn mar´o]	The soft, spongy material in the middle of bones.
Buffy coat [bufé kōt]	When blood is centrifuged, spun in a test tube in a machine, the blood separates into three parts. This middle part is composed of white blood cells and platelets
Capillary [kap´ĭ-lar˝e]	Smallest arterial blood vessel; connects the arterioles with the venules.
Centrifuge [cen´trĭ-fūj]	To spin around; a machine used to spin test tubes of blood at high speeds in order to cause the parts of blood to separate.
Closed circulatory system	A blood system composed of vessels of different sizes that encloses the blood at all times. The blood is pumped by the heart and does not fill body cavities.
Chordae tendineae [kor´dah ten di nee a]	Fibrous strings that connect to the edges of the heart valves. They keep the valves from inverting or flipping backwards. Also known as the "heart strings."

Unit 3: The Complex Circulatory System

Word [Pronunciation]	Definition
Coronary [kôrʹə-nĕrʹē,]	The blood vessels that line the outside of the heart.
Diastole [dī-ăsʹtə-lē]	The phase in the heartbeat when the heart muscle relaxes and allows the heart chambers to fill with blood.
Electrocardiogram [ĭ-lĕkʹtrō-kärʹdē-ə-grămʹ]	A machine that graphically records the heart's electrical activity.
Endocardium [ĕnʹdō-kärʹdē-əm]	The inner muscle layer of the heart; the muscle that lines the inside of the heart.
Epicardium [ĕpʹĭ-kärʹdē-əm]	The outer muscle layer of the heart that lies under the pericardial sac.
Erythrocytes [ē•rith•rō•sits]	A red blood cell that contains hemoglobin and transports oxygen.
Fetus [fēʹtəs]	An unborn baby.
Hematophagic [hĕʹmă-tō-făʹjē-ă]	The act of an animal or insect like a mosquito drinking blood.
Hematopoiesis [heʺmah-to-poi-eʹsis]	The formation of blood cells. In the fetus, it takes place at sites including the liver, spleen, and thymus. From birth throughout the rest of life, it is mainly in the bone marrow.
Hemoglobin [heʹmo-gloʺbin]	A protein housed in red blood cells that contain iron. Hemoglobin facilitates in carrying oxygen.
Hemophilia [*hee-muh-fil-ee*-uh]	Any of several X-linked genetic disorders transmitted from the mother's genes, is a disease that occurs mainly in males. Excessive bleeding occurs due to the absence or abnormality of a clotting factor in the blood.
Hemostasis [heʺmo-staʹsis]	Stopping the escape of blood by natural means (either clot formation or vessel spasm).
Malaria [muh-lair-ee-uh]	A disease transmitted by mosquitos in which a parasite infects the red blood cells; can be deadly.
Myocardial infarction [miʺo-kahrʹde-al in-farkʹ shun]	A heart attack.
Myocardium [miʺo-karʹde-um]	The middle and thickest layer of the heart wall muscle.
Open circulatory system	System in which the blood is pumped by the heart and fills the body cavities. The blood does not stay within the vessels.

God's Wondrous Machine

Word [Pronunciation]	Definition
Pericardial sac [per″ĭ-kahr´de-al sak]	Fibrous double-layered sac that surrounds the heart. It is filled with a lubricant that allows the heart to move without friction.
Platelets [plat´lits]	Small cells in the blood that are important in hemostasis, forming blood clots.
Prothrombin [pro-throm´bin]	A clotting factor, made in the liver, that is in the blood. It is activated to thrombin for clot formation.
Red blood cells	Cells in the blood that contain hemoglobin, an iron that carries oxygen.
Sickle cell anemia [ah-ne´me-ah]	A blood disease that is inherited in which the red blood cells become misshaped to a sickle-like appearance. Causes long-term problems.
Sinoatrial node [sahy-noh-ey-tree-uh]	A mass of muscle tissue on the top of the right atrium that is the electrical pacemaker of the heart.
Stem cell	A cell that has the ability to differentiate to other specialized cells.
Stethoscope [steth´o-skōp]	A medical device used to listen and magnify the sounds heard in the body.
Syncope [sing´kah-pe]	To lose consciousness; pass out.
Systole [sis´to-le]	The phase in the heart cycle of beating in which the heart chambers contract to expel blood out of the heart.
Tachycardia [tak″e-kahr´de-ah]	A fast heartbeat that typically is over 100 beats a minute in an adult.
Tricuspid valve	The heart valve between the right atrium and right ventricle.
Universal donor	A person who has type O blood.
Universal receiver	A person who has type AB blood.
Valves [valv]	The "door" between the chambers of the heart that prevents blood from flowing backwards.
Veins [vān]	Blood vessels in the body that carry deoxygenated blood. They transport blood to the heart.
Ventricles [ven´trĭ-k'l]	The lower chambers of the heart.
Venules [ven´ūl]	Small blood vessels that carry deoxygenated blood toward the heart. They connect the capillaries to the veins.
White blood cells	Blood cells that are part of the immune system that fight invaders that attack the body.

*Pronunciation Keys from http://medical-dictionary.thefreedictionary.com

Introduction

Lightning flashed. The cloud hurled its pellets downward. A blood-curdling scream resonated through the cold, dank, and dreary marble halls . . . a suspenseful way to begin a book on *The Complex Circulatory System*, right? Just the mention of the word or seeing blood causes some people to feel woozy and go wobbly in the knees. Some people will even pass out at the very sight of blood. Take heart. There will be no need to be faint of heart.

Our heart beats passionately. It never stops. It never rests. It works around the clock, day and night. It starts to beat after you were conceived in your mother's womb at 3 to 4 weeks (a full-term pregnancy is 40 weeks), and continues until the day God calls you heavenward. Aside from our Heavenly Father, Lord, God, and Jesus, no two words are more heavily mentioned in the Bible than "blood" and "heart." The word blood is mentioned in the Bible over 400 times. Heart is mentioned over a staggering 900 times. We will take a look at some of the powerful images illustrated and represented by these words.

The Complex Circulatory System will catapult you into a whole new dimension. First, we will take an historical excursion through the pages of time and see how our knowledge of the circulatory system has expanded. We will learn all about blood, where it comes from, and how clots develop. Next, we will wade through the life-giving fluid that courses through the highways of your body. We will explore bloodsucking critters and enter the atrium of the heart and peer into the heart's many rooms. My prayer is that as we journey through the tributaries of your body, you will gain a deeper understanding of the magnificent artistry God has fashioned in you.

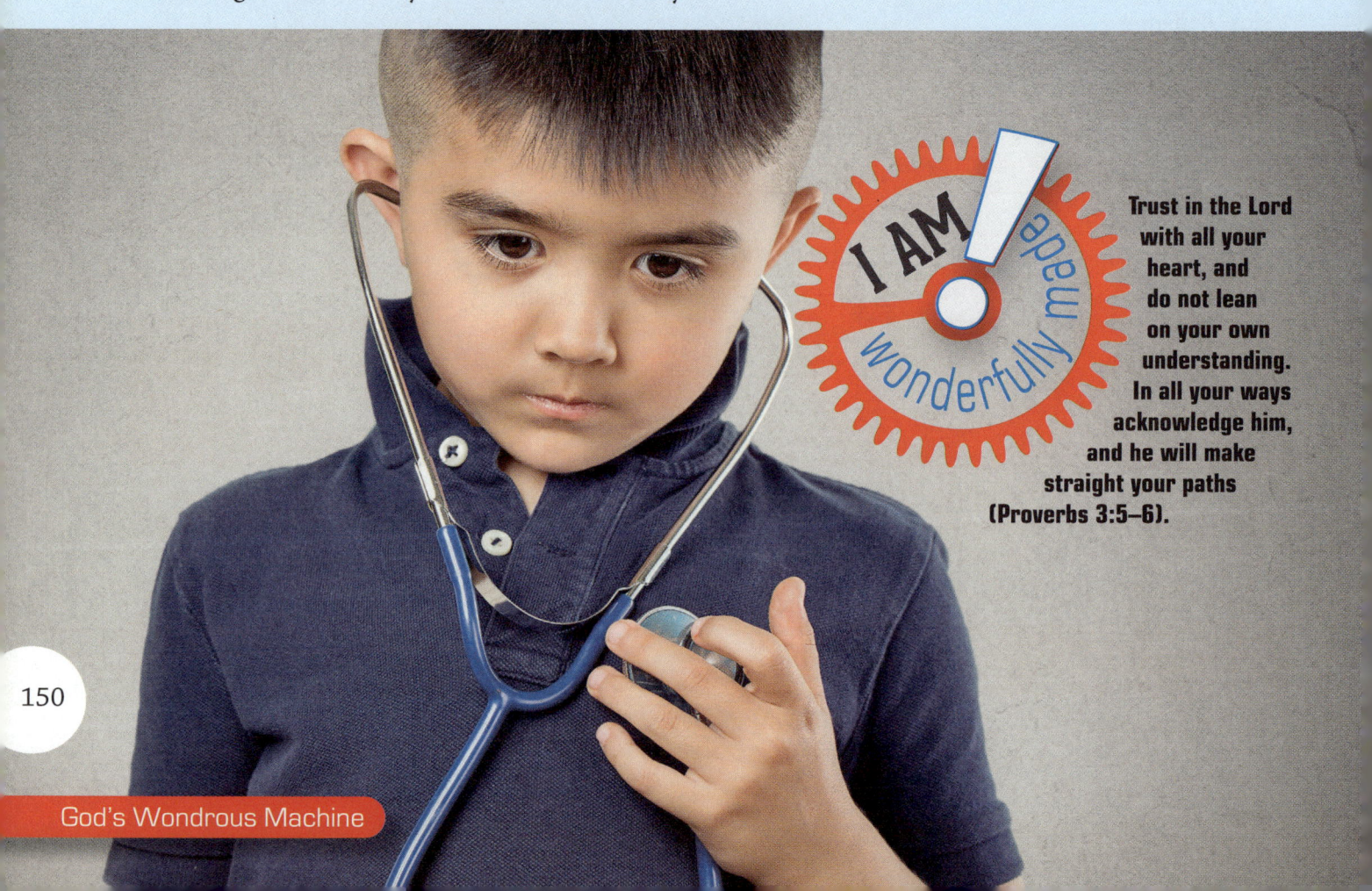

I AM wonderfully made!

Trust in the Lord with all your heart, and do not lean on your own understanding. In all your ways acknowledge him, and he will make straight your paths (Proverbs 3:5–6).

God's Wondrous Machine

Biblical References to the Heart

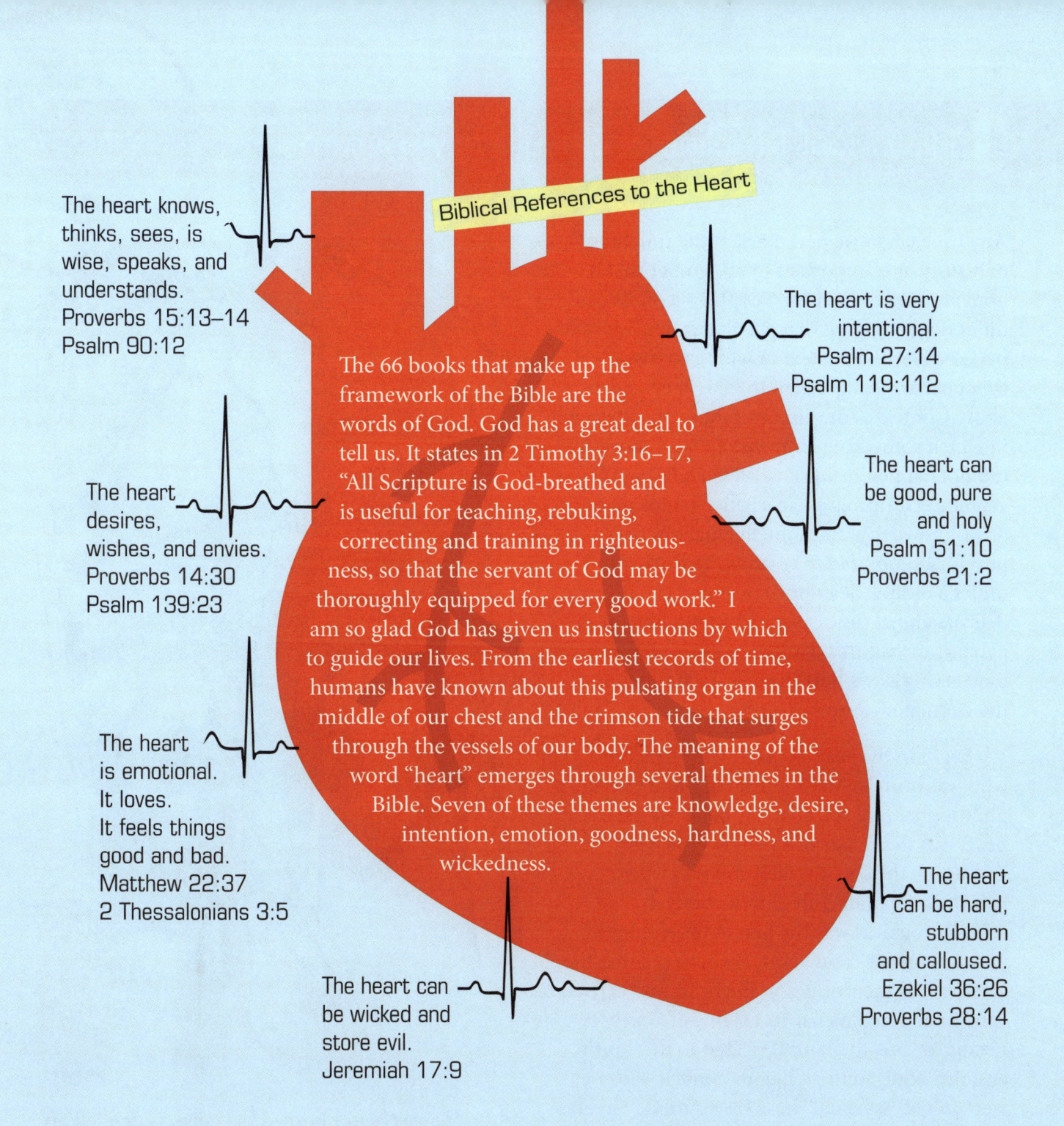

The heart knows, thinks, sees, is wise, speaks, and understands.
Proverbs 15:13–14
Psalm 90:12

The heart is very intentional.
Psalm 27:14
Psalm 119:112

The heart desires, wishes, and envies.
Proverbs 14:30
Psalm 139:23

The heart can be good, pure and holy
Psalm 51:10
Proverbs 21:2

The heart is emotional. It loves. It feels things good and bad.
Matthew 22:37
2 Thessalonians 3:5

The heart can be wicked and store evil.
Jeremiah 17:9

The heart can be hard, stubborn and calloused.
Ezekiel 36:26
Proverbs 28:14

The 66 books that make up the framework of the Bible are the words of God. God has a great deal to tell us. It states in 2 Timothy 3:16–17, "All Scripture is God-breathed and is useful for teaching, rebuking, correcting and training in righteousness, so that the servant of God may be thoroughly equipped for every good work." I am so glad God has given us instructions by which to guide our lives. From the earliest records of time, humans have known about this pulsating organ in the middle of our chest and the crimson tide that surges through the vessels of our body. The meaning of the word "heart" emerges through several themes in the Bible. Seven of these themes are knowledge, desire, intention, emotion, goodness, hardness, and wickedness.

It has taken us many generations to acquire the understanding of the heart in the context of our biological processes. Our Lord amazes me. Before man made these "great" discoveries, God's creation and order already existed. We have just begun to understand some of the complexities of His handiwork, to put words and descriptions to this order. We continue to gain increasing understanding of this order. Never will our understanding and intellect put us on equal footing with our Lord. May our hearts become tender to the soothing words and guidance of our Heavenly Father.

Unit 3: The Complex Circulatory System

1 Historical Timeline of Circulatory System

Any time when we peek back at the timelines of history, it is important to remember that it is an account of the past. People's accounts can differ depending on that particular person's perspective. The context in which an historical event occurs is important to take in consideration. Context is the circumstances or situation in which something happens. These discoveries did not happen inside an airless and weightless vacuum. Our progress in science builds on our prior knowledge. Each intellectual discovery provides a foothold to reach up to further our understanding. Scientific reasoning can be very delicate and at times silenced depending on a person's or culture's worldview. We will take a look at this as we tour the historical timeline of the circulatory system.

We begin in the year 384 B.C. with Aristotle who was born in Macedonia. He was a Greek philosopher and scientist. He believed the heart was the center of a person. The heart was where the soul dwelled and was where blood was manufactured in the body. In 340 B.C., Praxagoras was the first to differentiate between arteries and veins. He believed that the arteries had their origin in the heart and carried "pneuma." Pneuma has its origins in Greek. It means to "breathe" and is related to the "spirit" and the "soul" in the religious context. Arteries were full of "spiritual" air. Erasistratus, a Greek anatomist (one who studies the body) and royal physician, described the heart as being a pump. He also in 250s B.C. saw the heart as a source of both arteries and veins. This was the wisdom of the times. This set the stage for one of the most influential physicians of the middle ages. Claudius Galenus, was born in Pergamum, Asia Minor (Western Turkey), during the peak of the Roman Empire in the approximate year of A.D. 129. He was better known as Galen. Galen left an indelible mark on the anatomical world. So deep was his impact that his view of the circulatory system was believed for 15 centuries!

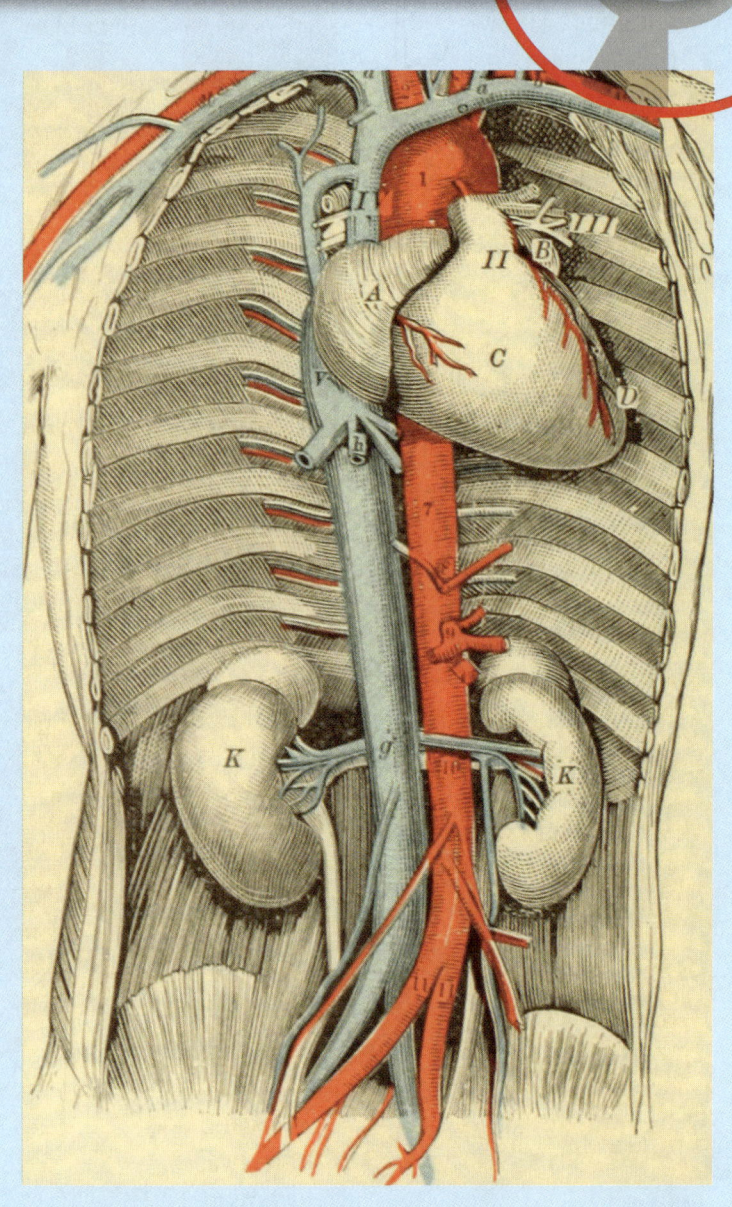

> **Word Wise!**
> TOURNIQUET is any device that uses pressure to stop the flow of blood, usually through the arteries of an arm or leg, as after a serious injury.

152

God's Wondrous Machine

If you lived in these times you would believe the following about the body:

The body's function was to refine the food you ate. Natural spirits had their beginnings in the food and drink you consumed. Vital spirits were derived from the air. Veins carried natural spirits. Arteries carried vital spirits.

Food was transformed in the liver. Veins originated at the liver. These veins contained the four humors or liquids of the body: yellow and black bile, blood, and phlegm. The blood of the veins went to the heart, and air and blood mixed in the left side of the heart. The heart was like a burning cauldron that produced heat and provided body warmth. (The brain cooled the body.) The humors naturally flowed around the body and went only where they were needed. The blood was consumed.

Why was this view so important? This theory guided the ideas about the origin of disease. Illness and disease were seen as functions of an imbalance of humors or a shift in its flow in the body. Treatment was aimed at restoration of this natural balance. Bloodletting was the practice of bleeding someone to restore this "healthy" balance. (We will talk a bit more about this later.) Tourniquets, which stop blood flow in an artery or vein, were also applied to parts of the body in attempts to redirect the flow of blood to other areas of the body. Today, we only use tourniquets in emergency situations to stop the bleeding from a wound.

Galen began his study of medicine at the age of 16. At the age of 28, he was appointed to the post of surgeon to the gladiators. He received a great deal of on-the-job training patching up wounded gladiators. In the year A.D. 162, he became the leading authority on medical knowledge and was appointed to the position of physician to the emperor. Galen left the world a legacy of these essential views:

	Galen's View	Modern View
1.	Veins contained blood. These veins were open ended, and the blood bathed the organs.	Veins do in fact carry blood. They are not open ended or bathe the organs. They carry deoxygenated blood.
2.	A small amount of the blood provided nourishment to the lungs.	All the blood in the body is transported to the lungs to obtain oxygen.
3.	The heart pulsated.	The heart does beat and therefore it could be considered to "pulsate."
4.	Breathing cooled the heated body and yielded the vital spirits.	Breathing is not the essential way that the body cools itself. "Vital" spirits are not taken up by the lungs.
5.	Arteries contained air and blood.	Arteries do contain blood. Oxygen is dissolved in the blood and is transported on hemoglobin in the red blood cells.
6.	Arteries were located deep in the body and pulsated. The blood in the arteries was hotter, thinner, and more "spirituous." Veins were located close to the surface.	Arteries can lay deep and superficially in the body. They do pulsate with each beat of the heart.
7.	The whole body breathes in and out.	The lungs do the breathing.

Unit 3: The Complex Circulatory System

This accepted view of the body did not advance for nearly 15 centuries. History and science discovery was guided by the worldview of the times. Over the course of these 15 centuries, the Roman Catholic Church dominated the attitudes and direction of the world of medicine. In essence, anyone who disagreed with the established church was labeled a heretic and was severally punished. A heretic is someone who dissents or disagrees from the established views or what is thought as the revealed truth. Illness was seen strictly as punishment from God. Today we have a process called the scientific method in which one asks questions, develops a hypothesis, and tests this hypothesis through experimentation. During this time, there was no tradition in the way scientific knowledge was acquired. People feared testing commonly held beliefs proposed by Galen. They also feared the church. It wasn't until the Reformation, among other events, when Martin Luther on October 31, 1517, nailed his *95 Theses* on the door of the All Saints' Church in Wittenberg. He challenged the church. The two over-arching points of his theses were that the Bible was the center of religious authority and that we reach salvation by our faith and not just by our deeds.

Fast forward hundreds of years to modern times, and we still have a battle of worldviews. Faith and belief in the Bible do not suppress scientific ideas and advancement. In fact, they are supported more and more with each new discovery, which furthers us to magnify the great designer in our Heavenly Father.

Galen's open-ended vascular system

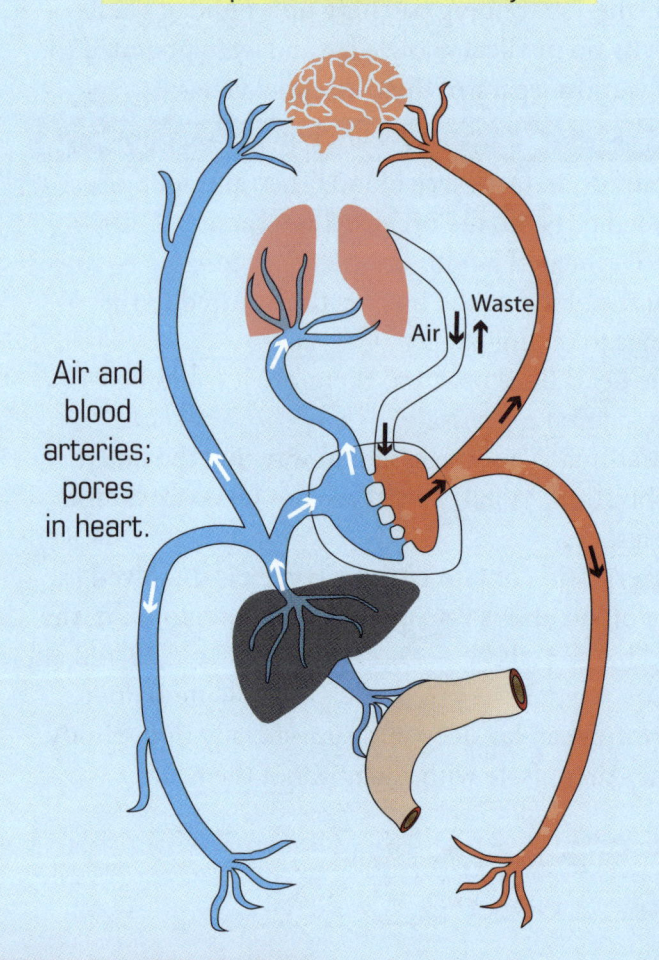

Air and blood arteries; pores in heart.

Harvey's closed circulatory system

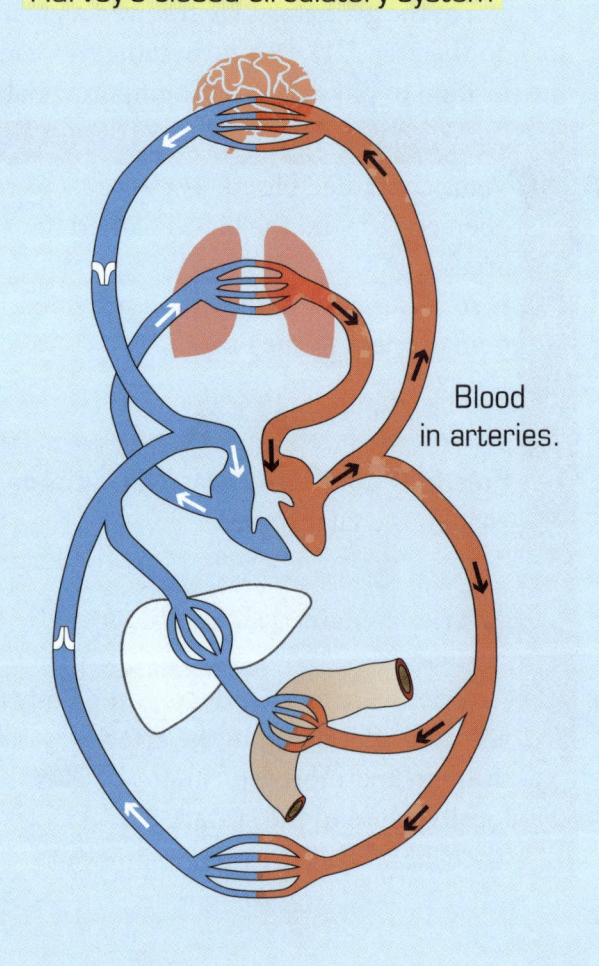

Blood in arteries.

God's Wondrous Machine

we got the beat

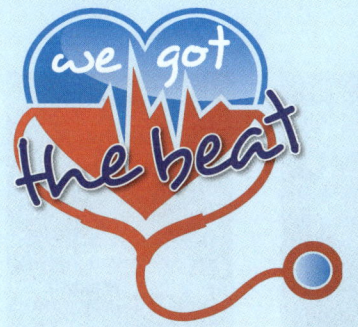

This symbol for the barber's pole began during the Dark Ages; the red represented the bloody bandages wrapped around a pole. Early versions had a brass wash basin on the top and bottom. The top basin was a representation of where the leeches were kept. The bottom one was the symbol for the basin used to collect the blood. The staff was the item that a patient would grasp to encourage the flow of blood after a bloodletting procedure.

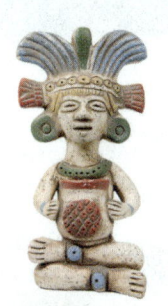

2000 B.C. to A.D. 1500

Mayan kings and queens who ruled in Central America would open their own veins so that their blood could be used in ceremonies.

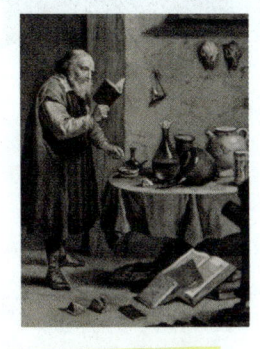

460-370 B.C.

Ancient Greek doctor Hippocrates (460–370 B.C.), was considered the father of medicine. He is credited with the idea of the four humors.

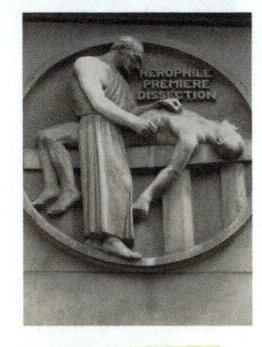

335 B.C.

Herophilus (335–280 B.C.), a Greek doctor, was considered to be the father of anatomy.

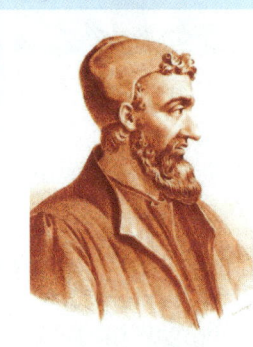

129-200

Claudius Galen of Pergamon (129–200) operated on gladiators. He greatly influenced the understanding of medicine and anatomy in the middle ages based on Hippocrates theory of the four humors.

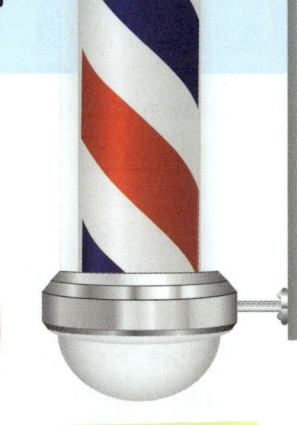

410-1095

In medieval times, barbers were also surgeons. Doctors of the time considered surgery messy and beneath them. Barbers were good with a sharp blade, not only could they cut hair, but they would practice procedures from bloodletting to amputation of limbs. The barber pole was originally red and white striped.

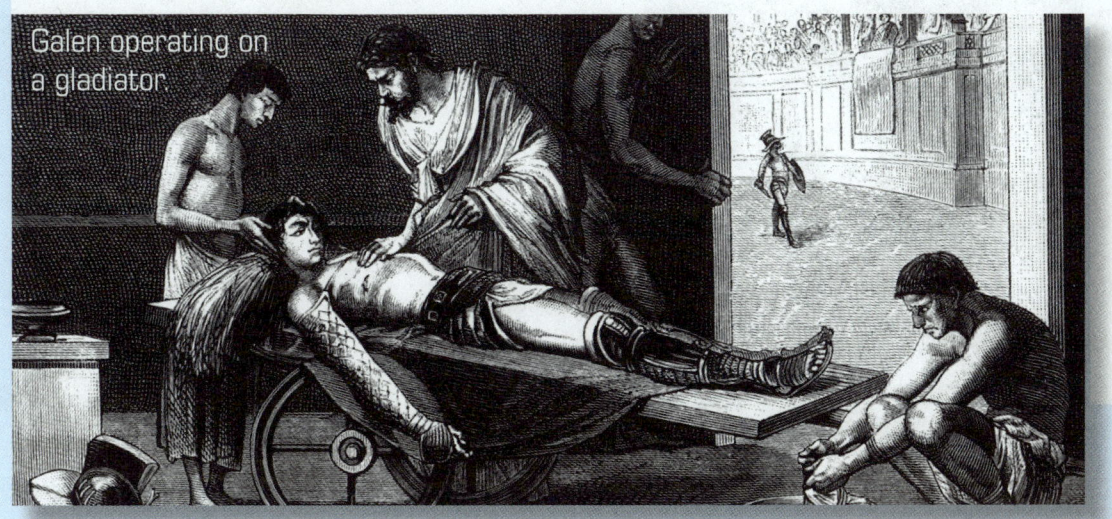

Galen operating on a gladiator

Unit 3: The Complex Circulatory System

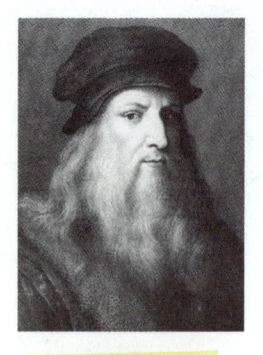

1500

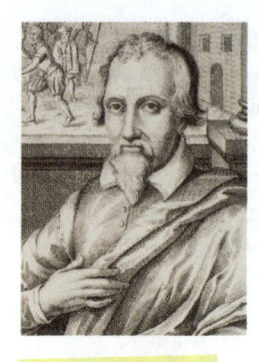

Leonardo Da Vinci (1452–1519) noted tiny "hairs" in tissues. He was interested in the link between form and action of the body. He made the first accurate drawing of the body as well as the heart and its valves.

1553

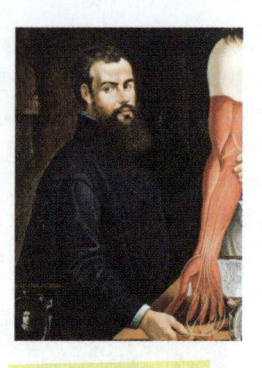

Michael Servetus (1511?–1553) was a theologian and physician who was burned at the stake. He was considered a heretic for his description of the circulation of the blood through the lungs.

1543

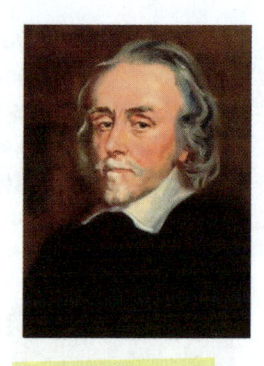

Andreas Vesalius (1514–1564) wrote one of the first books on the human anatomy entitled *De Humani Corporis Fabrica (On the Fabric of the Human Body)*.

1578

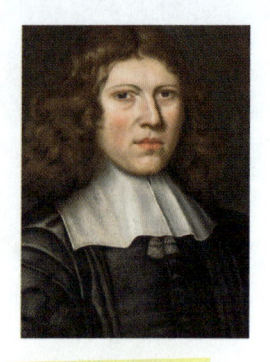

William Harvey (1578–1657), an English physician, was the first to describe blood circulation in the body. He stated that blood flowed in a closed circuit — it was conserved, which means that the blood was not consumed by the organs. His discovery caused him much concern because it went against centuries of medical thought. He said, "Not only do I fear danger to myself from malice of a few, but I dread lest I have all men as enemies."

1666

Richard Lower (1631–1691), a physician, followed the works of William Harvey. He pioneered the idea of blood transfusions. He experimented on transfusing dogs. He even transfused a lamb's blood into a human — but such practices were very dangerous so laws in both England and France were created to stop it!

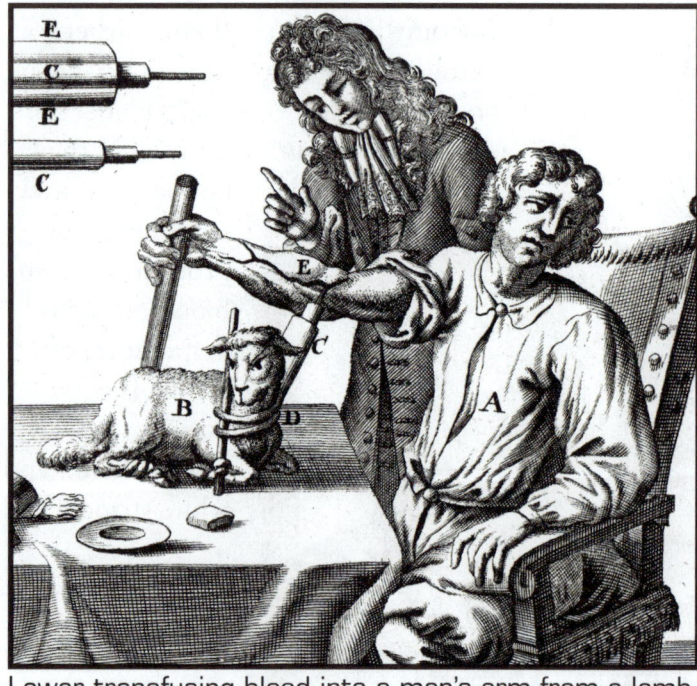

Lower transfusing blood into a man's arm from a lamb.

God's Wondrous Machine

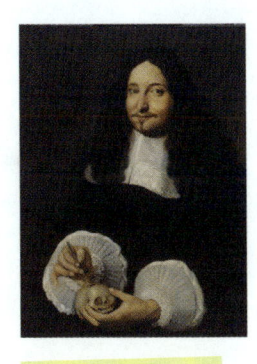

1670

Marcello Malpighi of Bologna (1628–1691), a biologist and physician, utilized a primitive microscope and discovered a network of tiny vessels called capillaries in the lung of a frog. This discovery linked the arteries and veins.

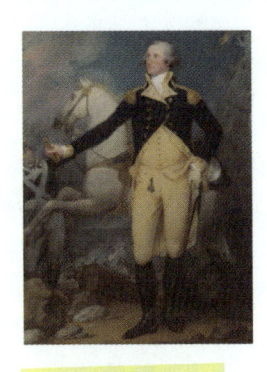

1799

George Washington (1732–1799) died due to bloodletting. After a day of riding his horse out in the cold, he returned to find his throat sore. Soreness and the swelling in his throat advanced. He became short of breath, and a team of doctors were called. They utilized the most "effective" treatment of the times, bloodletting. It is said nearly 40 percent of his blood volume was removed, and he died. Before dying, George Washington thanked the doctors for their excellent care.

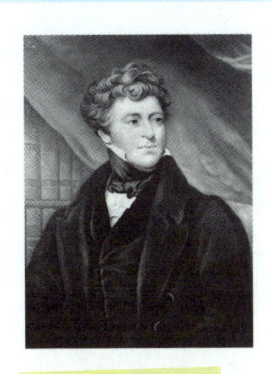

1818

James Blundell (1791–1878) became the first in the United States to perform a successful blood transfusion. The transfusion was performed on a woman who had just delivered a baby. She immediately suffered from severe bleeding. He took 4 ounces from the woman's husband and transfused it into her. Today we know it's not that simple. People have one of four different types of blood, and it can be deadly if you receive the wrong kind during a transfusion.

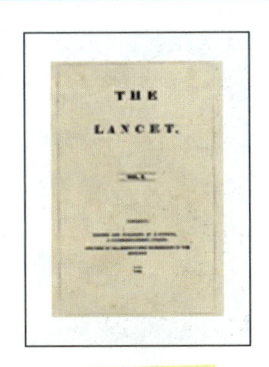

1823

The first medical journal, *The Lancet*, was published. *The Lancet* still exists today. It is one of the leading medical journals. Thomas Wakley (1792–1862) first published it on October 5, 1823. As the journal was going to press he stated, "A lancet can be an arched window to let in the light or it can be a sharp surgical instrument to cut out the dross and I intend to use it in both senses." A lancet was the indispensable tool utilized in bloodletting. It was used to cut the skin and blood vessels.

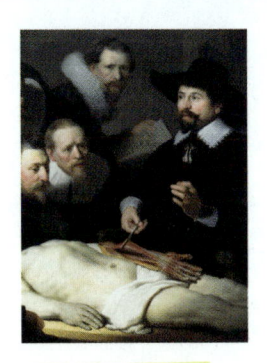

1832

The laws were changed, and medical professionals could legally use donated bodies for study and dissection.

The picture above is Rembrandt van Rijn's *The Anatomy Lesson of Dr. Nicolaes Tulp*, completed in 1632. Dissection was not limited to the eager learning eyes of apprentice doctors of the day; dissections were also held for public "amusement." You could even buy tickets for these events.

157

Unit 3: The Complex Circulatory System

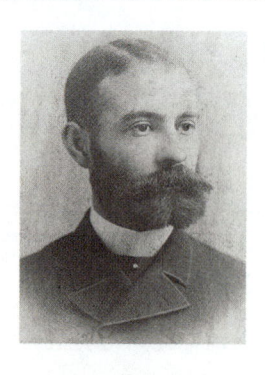

1893

Daniel Hale Williams (1856–1931) was an African American general surgeon who performed the first successful open heart surgery and founded the first non-segregated hospital in the United States. He operated on James Cornish at Provident Hospital in Chicago. Mr. Cornish had been stabbed in the heart. Today's common practice of blood transfusion and the use of blood products was not safely utilized at that time. Even without this life-saving practice, he was able to suture (sew) the covering around Cornish's heart, saving his life.

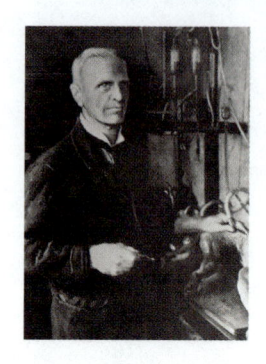

1896

Ernest Henry Starling (1866–1927), an English physiologist (a person who studies the body's processes), was the first to explain the maintenance of a fluid balance in the body. It is called Starling's Law. The law states that the stroke volume (the amount of blood pumped into the left ventricle per a heartbeat) of the heart will increase with additional blood filling into the ventricle. The more the heart wall stretches due to increased blood flow, the more force the heart muscle will use to contract.

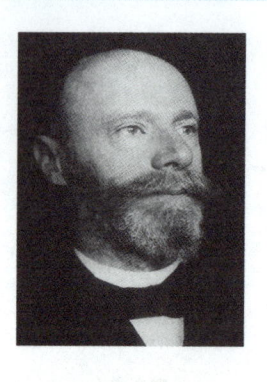

1903

Willem Einthoven (1860–1927) was a Dutch doctor and physiologist who invented the first electrocardiogram (EKG or ECG). It was already understood and accepted in medicine that the heart generated electrical activity. However, prior to Einthoven's invention, the only way to record this activity was placing electrodes directly on the heart muscle. This was impractical. He won the Nobel Prize in Physiology or Medicine in 1924.

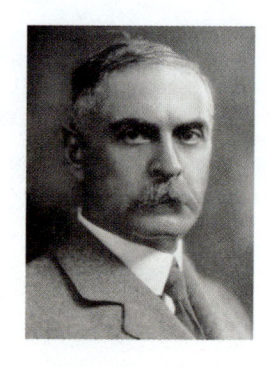

1900's

Karl Landsteiner (1868–1943) an Austrian-born biologist and physician was the first to identify the major blood groups: A, B, AB, and O. He discovered that agglutinins were found on blood red blood cells that caused an immune reaction in which blood clumps when two different types of blood are mixed.

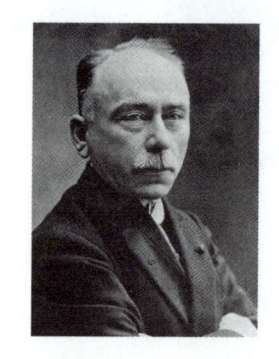

1919

Jules Bordet (1870–1961), physician, was awarded the Nobel Prize in Physiology or Medicine for his discovery of factors in blood that destroy bacteria and how the blood breaks apart (called hemolysis) due to foreign blood cells in the body.

God's Wondrous Machine

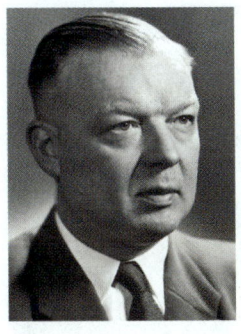

1920s

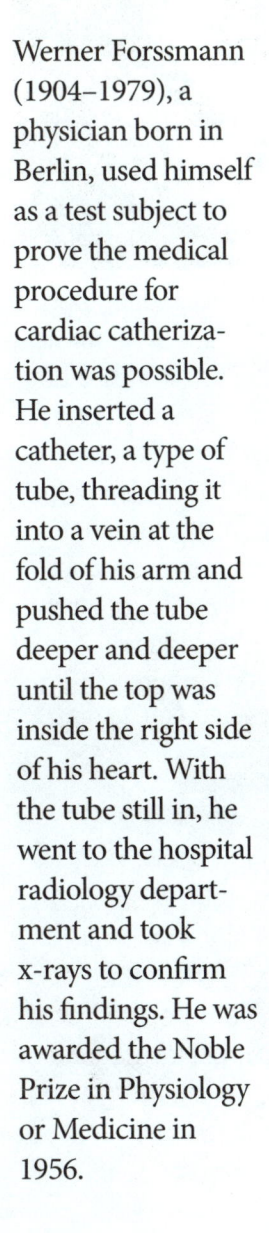

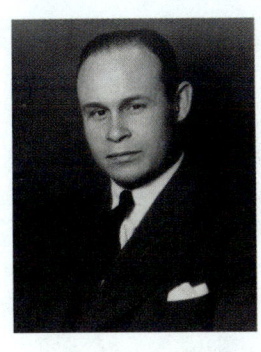

Werner Forssmann (1904–1979), a physician born in Berlin, used himself as a test subject to prove the medical procedure for cardiac catherization was possible. He inserted a catheter, a type of tube, threading it into a vein at the fold of his arm and pushed the tube deeper and deeper until the top was inside the right side of his heart. With the tube still in, he went to the hospital radiology department and took x-rays to confirm his findings. He was awarded the Noble Prize in Physiology or Medicine in 1956.

1930s

Charles Richard Drew (1904–1950), was an African American physician and surgeon who is credited for blood banks. He studied how blood transfusions were given, and invented better techniques for storing blood. During World War II, he utilized this new knowledge to help provide life-saving blood storage to help wounded soldiers in the field.

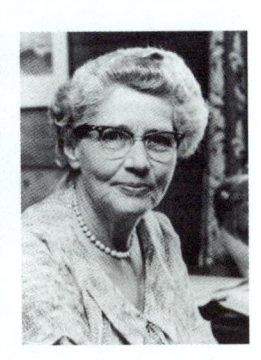

1944

Helen Brooke Taussig (1898–1986), physician, is credited with being the founder of pediatric cardiology. She assisted in the development of the Blalock-Taussig Shunt. This is a surgical procedure that helps children born with heart defects, "blue baby syndrome," that cause them to be blue. She was awarded the Medal of Freedom from President Lyndon Johnson. In 1965, she became the first woman president of the American Heart Association.

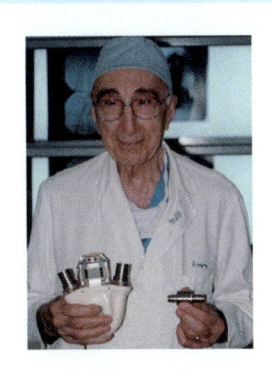

1952

Michael DeBakey (1908–2008) invented a new kind of graft for repairing torn arteries. In 1932, he invented a part for the first heart-lung machines. These machines are utilized for heart surgery. He was the first person to identify the smoking of cigarettes as a connection to lung cancer. In the 1950s, the DeBakey Dacron Graft was used in repairing damaged blood vessels.

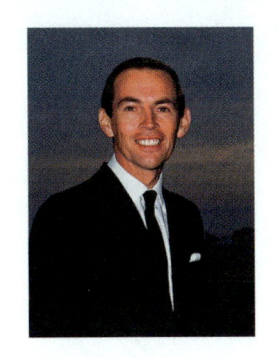

1967

Christiaan N. Barnard (1922–2001), a South African cardiac surgeon, was a pioneer who performed the first successful human heart transplant. Although his patient lived only 21 days after, it was still considered a great success.

Unit 3: The Complex Circulatory System

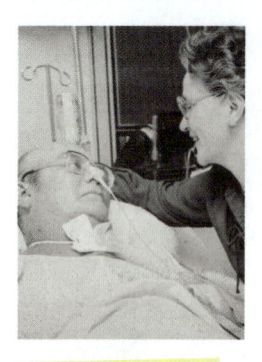

1982

Barney Clark at 61 years of age survived a Jarvik-7 artificial heart for 112 days. Dr. William DeVries (1943–) performed the surgery. Clark knew that his chances for long-term survival were not likely, but he agreed to the heart to help further medicine.

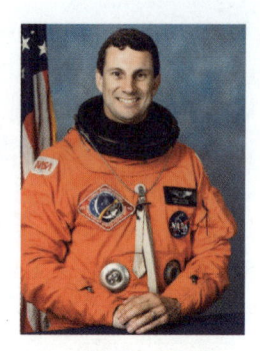

1991

Dr. Drew Gaffney (1946–), physician, flew on NASA's space shuttle as a "payload specialist." A payload specialist is someone who rides as an expert in a particular field. While on board, he studied how the heart and the circulatory system adapted to flight in space. This was the first mission to explore the human body in space. A catheter, a long tube, was inserted into his elbow prior to lift off and threaded to his heart. This allowed close measurement of his heart functions.

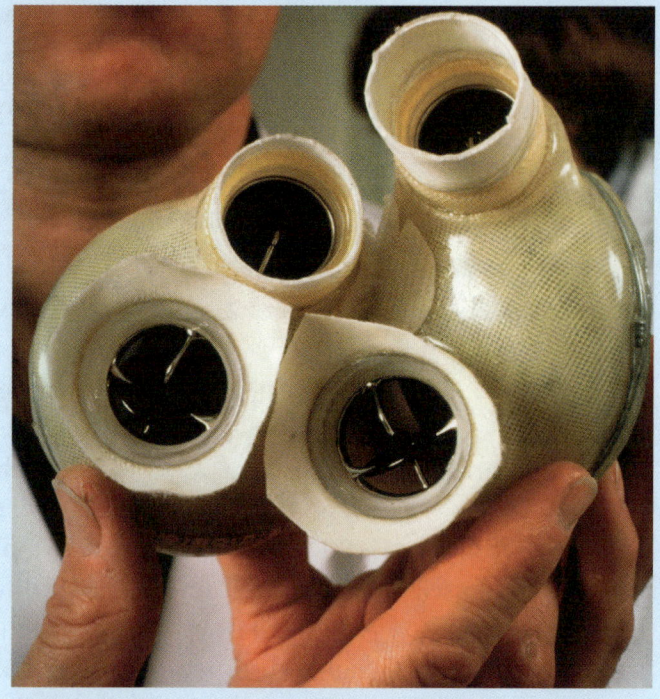

A number of artificial hearts were proposed and experimented with since the first one by Vladimir Demikhov in 1937, who transplanted it into a dog. There were limited successes in tests with animals, but this helped to advance understanding of the challenges. Here you can see the major blood vessels on the Jarvik-7, an aluminum and plastic artificial heart used during the first successful human implant in 1982 at the University of Utah Medical Centre in Salt Lake City. The Jarvik-7 heart relied on external power for compressed air and electricity. The patient had a six-foot lifeline to the support equipment.

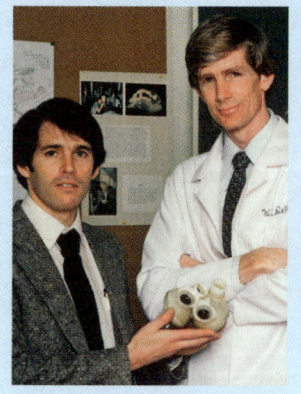

Dr. Robert Jarvik, developer of the Jarvik-7 artificial heart, and Dr. William DeVries who, with Dr. Tom Kessler (not pictured), performed the first successful permanent artificial heart surgery.

God's Wondrous Machine

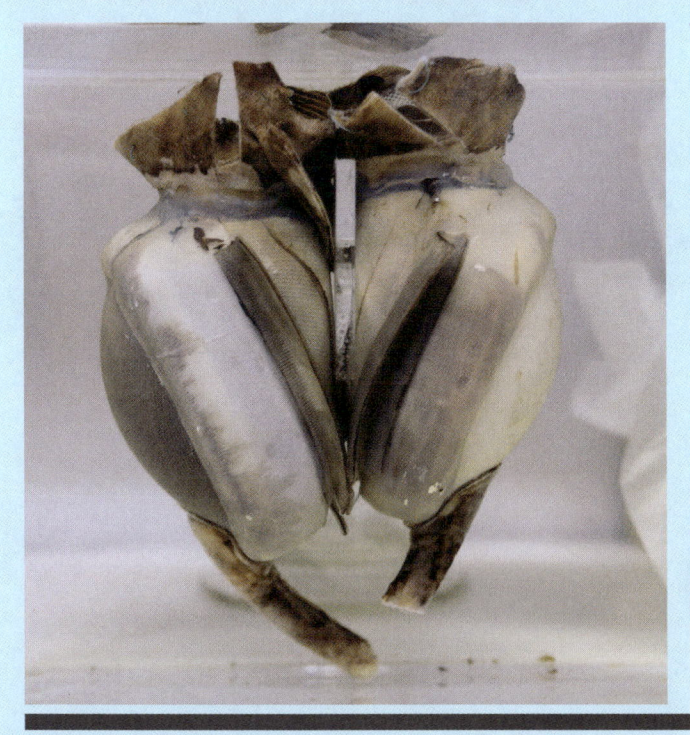

The first total artificial heart implanted in a human body was developed by Domingo Liotta and placed by surgeon Dr. Denton Cooley in 1969 at St. Luke's Episcopal Hospital in Houston. (Dr. Liotta joined the staff at the hospital in Texas in 1961 as the director of the Artificial Heart Program. He was hired by Dr. Michael DeBakey.) The patient lived for sixty-four hours with the artificial heart pumping oxygenated blood through his body until a human heart could be available for transplant. The patient died soon after receiving a real heart, and there was criticism about the use of the Liotta-Cooley plastic heart. However, it did show how artificial hearts could be used until real hearts were donated.

Word Wise!

The HIPPOCRATIC OATH, named after Hippocrates, is an oath that doctors are required to swear upon upholding professional standards in practicing medicine and the care of the patients.

Our knowledge of medicine continues to march on.

Today, we are looking at new ways to diagnose heart disease much earlier. An item with great promise is the Computed Tomography Angiography or CTA. It helps to find small blocks in the arteries that surround the heart. A dye is injected in a vessel in a patient's arm. A special x-ray machine called a CT scanner takes images of the heart and the dye flowing through the blood vessels. It can show where blockage exists in the vessels.

A new artificial blood is being tested in the United Kingdom. If successful, it could provide an answer to blood shortages. Perhaps it can be used in patients who refuse blood transfusion on the grounds of religious objection.

Maybe God has a plan for you to make contributions to the field of cardiology. He has given you unlimited potential. Walk boldly. Keep your eyes on Him. Look for ways to magnify His wonder.

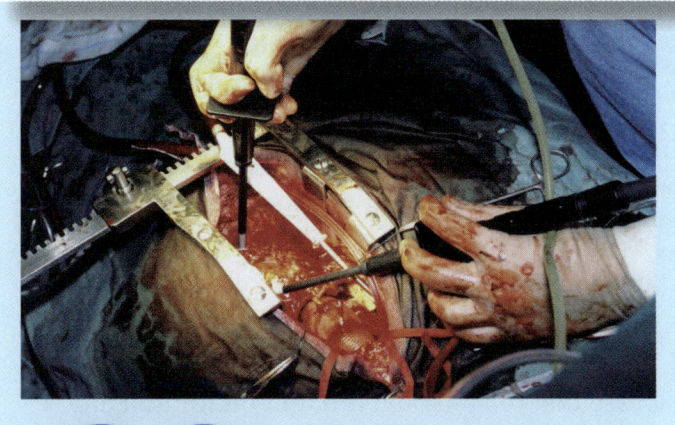

we got the beat

Racial segregation existed in the United States and even existed in the donation of blood. Charles Richard Drew resigned from his position with the American Red Cross over this issue. The American Red Cross did not change its position on this policy of segregation until 1950.

Unit 3: The Complex Circulatory System

2 Blood

Blood brothers, bad blood, blood oath, cold-blooded, blood-thirsty, blood bath and blood ties are just a few idioms that you may have encountered in reference to blood. An idiom is an expression that has a meaning that is not obvious from the traditional definition of the words used. Blood can have many colorful meanings.

In the Bible, three of the biggest themes central to blood are references to life, sacrifice, and salvation. In the Old Testament, animal sacrifice was a common practice. The best of the best animals were selected for the offering to God. The animals provided a way to atone, or make right, wrongdoings. In Exodus 12, blood from an unblemished lamb was placed on the top and the two sides of the door frame to protect the firstborn of the Israelites during the Passover. An angel passed through the lands of Egypt destroying the firstborn. Those that had marked their door frames with blood were protected. It was a curse that the pharaoh brought on himself and his land when he refused to release the Israelites from slavery.

The ultimate sacrifice was the blood Jesus shed for us on the Cross. During the Last Supper with His disciples in Mark 14:23–24 it states:

Then he took a cup, and when he had given thanks, he gave it to them, and they all drank from it. "This is my blood of the covenant, which is poured out for many," he said to them.

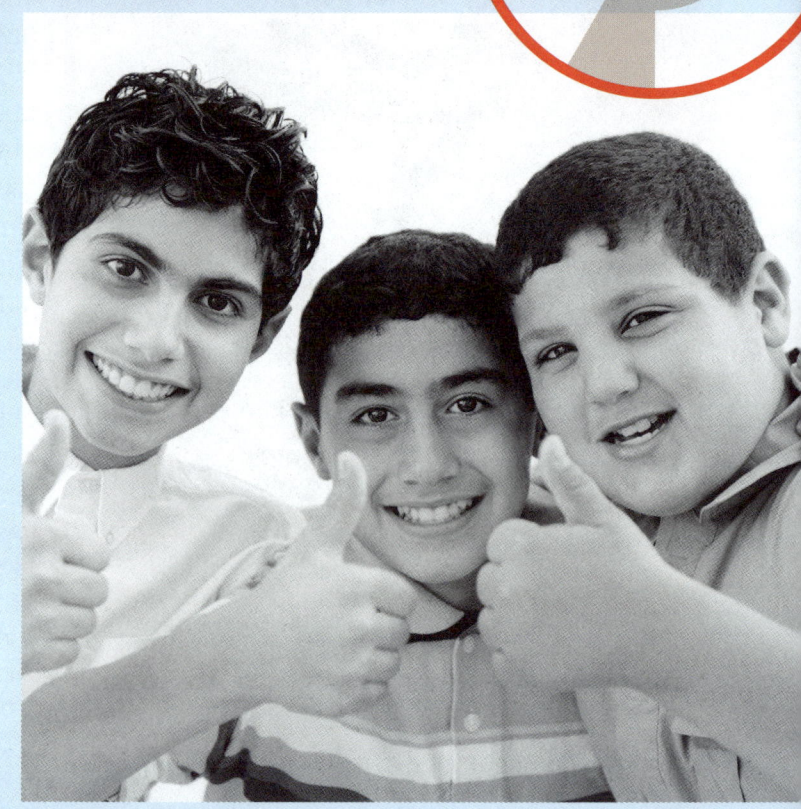

Functions of Blood

Blood is important. It has great significance in keeping us alive, not only spiritually but also physically. There is an average of 4–5 liters of blood in an adult. That is the total of 2 to 2½ two-liter bottles of soda pop.

Word Wise!
BLOOD is the liquid that flows through arteries and veins within the body. The word is related to blut in German, *blōd* in Old English, and *bloed* in Dutch.

God's Wondrous Machine

What is the function of blood? Of course, we all know it is better for it to be in our body instead of flowing out of our body. Let's dig a bit deeper. Following are the functions of blood:

1.	Blood acts as a delivery man.	As the blood flows through the miles and miles of highways of blood vessels, it delivers gases like oxygen, nutrients, and hormones. These items are essential for our cells to work efficiently.
2.	Blood acts as a garbage man.	As the cells complete their multitude of biological activities, waste products are generated. The waste is transported out of the cells and thrown into the blood stream where it can be transported for disposal by our kidneys.
3.	Blood helps control the heat in our bodies.	When you go out for a run, your body heats up. You may notice that your skin may become red, sweaty, and flushed. The blood vessels under your skin dilate (become larger) to allow the heat to be more effectively released from your body. This helps you to cool off.
4.	Blood controls the pH balance in your body	pH is a number scale that rates the level of acid vs. base in a substance. Scratching your head, still not clear? Okay, let's look at it another way. Your body likes a pH of 7. This is considered in the middle of the road on the pH scale. (The scale has a range from 0-14.) If the value is higher than 7, the solution is considered in the basic range. The higher you go the more "basic" it is. Milk of Magnesia® has a basic pH and is a medicine that can help settle an upset stomach. Less than 7 is considered to be acidic. The lower the number, the more acidic it is. Lemon juice has a pH of 3. This gives it its sour taste. Your blood helps to keep the pH in a tight range because your body works best at a neutral level of 7.
5.	Blood is comprised of elements that protect us against blood loss.	There is a special chain of events that happens in the blood that helps you to form clots. This keeps us from bleeding excessively. We will look deeper into this shortly.
6.	Blood protects us from foreign invaders like bacteria and diseases.	There are special cells in the blood to help us fight infection.

It is interesting to note that if you ever were to have the unfortunate accident of knocking out a permanent tooth, it is recommended that the tooth be put in milk when you are in transport to the dentist. Milk is a substance that has a neutral pH of 7, just like your body.

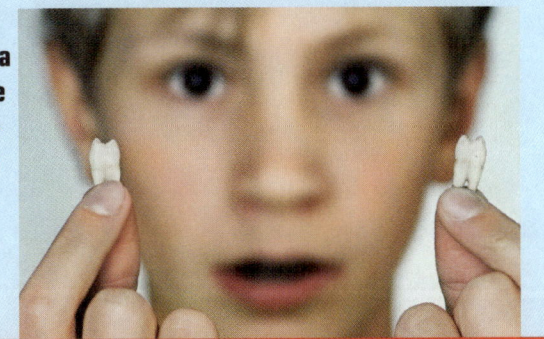

Unit 3: The Complex Circulatory System

The Parts of Blood

Blood serves many functions. This versatile liquid has many components. These components assist in helping blood perform its many jobs. You may have had an experience in which you went to a lab or the hospital where they took a sample of your blood for testing. A small needle was inserted just under your skin into a vein. Your blood would have been collected in a clear tube. Once the blood was collected, it is placed in a machine called a centrifuge. The machine spins the blood around and around. This allows the components of the blood to separate from each other. Each component can be easily sampled and tested once separated.

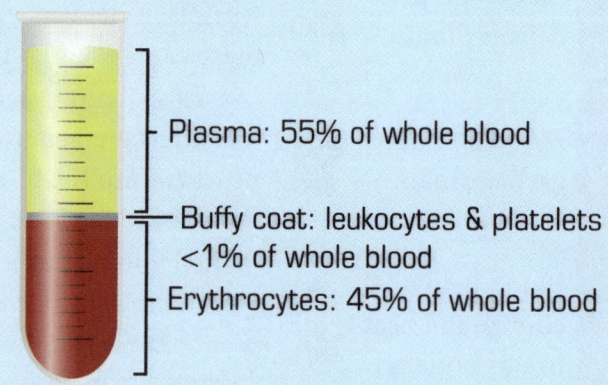

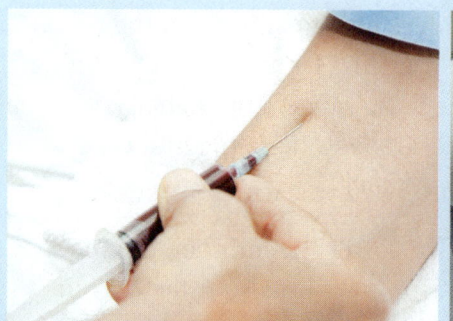

- Plasma: 55% of whole blood
- Buffy coat: leukocytes & platelets <1% of whole blood
- Erythrocytes: 45% of whole blood

Withdraw blood and place in tube

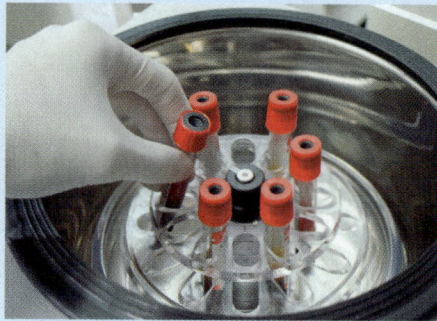

Place tube in Centrifuge Machine

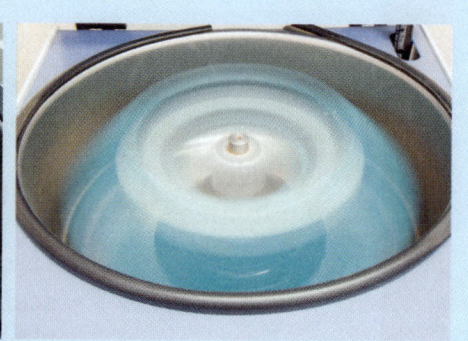

The machine spins the blood around to separate

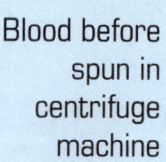

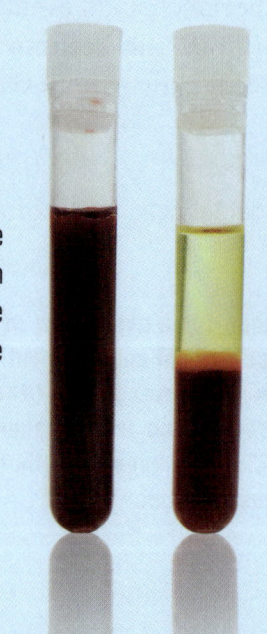

Blood before spun in centrifuge machine

After separation, each component of the blood can be easily seen and tested.

God's Wondrous Machine

Plasma

Three visual layers are seen after the blood is spun in the centrifuge. The top layer is a yellow straw-like color called plasma. Over half of your blood, 55 percent to be exact, is composed of plasma. Have you ever skinned your knee? After the bleeding stops, you may have noticed a clear to yellow watery substance oozing from your scraped knee. That is plasma!

Plasma is predominantly water. Dissolved in this watery substance are electrolytes like sodium, potassium, calcium, and others. Plasma also contains vital proteins like albumin (helps maintain a type of fluid pressure inside the vessels), fibrinogen (helps in clot formation) and globulins (there are many different types to help in processes like immunity). Plasma contains dissolved nutrients like sugar and vitamins as well as gases like oxygen and carbon dioxide.

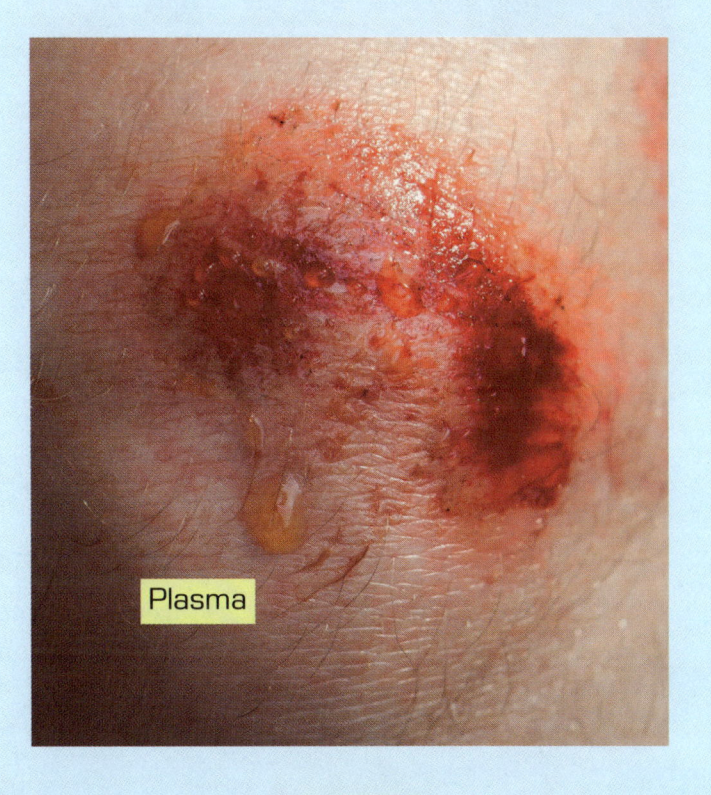

Plasma

Buffy Coat

Under the plasma level, you will find the buffy coat. When most grown-ups think of "buffy" coat they may think of the nice shiny, waxy coat given to their car to restore its luster. The buffy coat is only 1 percent of your blood. It contains your white blood cells (WBC) and platelets. The white blood cells are important in your immunity. They help you to fight illness and disease by producing antibodies, special biological heat-seeking missiles that are launched to attack unwelcome guests in your body.

Platelets contribute to the process of hemostasis. Whew, now there is a word. Scientific jargon comes much easier when you know some of the roots of words. Hemo means blood. Stasis means "to stand still" or stop. So when you put these two roots together, hemostasis is the process in which the body stops bleeding.

MED+MOMENT

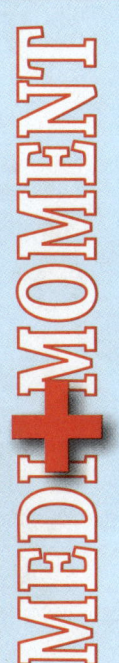

Centrifuges came from an 1850 invention of a practical machine developed by Antonin Prandtl to separate cream from cows' milk. In 1869, scientist Friedrich Miescher used this device in a lab. Other scientists quickly saw the potential and began using it as well. Within 10 years of Miescher using the machine, a commercial centrifuge was developed by Gustaf de Laval.

Unit 3: The Complex Circulatory System

Preparation of a Blood Smear for Examination

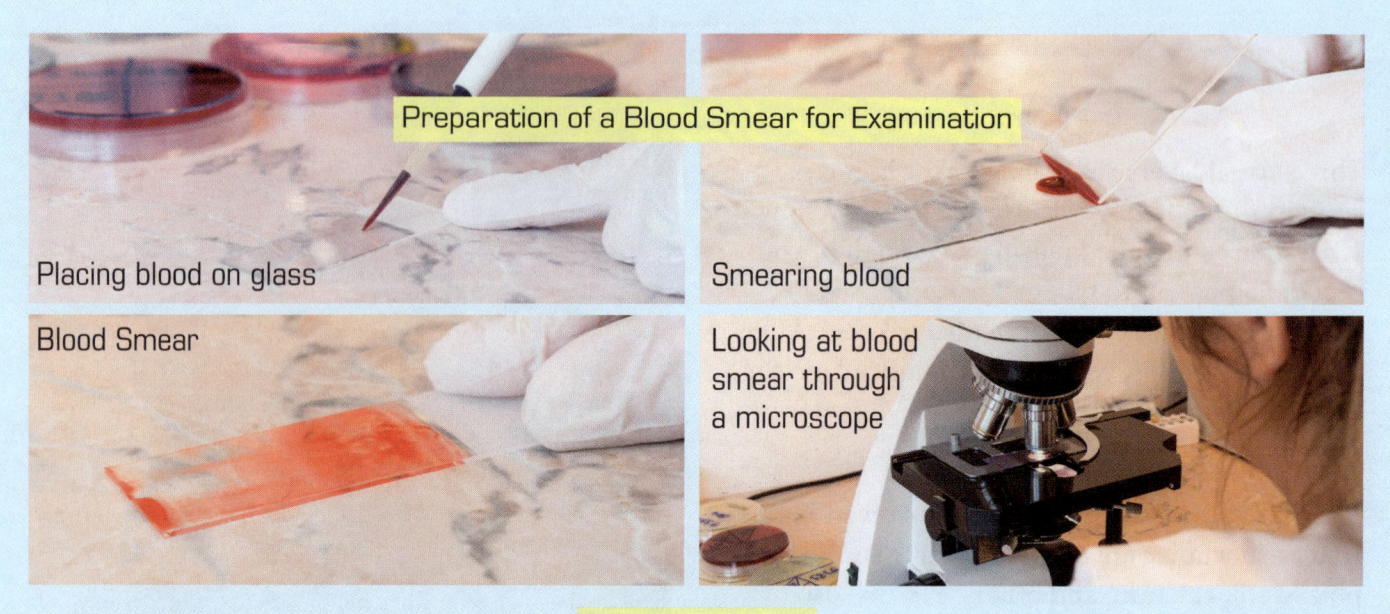

Placing blood on glass

Smearing blood

Blood Smear

Looking at blood smear through a microscope

The Bottom Layer

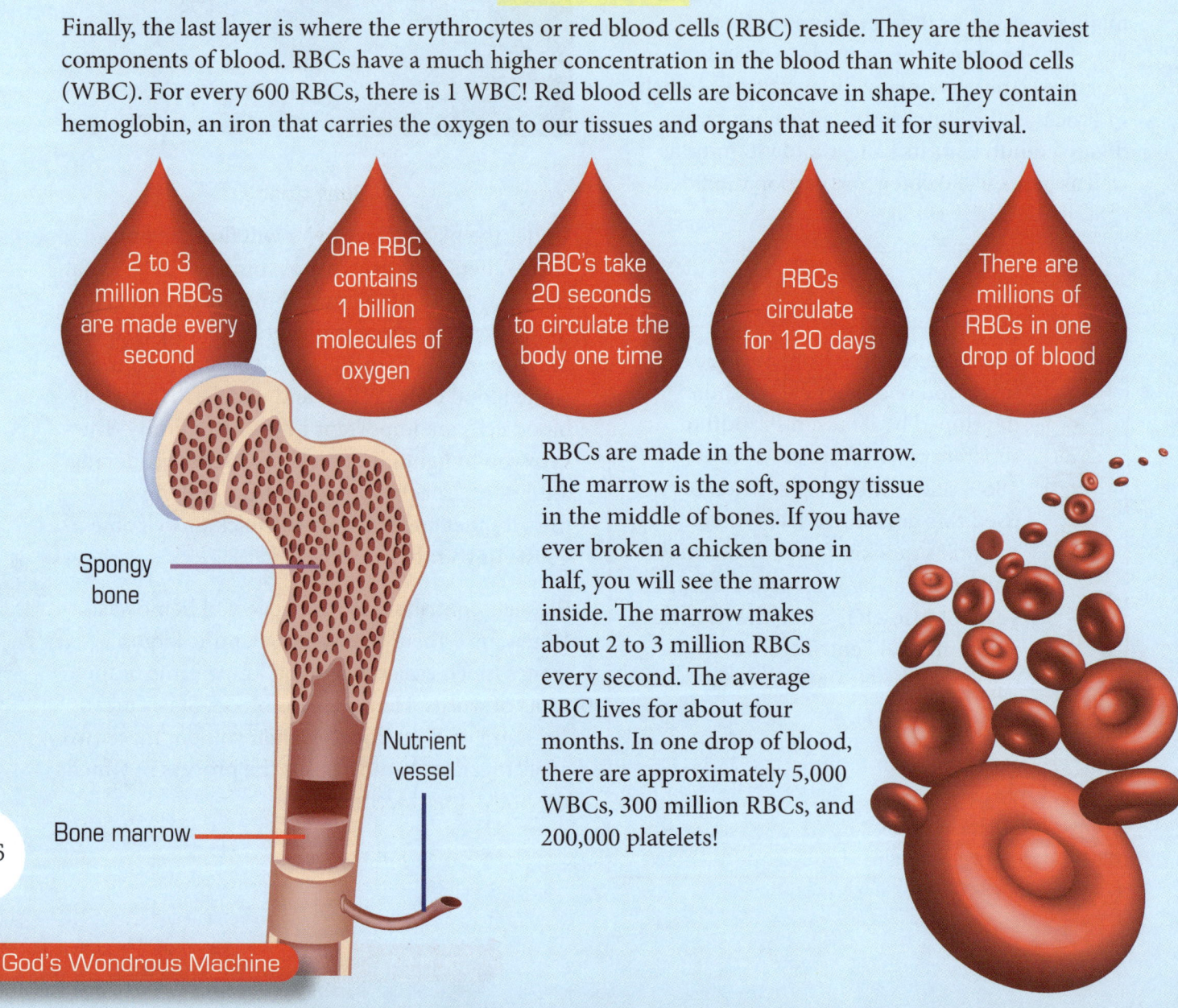

Finally, the last layer is where the erythrocytes or red blood cells (RBC) reside. They are the heaviest components of blood. RBCs have a much higher concentration in the blood than white blood cells (WBC). For every 600 RBCs, there is 1 WBC! Red blood cells are biconcave in shape. They contain hemoglobin, an iron that carries the oxygen to our tissues and organs that need it for survival.

- 2 to 3 million RBCs are made every second
- One RBC contains 1 billion molecules of oxygen
- RBC's take 20 seconds to circulate the body one time
- RBCs circulate for 120 days
- There are millions of RBCs in one drop of blood

Spongy bone

Nutrient vessel

Bone marrow

RBCs are made in the bone marrow. The marrow is the soft, spongy tissue in the middle of bones. If you have ever broken a chicken bone in half, you will see the marrow inside. The marrow makes about 2 to 3 million RBCs every second. The average RBC lives for about four months. In one drop of blood, there are approximately 5,000 WBCs, 300 million RBCs, and 200,000 platelets!

God's Wondrous Machine

Seeing Red

What is the color of your blood? That's an obvious question, right? Not so fast. There are many misconceptions that seem to continue to "circulate" in regard to this question. Most people, kids and adults alike, will say it is blue when it does not have much oxygen and when it hits the air or is rich with oxygen the color is red. Sound familiar? Many people believe this. After all, when you look at most books on the body, deoxygenated blood (blood with lower content of oxygen) in the illustrations is depicted blue. Blood rich in oxygen is depicted red. This is for illustration purposes only. Okay, how about this . . . if your skin is fair in color, why do the veins appear blue? All great observations! The actual lining of the blood vessels filters out certain light waves, and the color appears blue. Deoxygenated blood is actually a dark maroon color. It is never blue. The substance hemoglobin is an iron contained in RBCs that carries oxygen and gives our blood the familiar color red. Depending on the region of the country you live, you may be familiar to this process of oxygen reacting with a metal. The iron in a car can combine with oxygen in the air and form iron oxide. This causes the car to rust in areas. The mixture of iron and oxygen causes this familiar red color.

Hematopoiesis

Now that we have established the "recipe" for blood, how does our body "cook" up this wonderful thick substance? The process of making blood in our body is called hematopoiesis. Let's break that word down. Hemato comes from the Greek language meaning "blood." Poiesis has its origin in the Greek which means "the act of making or producing" something. Hematopoiesis is the formation of blood. When you were growing in your mother's womb, your blood was made in your spleen and liver. By the time you were born, your bone marrow in your long bones, such as your femur and tibia, had taken over the job of blood manufacturing. Blood cells are formed in the bones of the pelvis, skull, vertebrae (bones of the spine), and sternum (the breast bone) in adults.

we got the beat

Not all animals have red blood. There are creatures that do have blue blood. Can you think of any? Here is a hint. Animals that have blue blood have copper instead of iron in their blood.

The animals that have blue blood are horseshoe crabs, mollusks (snails, octopus, and squid), crustaceans (crabs, shrimp, and crayfish) and arachnids (spiders, scorpions, and tarantulas).

Hematopoiesis blood cells are formed:
- Pelvis and Vertebra
- Sternum
- Ribs
- Lymph nodes
- Femur

Unit 3: The Complex Circulatory System

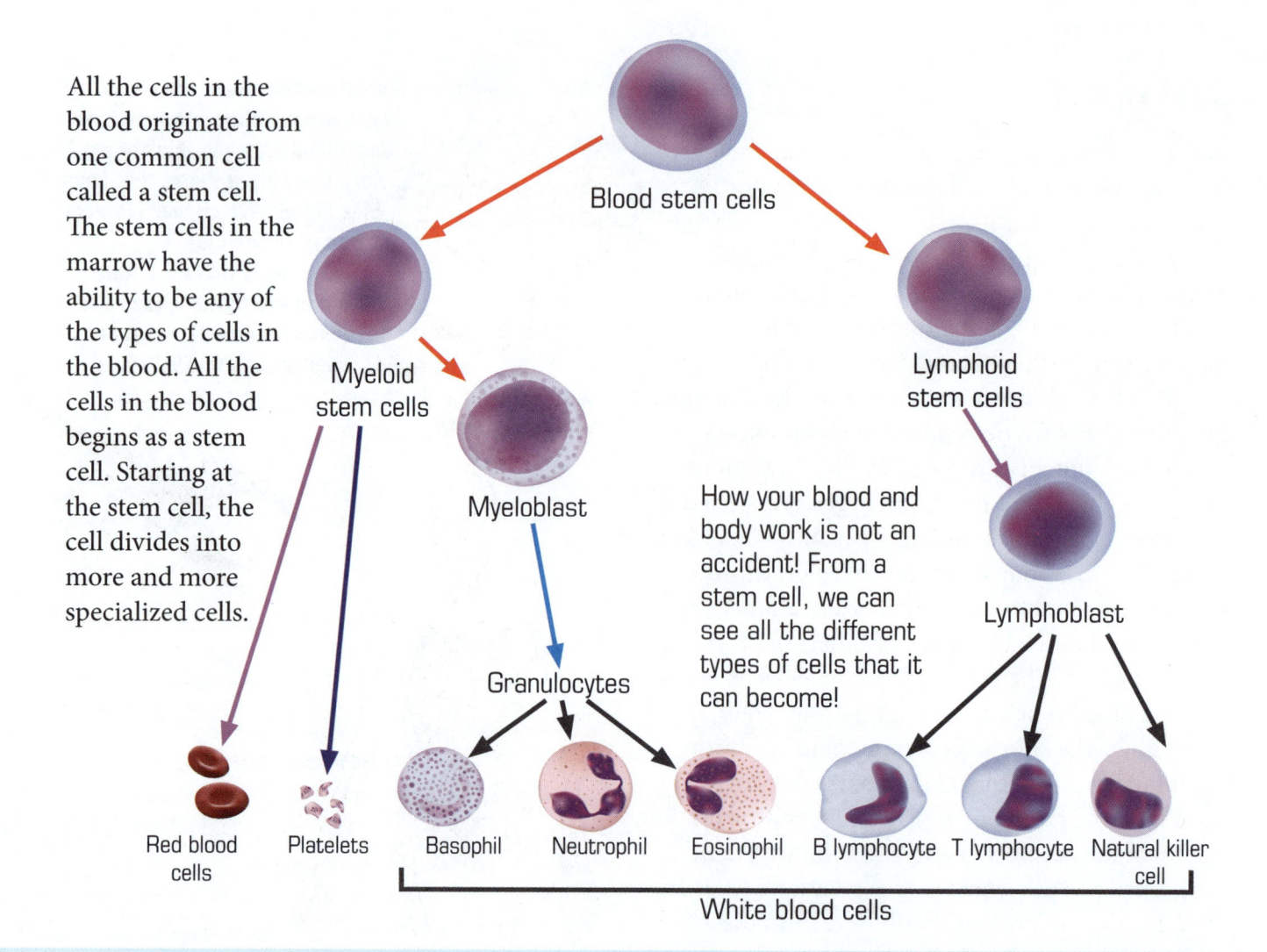

All the cells in the blood originate from one common cell called a stem cell. The stem cells in the marrow have the ability to be any of the types of cells in the blood. All the cells in the blood begins as a stem cell. Starting at the stem cell, the cell divides into more and more specialized cells.

Blood stem cells

Myeloid stem cells

Myeloblast

Lymphoid stem cells

How your blood and body work is not an accident! From a stem cell, we can see all the different types of cells that it can become!

Lymphoblast

Granulocytes

Red blood cells | Platelets | Basophil | Neutrophil | Eosinophil | B lymphocyte | T lymphocyte | Natural killer cell

White blood cells

Bad Blood

One of the most common blood problems is anemia. Anemia occurs when you do not have enough red blood cells or the cells do not function properly. If you remember, red blood cells contain hemoglobin. This hemoglobin is important for the transport of oxygen throughout the body. People who suffer from anemia may experience tiredness, shortness of breath, dizziness, and pale skin. Anemia can be caused by things such as poor diet, intestine problems, and many diseases.

There are many types of anemia. Sickle cell anemia is one type of anemia. You cannot "catch" sickle cell anemia like a cold. It is a genetic disease that runs in families. Normally, a red blood cell has a nice flexible, smooth, and round contour. This allows the cells to glide through our vessels. In a person who suffers from sickle cell anemia, the red blood cell is rigid and sticky, and shaped like crescent moons. During a sickle cell crisis, a person will experience extreme pain. The sickled cells clump together. The cells will stick to the very walls of the blood vessels. These clumped cells block blood flow and cause damage to their organs like the brain, heart, bones, kidneys, and spleen to name a few.

Sickle cell is a disease that can be passed on in families whose origins began in Africa, India, and the Middle East. Interestingly, the disease is found more often on the continents where

Normal red blood cells

normal hemoglobin

sickle cells blocking blood flow

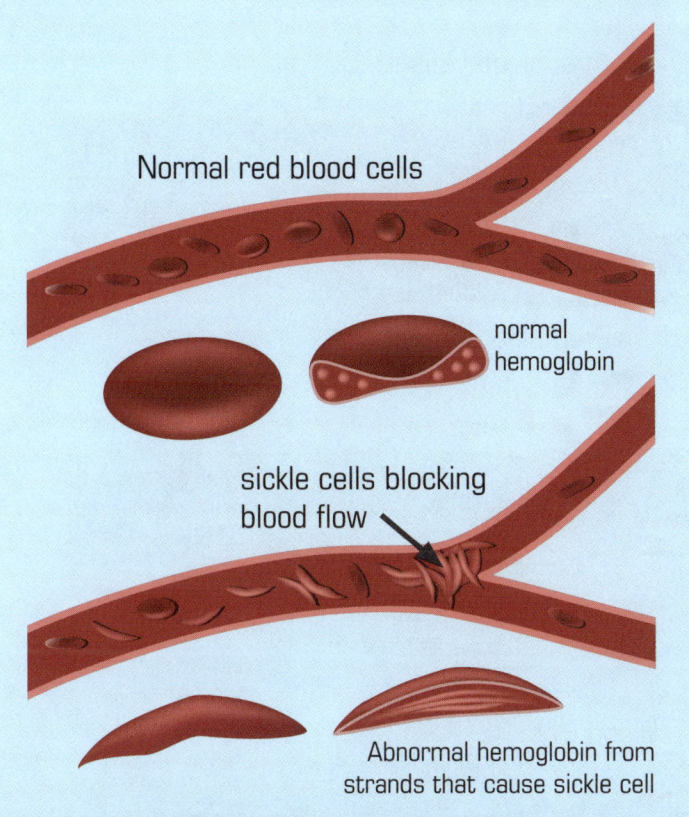

Abnormal hemoglobin from strands that cause sickle cell

Abnormal, sickled, red blood cells (sickle cells)

the disease malaria is found. Malaria is a deadly disease transmitted by mosquitos. The malaria parasite, a small microscopic organism, is transmitted by mosquitos when they bite. Normally, this transmitted parasite will take residence in red blood cells. This parasite does not like sickle cells. In areas of the world where malaria is a problem, people born with sickle-cell anemia have an advantage in surviving malaria outbreaks. Two famous people who had or do have sickle cell anemia are Tiki Barber (a former NFL running back who played for the New York Giants) and Miles Davis (legendary jazz musician).

Put a Plug in It

Our blood tends to flow freely. When you skin your knee, this precious fluid leaks out. Have you ever stopped to wonder how your body stops the bleeding? This process is called hemostasis. It is the way the body stops you from bleeding. Let's take a look at this from the inside. Pretend you are a platelet floating along in the blood stream. Suddenly, as you approach the area of the knee, a small opening occurs in the blood vessels closest to the skin. The ragged edges expose collagen fibers that are connective tissue, usually confined within the vessel walls.

1. Spasms and Narrows: This damaged tissue of the blood vessel alerts the body to spring into action. Instantly, the blood vessel you are traveling in becomes narrowed. This is called vascular spasm. The body's response to narrowing the vessels in that area decreases the blood flowing out.

2. Plug the Hole: You move closer to the opening. Once you arrive at the opening, you stick to the edges of the open wound. Other friendly platelets join in, and you all stick together to plug up the opening. You all are held together by fibrin strands. You stick to the wound edges and wait for reinforcements. You release a protein called tissue factor (thromboplastin). Tissue factor is your mayday, a call for help to enlist help from prothrombin. The last stage occurs when the blood begins to clot.

3. Clotting Cascade: Prothrombin springs into action. Prothrombin is a special protein that is made in the liver. It circulates in the blood. It is not active but is ready to go to work when it is called into action by tissue factor. Prothrombin is activated and becomes thrombin. Red blood cells and white blood cells join the party. They stick close by you and your platelet friends. A cascade of events is triggered at this time. A cascade is like a stream or sequence of events occurring one after the other. Many other supporting factors spring into action in this miraculous cascade.

Unit 3: The Complex Circulatory System

The blood in the area becomes gel-like, and a clot is formed. The hole is plugged up. Healing begins. The clot hardens and becomes a scab. New cells begin to grow and repair the wound area. Last, once the healing is complete, an enzyme is released to dissolve the clot.

Presto! The scab falls off, and you are healed! This is why you should not pick a scab. The scab is aiding in the healing process. The wound is not healed yet. If you pick the scab, you will begin to bleed a bit again.

In summary, the process of hemostasis occurs in three stages. First, the vessel spasms and narrows to slow down bleeding. Second, the platelets form a plug. Third, the blood-clotting cascade occurs. Crazy, right? The complexity of your body is amazing… even at levels you cannot see. The blood-clotting process truly demonstrates the genius of our great God.

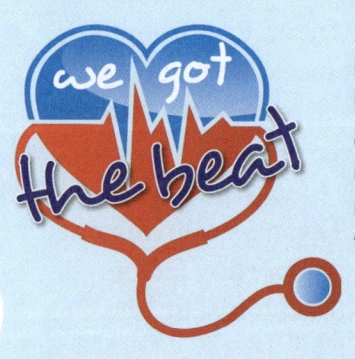

How your blood and body work is not an accident! From a stem cell, we can see all the different types of cells that it can become!

Hemophilia: The Royal Disease

Sometimes things can go wrong in the body. The clotting system can be overactive and form clots blocking blood flow to areas of the body. Sometimes the clotting system doesn't clot when an injury occurs in the case of a rare genetic condition called hemophilia. It is a disease that runs in families and is not contagious. People who suffer from hemophilia are lacking one of the items in the blood-clotting cascade that makes them unable to form a clot. Hemophilia has no cure. We do have ways to help a hemophilic in the face of an emergency. The item or factor that they are missing can be given to them intravenously (via a vein) and can be life-saving.

God's Wondrous Machine

Prince Leopold

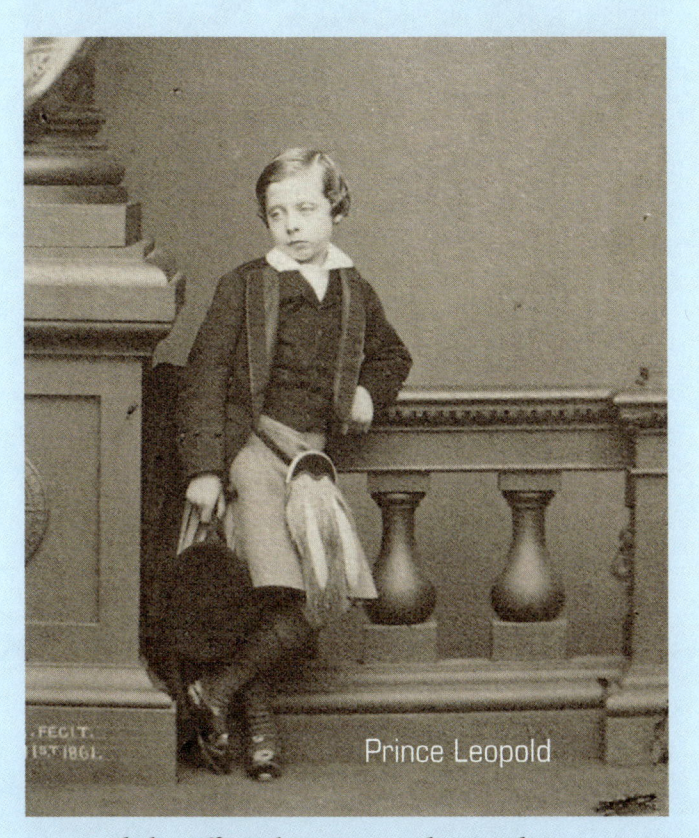

Hemophilia affects boys more than girls. Hemophilia has not always been understood. It has a debilitating history. In 19th-century Europe, during the rule of Great Britain's Queen Victoria (1819–1901), a disease was playing havoc with the royal family. The royal family felt it was important to keep their blood lines "pure." The royal family would marry other family members, like first cousins, so as not to taint the royal line with other blood. Due to this intermarrying of family members, diseases that could be passed on to other family members were more common and severe.

Prince Leopold, the Duke of Albany, was Queen Victoria's eighth child. He was considered to be "very delicate." He suffered many life-threatening bleeding episodes. Because of his fragile nature, he was constantly monitored by the royal staff. Unfortunately, Prince Leopold died when he was 31 years old due to a minor injury.

Darwin's Corner

Creationists and evolutionists are at odds with each other in regard to life's origins. Evolutionists believe that human life evolved from the simplest life forms to the complexity we see in our bodies today. In Genesis 1 it states God created plants and animals to reproduce according to their kinds. A turnip can not produce a grape. A single-celled microscopic organism does not produce a human.

Evolutionists have used the disease sickle cell anemia as one of their defenses for evolution. The illness of malaria is devastating. It kills approximately 2 million people a year. People who suffer from sickle cell anemia are "protected" from the malaria parasite transmitted by mosquitoes. Their blood cells are fragile and "sickle," crushing the parasite. Evolutionists defend that people who have this one amino acid mutation in their hemoglobin that causes the sickling are at an evolutional advantage over others. They cannot contract malaria, and therefore sickle cell is beneficial. I don't believe any of us would request this "minor" substitution in one of our amino acids to give us immunity from malaria. Sickle cell anemia is a extremely painful genetic disorder that causes life long problems. To sum it up, sickle cell anemia is caused due to a mutation that is not favorable for the recipient and not a defense for evolution.

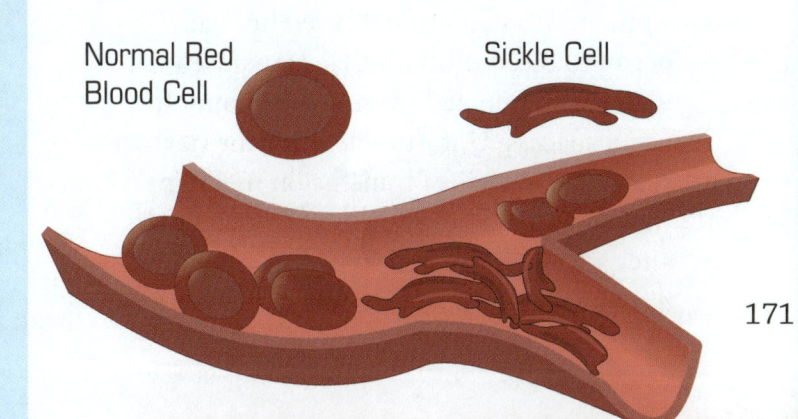

Normal Red Blood Cell   Sickle Cell

Unit 3: The Complex Circulatory System

You're Not My Type

Blood has always had an air of mystery about it. The earliest accounts of blood transfusion met with disastrous results. One of the earliest recorded transfusions was performed by Jean-Baptiste Denis (physician to Louis XIV of France) in 1667. His patient was a man who was considered "mad." The man would wander through the streets of Paris unclothed, was abusive to his wife, and set houses on fire during his fits. Dr. Denis thought if perhaps he transfused blood from a gentle lamb into the man that he would become calm. After a few transfusions, the man became very ill. He no longer had the energy to beat his wife or to set things ablaze. In the minds of everyone, this treatment was successful! After his recovery, the man returned to his old ways. His distressed wife begged Dr. Denis to redo his treatments. Dr. Denis refused. Sadly, the woman, feeling she could take no more, poisoned her husband. Due to this act, blood transfusions were banned in France and Great Britain, and by the pope.

The buzz about the ability to transfuse blood from one person to another began to resurface in the early 1820s. James Blundell, in 1828, is credited for introducing the concept of blood transfusions as a potentially life-saving procedure. He was an obstetrician, a doctor who cares for pregnant women, at Guy's Hospital in London. A woman who had just delivered her baby began to bleed profusely. He transfused her with blood donated from her husband. It was a success. Unfortunately, for the next 70 years, the success of transfusion medicine was unpredictable. Some people survived after a transfusion, but many people would die shortly after a transfusion.

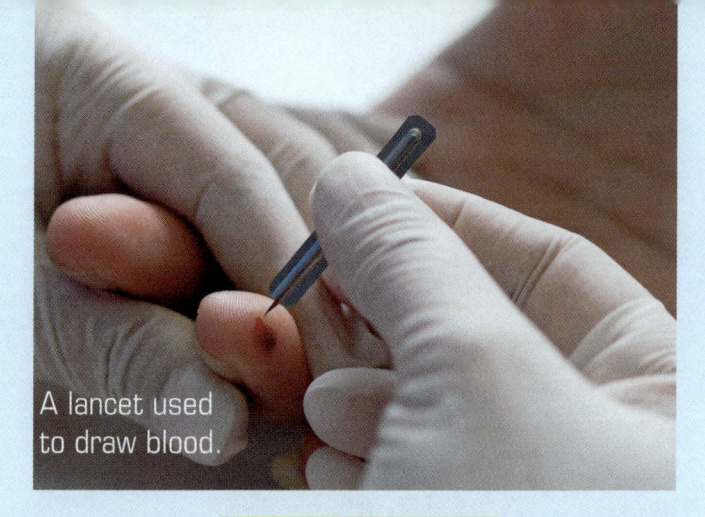

A lancet used to draw blood.

Solving the Mystery

Austrian born Karl Landsteiner was able to put the pieces together for the puzzling problems of blood transfusion. He identified that although blood from all people looked alike, that there were differences in blood types. He identified four major blood types: A, B, AB, and O. The differences lay in the presence or absence in A or B antigens. Antigens are substances found on cells. It can activate the immune system to produce antibodies against foreign invaders. Antibodies are a distress call that signals the body to send white blood cells to defend and protect the body from foreign invasion. When blood from a person is given to a person with a different blood type, then the body's immune system springs to action. The blood will clump and causes a reaction that can be deadly.

Group O can donate red blood cells to anybody. It's the universal donor.

Group A can donate red blood cells to A's and AB's

Group B can donate red blood cells to B's and AB's

Group AB can donate to other AB's, but can receive from all others.

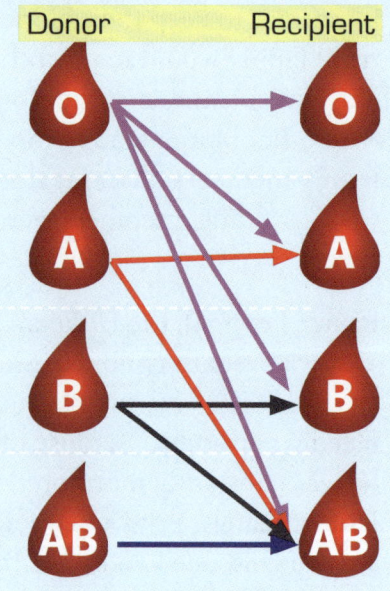

God's Wondrous Machine

People with blood type AB are called "universal" receivers. They can receive blood from any blood type. AB contains both A and B antigens but has no antibodies. A person with blood type O is called a "universal" donor. O contains no antigens but contains both anti-A and anti-B antibodies.

During World War II, plasma, one of the components of blood, was found to be vitally useful in treating wounded soldiers. It was easier to transport. The red blood cells were removed so there was no need to match blood types of the donor with the recipient. Dr. Charles Drew, developed these techniques. He worked with the American Red Cross to establish blood banks, or bloodmobiles, which were trucks serving as donation centers. In addition to the A and B antigens, there is a third antigen called the Rh (Rhesus) factor. When present it is marked with a plus (+), when not present it is negative (−). People with Rh negative blood can only receive blood from other Rh negative donors. People with Rh positive can receive Rh negative or Rh positive blood.

Your blood type was determined and passed onto you based on the genetic makeup of your parents.

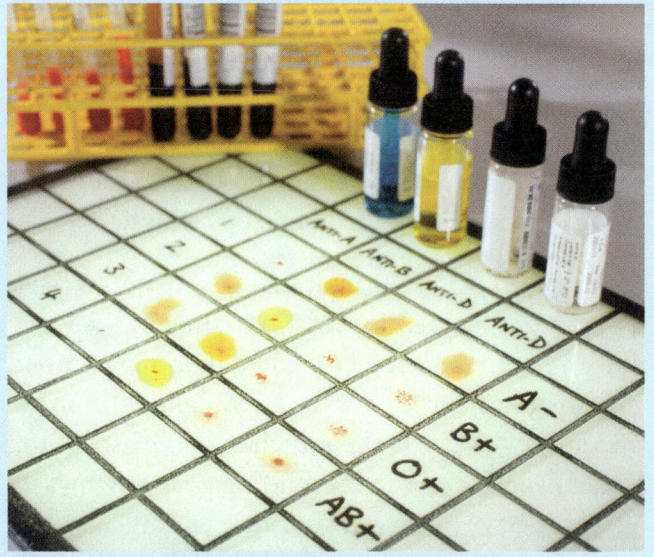

Blood typing tests (pictured) can occur before transfusions or during pregnancies. Results are determined though the reactions shown. Type A blood has type A antigens on its blood cells and anti-B antibodies in its serum. Type B blood is the reverse. Mixing type A blood with anti-A antibodies leads to a clumping reaction, which is seen as dense red dots. AB blood has both A and B antigens on its cells, but no antibodies. Type O blood has no antigens and both antibodies. Anti-D is an antibody used to test for Rhesus antigens (which point to some prenatal diseases), and it reacts with Rhesus positive blood.

Blood Type Percentages by Ethnicity

	Caucasians	African American	Hispanic	Asian
O+	37%	47%	53%	39%
O−	8%	4%	4%	1%
A+	33%	24%	29%	27%
A−	7%	2%	2%	0.5%
B+	9%	18%	9%	25%
B−	2%	1%	1%	0.4%
AB+	3%	4%	2%	7%
AB−	1%	0.3%	0.2%	0.1%

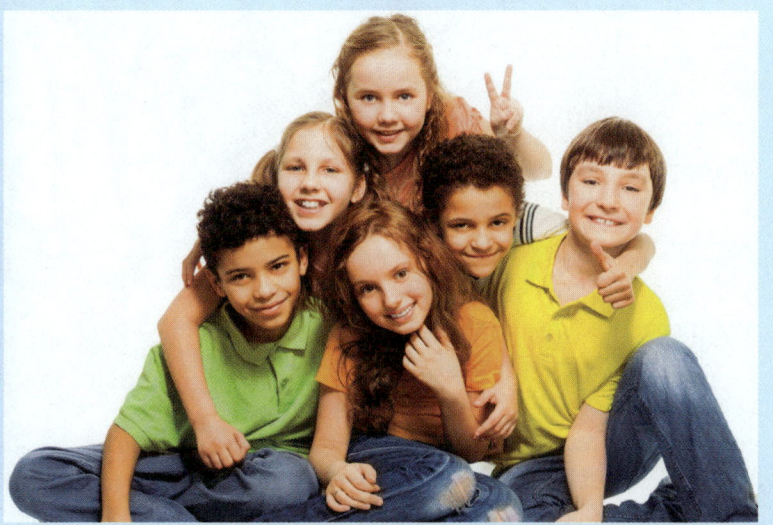

Unit 3: The Complex Circulatory System

3 Highways of Blood

Inside your body is a small universe. The blood vessels that travel to every nook and cranny in your body are impressive. If you were to take all the vessels and line them up end to end, they would expand a distance of 60,000 miles!

As you read this section, it may be helpful to have a picture of the heart nearby. Starting on the left side of the heart, the oxygenated blood is pumped into the largest artery of the body called the aorta. The aorta has two large branches — the ascending goes upward, and the descending goes downward. You may have observed your descending aorta pulsating. If you lie on your back and watch your stomach, you may see it slightly bouncing up and down at the same rate as your heart beats. This is your abdominal aorta artery.

Arteries in your body carry blood that is rich in oxygen. The blood in these vessels is bright red. The size of the arteries traveling through your body, run from largest to the smallest. The flow runs from the arteries to the arterioles, and then to the smallest, which are called capillaries. The aorta measures about an inch in diameter. The capillaries are tiny. They are about 1/3000th of an inch in diameter. That is about a tenth the diameter of a human hair! The capillaries are so small that blood cells have to line up in single file to pass. Sometimes the cells have to bend their shapes even to pass through the small orifice (opening). (Remember when we talked about sickle cell anemia earlier? This is why sickle cell anemia is so painful. The sickled cells are not flexible and have jagged edges. They tear the capillary walls. This blocks blood flow. This causes a very painful crisis.) Capillaries are extremely helpful. The blood flow slows down to pass. Your organs and cells are able to extract what they need from the blood, from oxygen to nutrients, and deposits waste products.

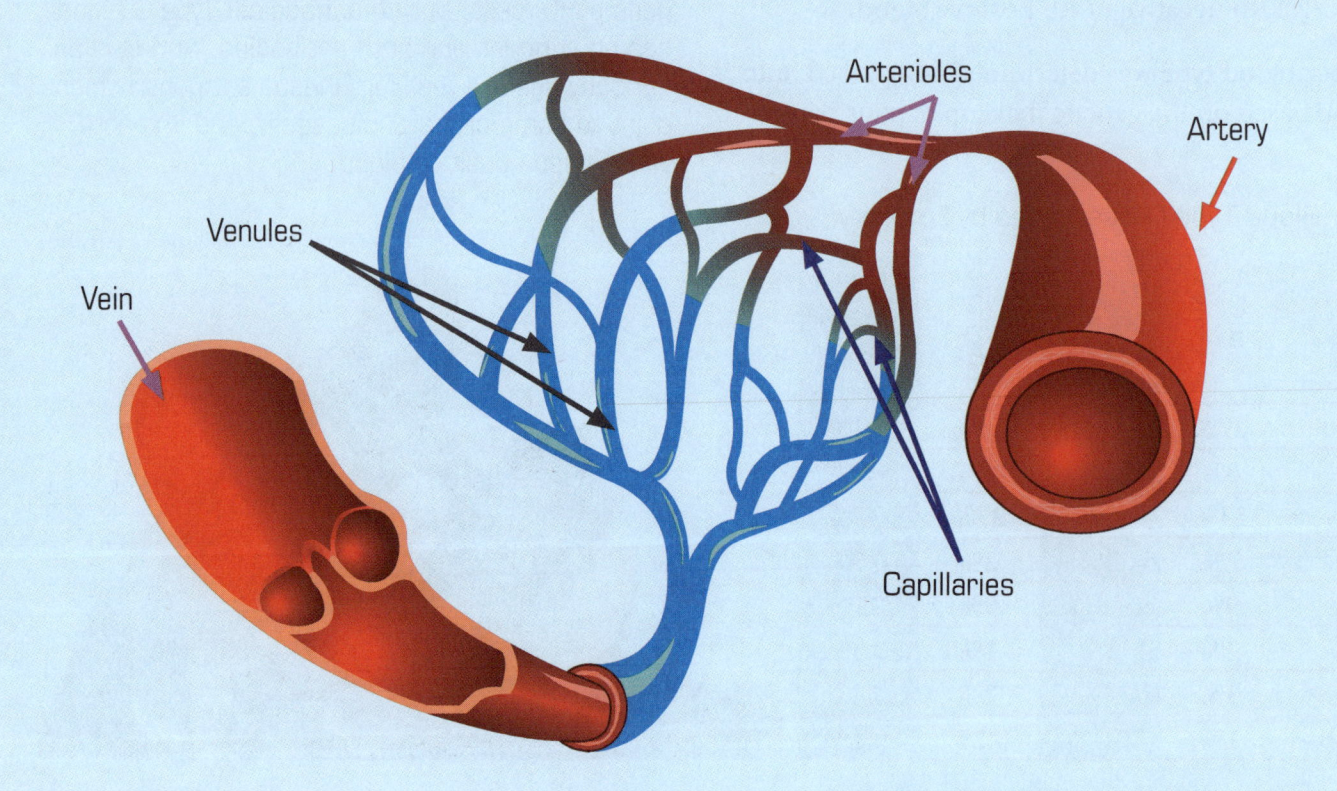

God's Wondrous Machine

we got the beat

Let's put that in perspective. The earth's circumference (the distance around) measures approximately 25,000 miles. Your blood vessels would wrap 2½ times around the earth!

The venous system vessels run from the small vessels to the large. The veins carry deoxygenated blood. The blood is maroon in color. The capillaries flow and connect to a network of vessels called the capillary network, which connect to the veins. The smallest veins are called venules. The venules expand to larger vessels called veins. The veins are the the ones that appear blue under your skin. The larger veins run to the right side of the heart.

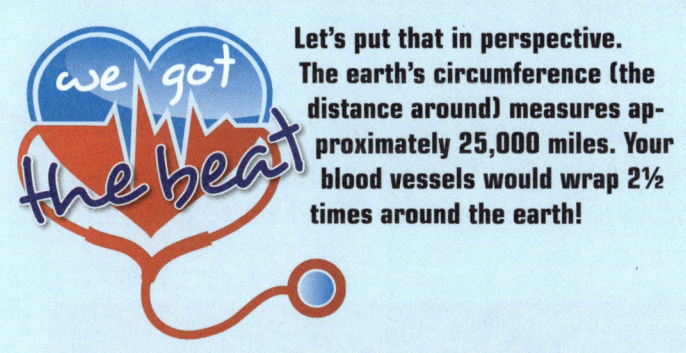

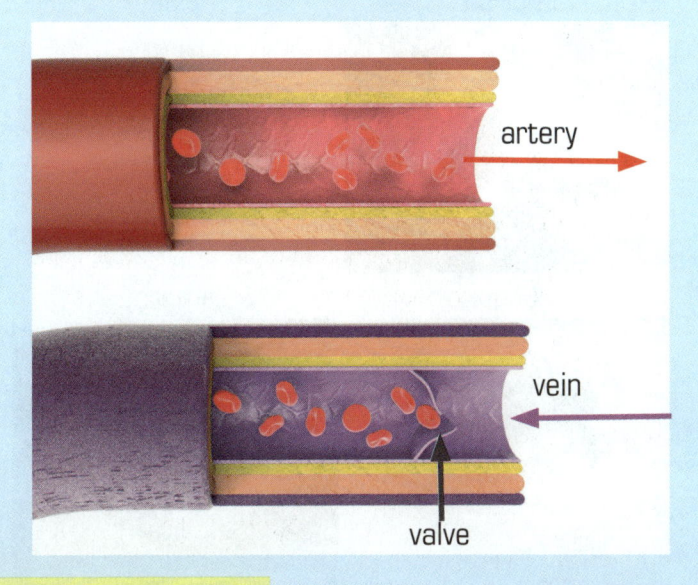

Once the blood clears the arterial system (arteries, arterioles, and capillaries), it needs to begin its journey back to the heart. The red blood cells need to be reloaded with oxygen. Your organs and cells throws out the "garbage" from all of its hard work. One of the garbage items that is thrown out is carbon dioxide. The red blood cells pick this up. They transport the garbage (carbon dioxide) to the lungs. This is where you breathe in oxygen and exhale carbon dioxide. The blood enters the venous system once it leaves the arterial system.

artery

vein

valve

Comparison of arteries to veins chart

Comparisons	Arteries	Veins
Oxygen content	Carries oxygenated blood	Carries deoxygenated blood
Direction of blood flow	Away from the heart	Toward the heart
Construction of the vessel	Thick and rubber-band like, which helps handle higher pressure and blood flow. Vessels are more rigid.	Thinner; vessels are easily compressible
Location	Can be deeper inside the body	Superficial in the body; lie closer to surface of the skin
Valves	Do not have valves	Have valves inside preventing the blood from flowing backward. Blood in veins works against gravity to get the blood back to the heart.

Unit 3: The Complex Circulatory System

4 Blood-Sucking Critters

Blood helps to keep us alive. There are creatures that not only have their own blood supply, but they feast on the blood of others. I know on many summer nights I have provided a tasty snack for hematophagic mosquitos. Hematophagy is the scientific name for the practice of animals feeding on blood. Hemato means blood; phagy means to eat or feed.

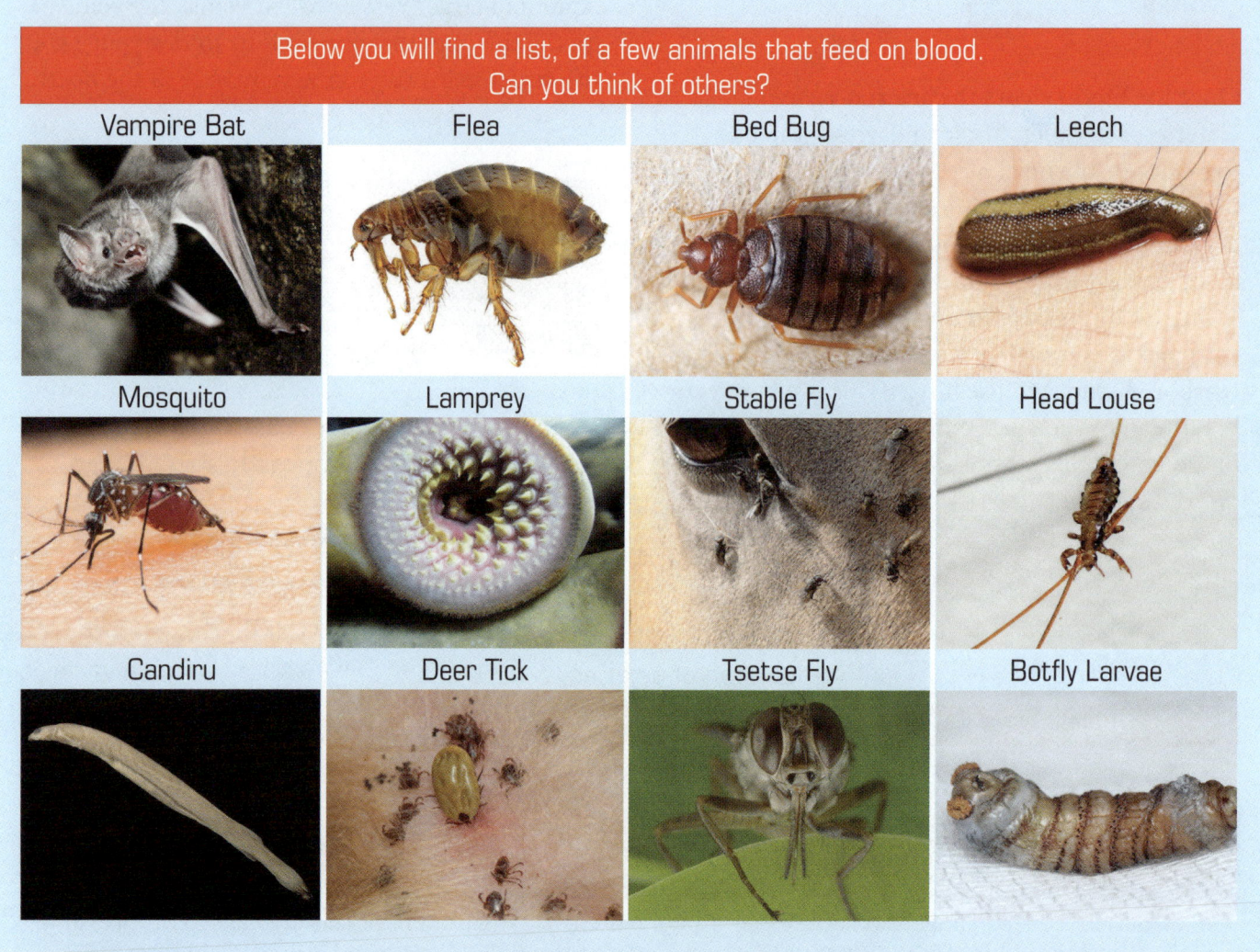

Below you will find a list, of a few animals that feed on blood. Can you think of others?

Vampire Bat	Flea	Bed Bug	Leech
Mosquito	Lamprey	Stable Fly	Head Louse
Candiru	Deer Tick	Tsetse Fly	Botfly Larvae

we got the beat

Mosquitos do have blood in their bodies. Whack! Have you ever caught a mosquito in the act of feeding on you? It is "kinda" messy after you forcefully "convince" the mosquito to stop their snacking. The blood you see does not belong to her! Mosquitos have clear blood! They do not have any metals in their blood to give it the red color.

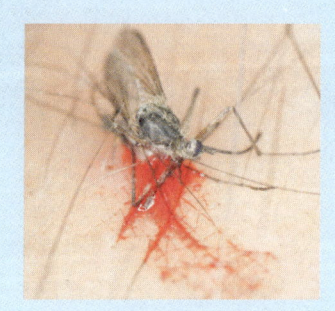

God's Wondrous Machine

I know everyone has their own favorite bloodsuckers, right? Here are three of my favorites:

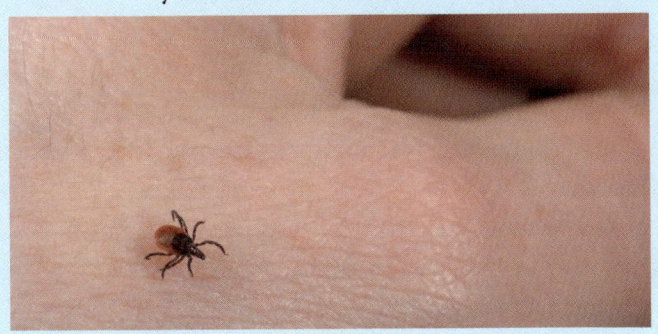

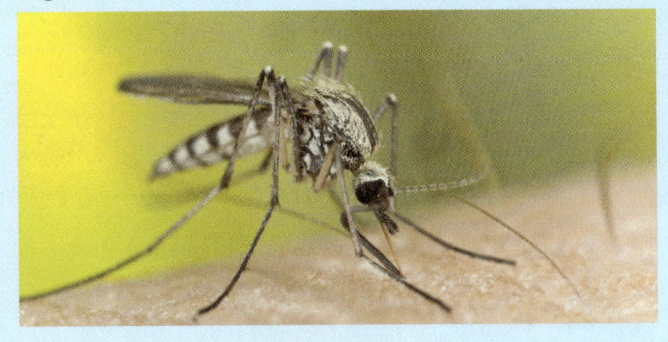

Ticks

There are more than 800 species in the tick family — it makes for quite a crowded family reunion. Some ticks are hard bodied. Some ticks are soft bodied. They inject a chemical that keeps their victim's blood from clotting. This allows them to get their "money's worth" when they go out to dinner. Their preferred dining location is biting around the head, neck, and ears of their blood "donors." Ticks need blood to grow and live. They normally reside in warmer climates that are humid, with wooded areas.

There are many tick-borne illnesses. Ticks transmit illness through their saliva. Some tick-borne illnesses are Rickettsia, Colorado tick fever, Rocky Mountain spotted fever, relapsing fever, and of course, Lyme disease, to name a few. Look out for the tick's close cousin, *Ixodes Scapularis*. He is known as the deer tick and is a known to be a carrier of Lyme disease.

Ticks track down mammals, like us, by sensing carbon dioxide. When we exhale carbon dioxide, the dinner bell rings for the tick and dinner is served. They utilize their mouth parts to clasp on and plunge their barb-like needle into the skin. They attach and commence dining. Ticks suck in the blood and dine for a few days until they become engorged and fall off.

Mosquitoes

Next up is the mosquito. Their name originates from the Spanish word *musketas,* which means little flies. A mosquito's wings flap 300 to 400 times each second. You may have encountered her annoying buzzing around your ears during a camping trip. The ladies of the mosquito family are the only ones who dine on blood. They love blood most when it is close to the time of egg laying. She only has a life span of about 14 days so she will probably have to eat and run.

The males of the family don't find blood palatable. They prefer the sweet taste of nectar from plants and flowers. Mosquitos can also be disease carriers. They can transmit diseases through their salvia, like yellow fever, West Nile, and malaria.

Mosquitos find some people's blood more "tasty" than others. Mosquitos prefer to feed more on people with type O blood, heavy breathers (lots of carbon dioxide attracts them), sweaty people, and women who are pregnant. A natural way to keep these insects away is to use lavender on your skin or eat lots of garlic. When you eat garlic, you sweat it, and mosquitos hate the smell. As a matter of fact, it may keep people away also.

Unit 3: The Complex Circulatory System

Leeches

Last, but not least, is the leech. They have a great family history that is as long as recorded time. Leeches are a type of worm. However, leeches are hermaphrodites, which means they are both male and female all rolled up in one.

Leeches, in early times, were used for bloodletting. They were considered easier to use than a lancet in Middle Ages to restore the "humors" back in order. They have suckers on both ends of their bodies that attach to the victim. They can grow five times their size with a good, filling meal. They do not let go until they have completed their meal.

Leeches are no longer used for bloodletting today, but they are used for "hirudotherapy." Hirudo is a type of leech. The Hirudo medicinalis leech is used in medicine. It has three jaws that cut like sharp razors into the skin. Once the skin is cut by the leech, it injects several substances. One substance is called hirudin. (This is where it gets its name.) This substance keeps the blood from clotting. Hirudin blocks fibrin from forming in a blood clot. Like the mosquito and tick, they inject an anesthetic, a substance that prohibits pain, into the wound. After all, they don't want their dining pleasure interrupted.

So the question remains — how on earth are they used in medicine? I am glad you asked. In the United States, leeches are considered a "medical device." Leeches are utilized after surgery in some cases for skin that has been reattached.

One of the problems with reattachment of skin from reconstructive surgery is that blood clots can form in the natural healing process and cause the area to die due to lack of blood supply. The leeches' talents are called into action. During a

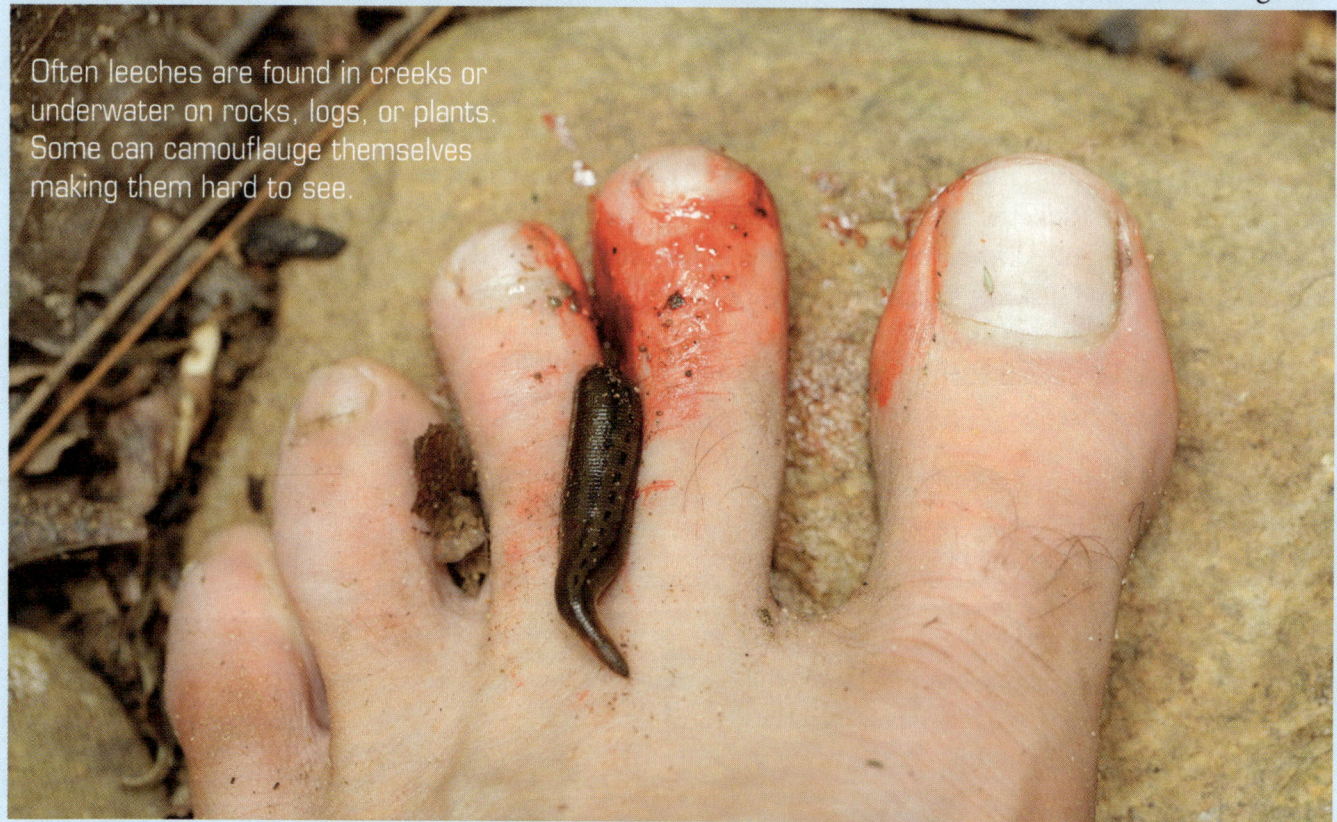

Often leeches are found in creeks or underwater on rocks, logs, or plants. Some can camouflauge themselves making them hard to see.

God's Wondrous Machine

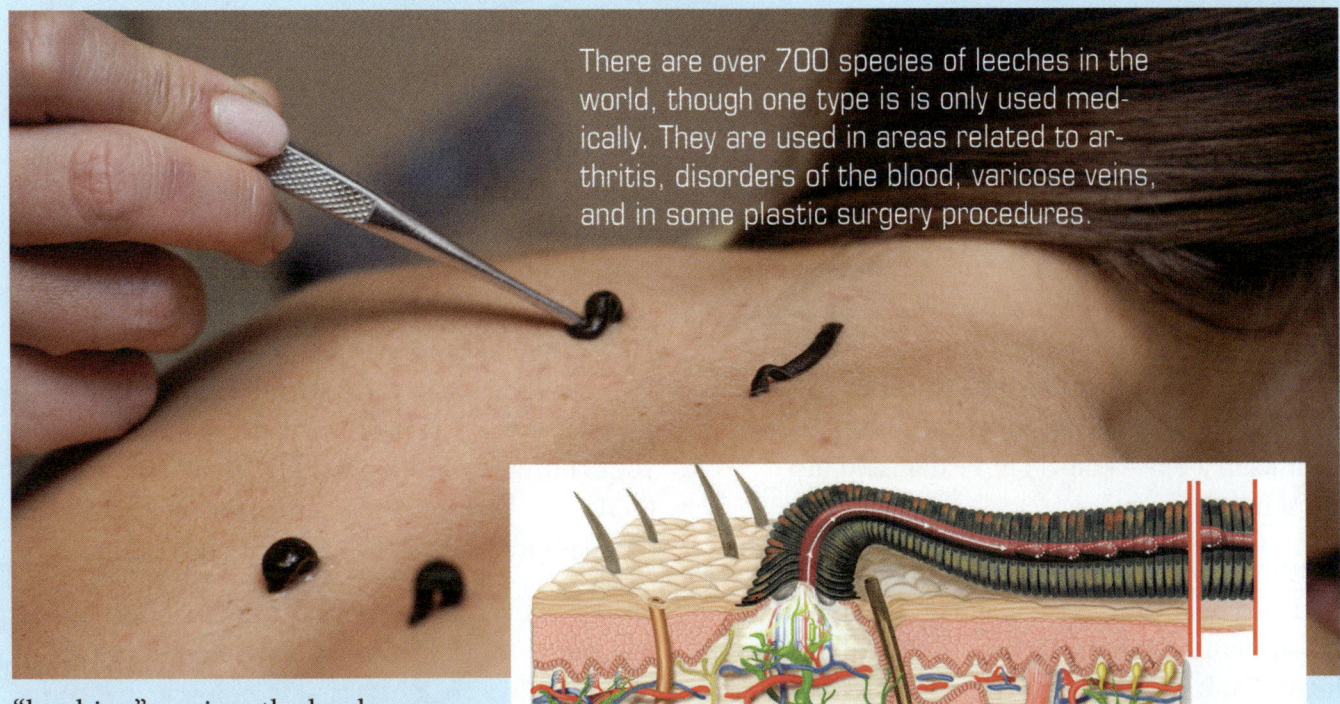

There are over 700 species of leeches in the world, though one type is is only used medically. They are used in areas related to arthritis, disorders of the blood, varicose veins, and in some plastic surgery procedures.

"leeching" session, the leeches are allowed to attach in the surgical area. They release into the skin the blood-thinning and clot-preventing chemicals. It gladly ingests the extra blood that accumulates in the area. The benefit is that it improves the blood circulation by breaking up the problematic clots, and this promotes healing.

Bloodsucking at its best. A leech attaching to the skin releases two chemicals into the local vessels that thins the blood and keeps it from clotting. This helps the leech enjoy a tasty meal longer.

Word Wise!
LEECHES used to be the common name given to people in Europe and North Americas who worked as healers or physicians centuries ago, and "to leech" meant to heal or cure someone. The use of leeches can be traced back to ancient India and Greece. Now, the term "leech" is used as to describe clinging to someone constantly or taking needed resources like money away from you.

Unit 3: The Complex Circulatory System

5 Take Heart: Getting to the Heart of the Matter

We now arrive at the "heart" of the matter. The blood and the vessels in our bodies could not work effectively if it weren't for our beating hearts. It weighs only about 11 ounces. (A pound is 16 ounces.) The largest heart known is that of the blue whale. It tips the scale at 1,500 pounds, which is the size of a small car. The aorta of the blue whale is large enough for an adult to crawl through. The average heart beats about 100,000 times a day. In an adult, the heart pumps 2,000 gallons in a day. Whew! I am exhausted just thinking about it.

We have what is called a closed circulatory system. A closed circulatory system means that blood travels only within the blood vessels and the heart. It does not ooze into our body cavities. An open circulatory system is seen in many insects, mollusks, and crustaceans. Blood in these animals is pumped by the heart into the body cavity where the organs are bathed. It is crazy, but it has been shown that if a cockroach's head is cut off, after the blood clots up the opening, that it can live up to one month! It ultimately dies due to starvation.

The Outside of the Heart

Let's take a look at the anatomy of the heart from the outside in. The heart lies in the chest underneath your sternum (breast bone). Your heart is about the size of your fist. It is encased in a double-layered sac called the pericardial sac. Peri means around. Cardi means heart. The sac's purpose is to cut down the friction generated by your constantly beating heart. A small amount of fluid exists between the layers of the sac that allows the membranes to slide freely without friction.

Have you ever had an opportunity to look at a real heart from a chicken or cow? Some people like to eat livestock hearts. It is a muscle that some find very tasty. Looking at the surface, you will notice blood vessels that travel on the outside of the heart. All the gallons of blood that run through the inside of the heart are for use by the whole body. The vessels outside of the heart are for the personal circulatory system of the heart. These are called the coronary arteries and veins. A heart attack (or medically speaking, a myocardial infarction) is the result of one or more of the coronary arteries becoming blocked. Once the

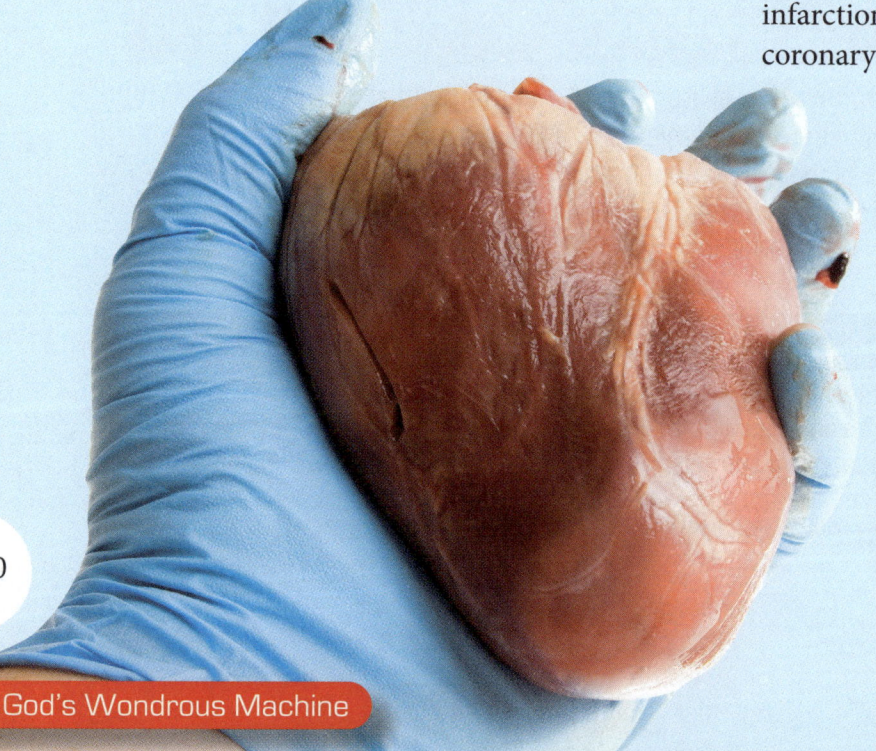

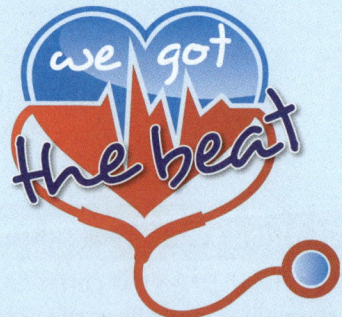

we got the beat

Your heart is about the size of your fist. It beats from 4-5 weeks of conception in your mother's womb until the day you take your last breath. It is without a doubt the strongest muscle in your body.

The Heart Wall

Pericardium

A heart attack occurs as a result of a blocked artery that supplies the muscle of the heart.

Myocardium

Epicardium

Pericardium cavity

Endocardium

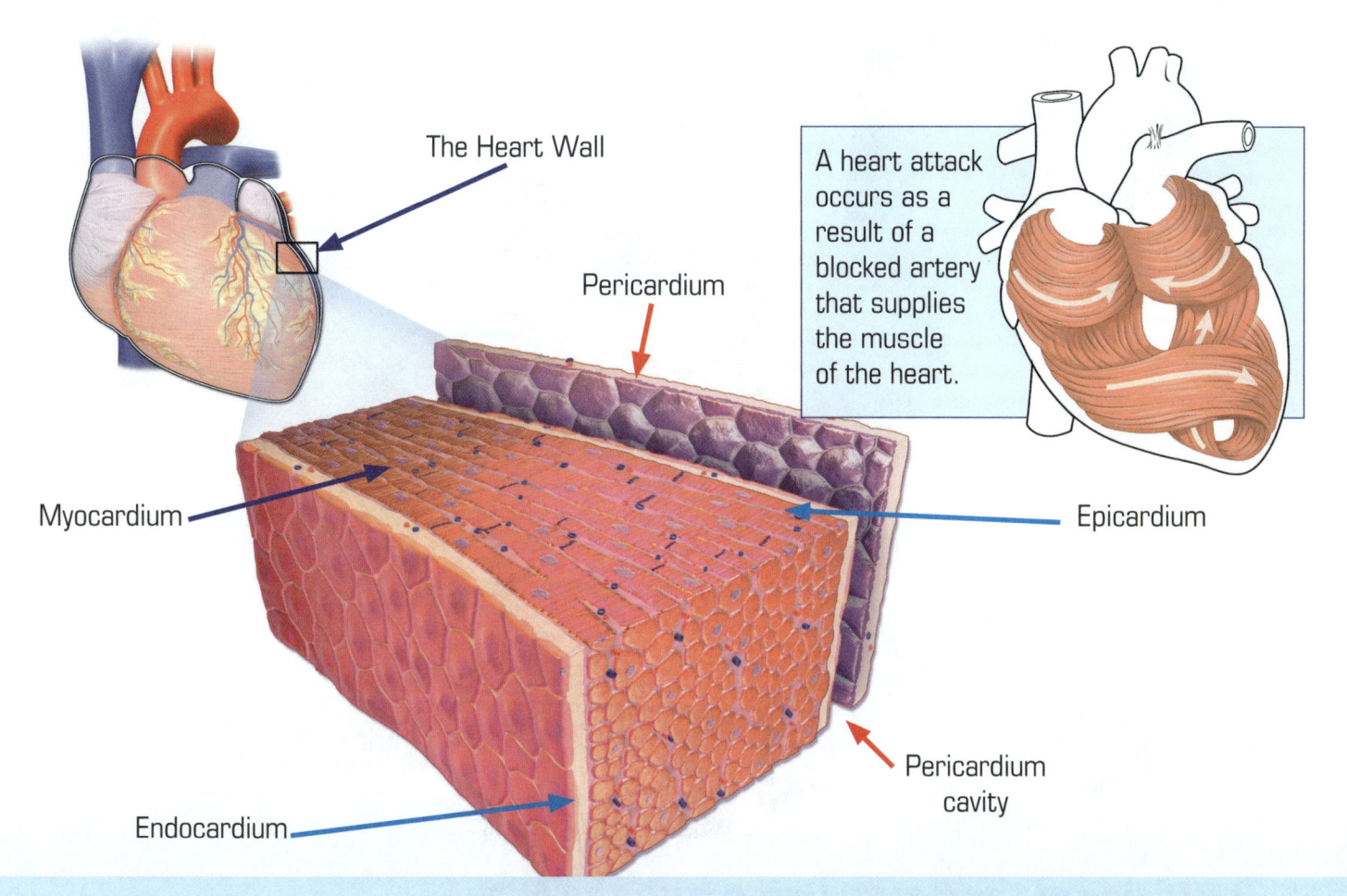

artery is blocked, the tissue lying downstream from the block does not receive blood. If it doesn't receive blood, it doesn't receive oxygen and nutrients. It begins to die.

The actual muscle of the heart is composed of three layers. The outer part of the muscle, lying under the pericardial sac, is called the epicardium. The epicardium literally means the outer part of the heart. The middle layer is called the myocardium. Myo means muscle. The most inner layer is called the endocardium (inside the heart).

I bet you will be amazed at how much you already know. I will give you three heart diseases. Can you tell me where each of them occur? Oh, yes, here is one more hint before you take a whack at it — any word that ends with "itis" means that something is inflamed or infected.

Are you ready? What do the words endocarditis, myocarditis, and pericarditis mean?

Endocarditis	An infection of the inner lining of the heart.
Myocarditis	is an infection of the myocardium, the middle layer of the heart wall. Myocarditis can affect both the heart's muscle cells and the heart's electrical system, leading to reduction in the heart's pumping function and to irregular heart rhythms.
Pericarditis	is swelling, irritation, or infection of the pericardium, the thin, sac-like membrane surrounding your heart.

181

Unit 3: The Complex Circulatory System

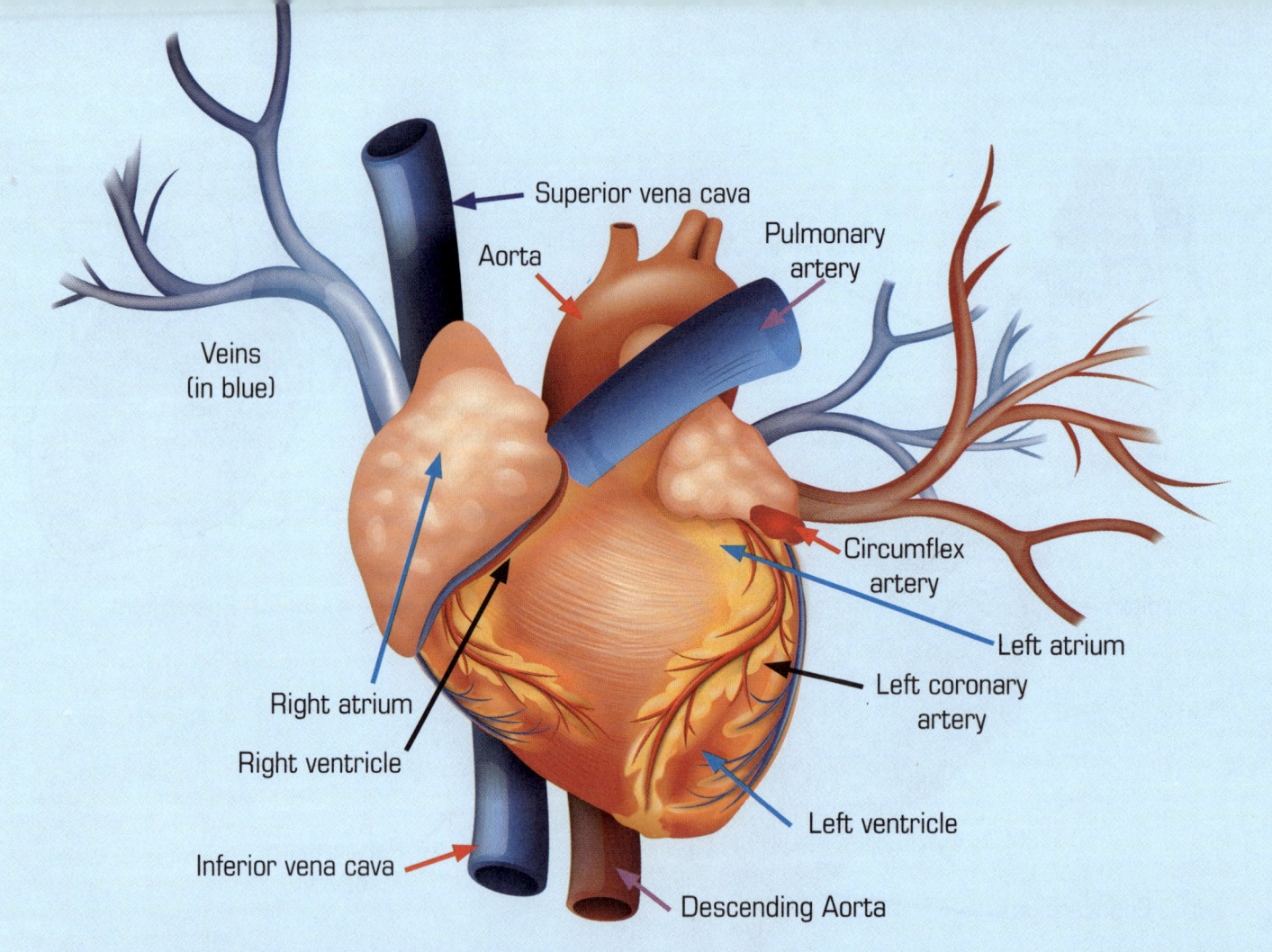

Diagram labels:
- Superior vena cava
- Aorta
- Pulmonary artery
- Veins (in blue)
- Circumflex artery
- Left atrium
- Left coronary artery
- Right atrium
- Right ventricle
- Left ventricle
- Inferior vena cava
- Descending Aorta

The Inside of the Heart: Going with the Flow

Allright, budding cardiologists, now we will take a look at the four chambers, or rooms, of the heart. There are two upper rooms and two lower rooms. The upper rooms are called atrium. Atrium means entrance in Latin. The lower rooms are called ventricles. Ventricles are derived from the Latin word meaning "little belly." The heart is similar to two pumps. The right side pumps the blood to the lungs. The left side pumps the blood to the entire body. Follow the numbers labeled on the heart diagram on the next page as you read the following descriptions.

Numbers 1–2: Deoxygenated blood (blood lower in oxygen concentration) enters the right side of the heart through the right atrium via two great veins. The superior vena cava brings blood from the upper part of the body. The inferior vena cava brings blood from the lower part of the body. The chambers and great vessels have "doors" separating them from the next room. These "doors" are called valves. The valves in the chambers are connected by cords to the floor of the heart. This ensures that the valves swing open in one direction and blood travels in one direction, forward. The cords are called the chordae tendineae. There is an old expression, "You're tugging on my heart strings," that may have originated from these cardiac strings. (It means to cause someone to feel more emotional.)

Numbers 3–4–5: From the right atrium, blood travels through the door of the tricuspid valve into the right ventricle. Blood is then pushed into the pulmonary artery past the pulmonary semilunar valves to be oxygenated in the lungs.

Numbers 6–7–8: Once oxygenated, it is returned to the left atrium of the heart via the pulmonary

God's Wondrous Machine

veins, by being pushed through the mitral valve (bicuspid valve) into the left ventricle.

Numbers 9–10: Finally, with great force, the blood is ejected out into the aorta artery past the aortic semilunar valve to the rest of the body. It takes approximately a minute when you are at rest for the blood to circumnavigate the full trip of the body. The time can be less, depending on the heart rate and size of the heart.

Did you notice any "errors" in that last paragraph? Take another look. You may have been savvy to pick up on something about the pulmonary artery and pulmonary vein. Normally, arteries carry oxygenated blood and veins carry deoxygenated blood. This is the only contradiction in the body. The pulmonary artery and vein carry the opposite. They are named this way because of how they are formed in fetal development.

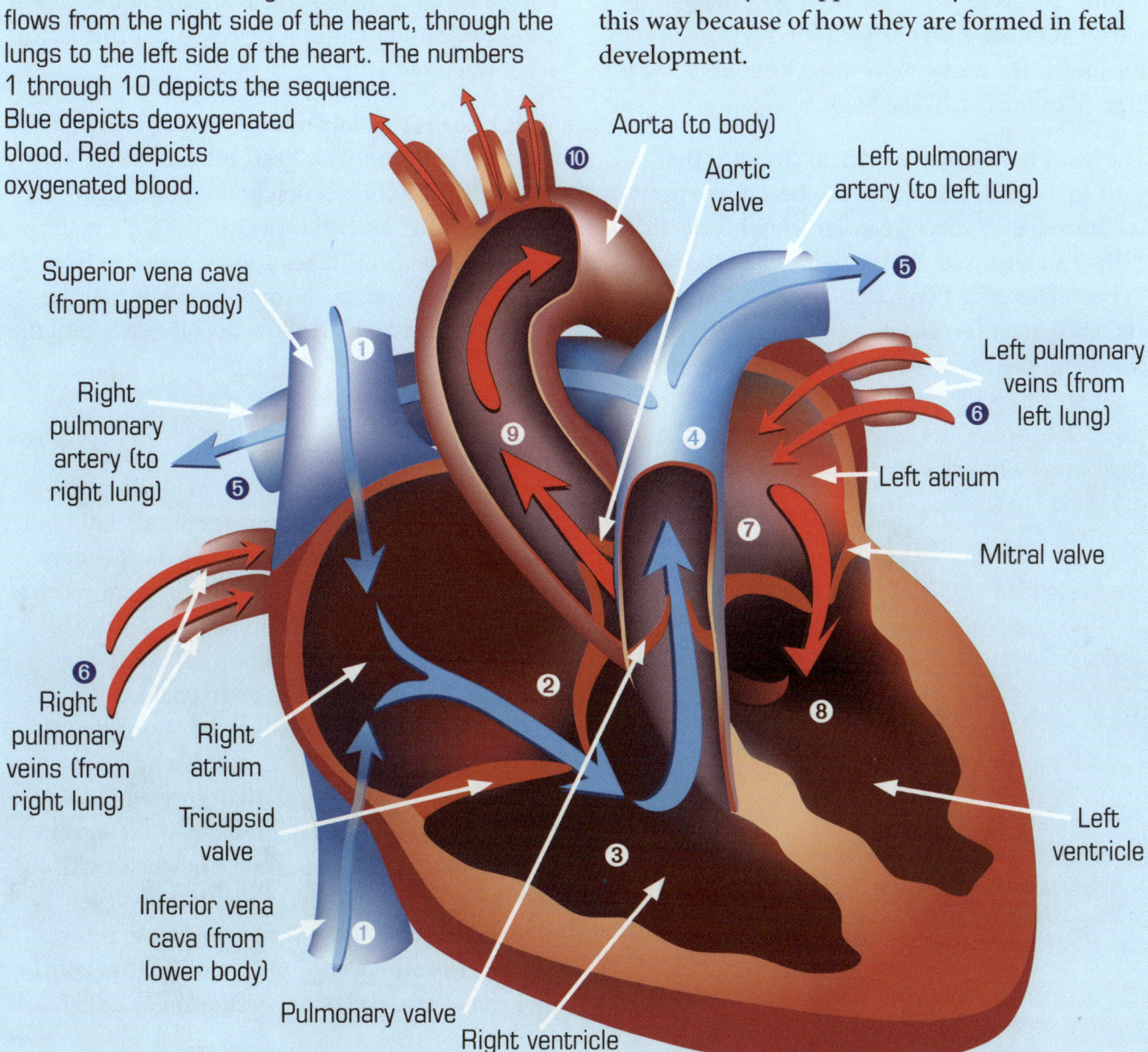

Flow of the Blood through the Heart: Follow the numbered arrows through the heart as the blood flows from the right side of the heart, through the lungs to the left side of the heart. The numbers 1 through 10 depicts the sequence. Blue depicts deoxygenated blood. Red depicts oxygenated blood.

Unit 3: The Complex Circulatory System

The Beat Goes On

"Lub-dub. Lub-dub. Lub-dub" is the characteristic sound heard when you listen to someone's heart. Lub is the first sound heard, dub is the second sound. The sounds that you hear when listening to a heart are actually the doors (valves) slamming shut in the heart. The first sound, lub, is the closure of the tricuspid and mitral valves between the atria and ventricles. The second sound, dub, is heard at the closure of the pulmonary semilunar valves as the blood is pushed into the lungs. The aortic valve also closes as blood is ejected to the rest of the body.

The heart has its own electrical circuitry that runs in its muscular walls. The beat of the heart is controlled by special cardiac muscle cells that deliver an electrical charge that causes the heart to beat. There are two special areas in the right atrium that trigger the beat of the heart. The sinoatrial (SA) node located on the top of the right atrium is the pacemaker. It controls the pace, or how fast the heart beats. It is like the pace car at a motor car race that goes ahead of the other cars to set the rate.

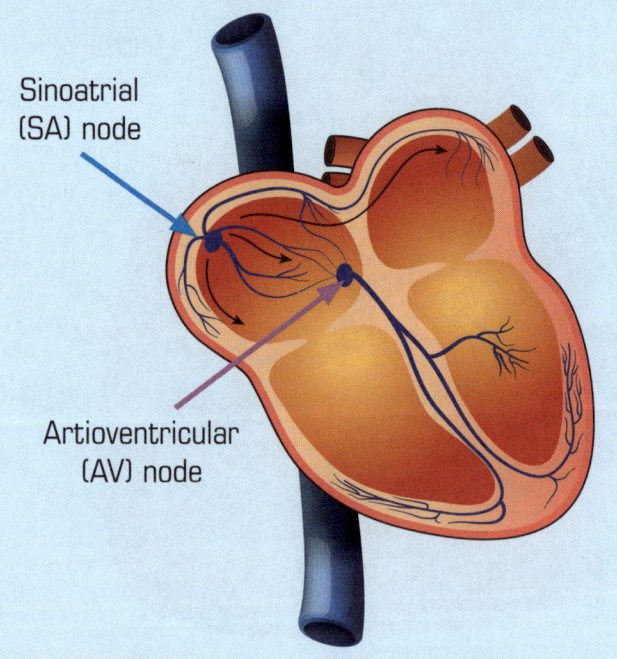

Sinoatrial (SA) node

Artioventricular (AV) node

The charge travels from the SA node down to the lower portion of the right atrium to the second area called the atrioventricular (AV) node. From here, the electrical impulse travels down the middle (intraventricular septum) between the right and left ventricles and travels around the outside walls of the heart. The heart has its own internal regulatory system. The heart will beat and continue to have some electrical activity for a couple of minutes after it is removed. (This is not recommended.)

Your heart is the only muscle in your body that does not get tired. The "rest" it takes is very short. Systole is the contraction phase of the heart when blood is pushed forward. Diastole is the only time the heart takes a small pause to "rest." What really happens during diastole is that the heart pauses briefly to allow the blood to refill the heart.

The heart also has a control system that can override the internal system. A nerve control system in the brain stem in the medulla oblongata is an essential partner in regulating the heart. Sometimes your heart needs to speed up or slow down. This area in the brain stem secretes chemicals that will speed up or slow down the heart, depending on the body's demands. For example, if you decided to go to Spain and participate in the event called the "Running of the Bulls," this will come in quite handy. You step out on the street with hundreds of your closest friends. The bulls are let loose down the streets. You begin to run for your life. Your heart will need to speed up to keep up with the oxygen demand of your body. Your legs start to pump. Your heart rate speeds up. Presto! You are able to dive out of the way of a snorting angry bull!

God's Wondrous Machine

The Electrocardiogram

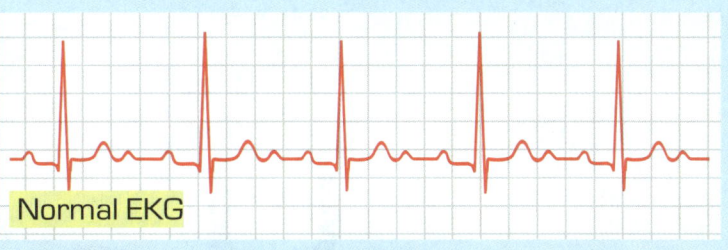

Have you ever seen these kind of images? They are a tracing from an electrocardiogram (ECG or EKG) machine. The electrical activity of the heart is present all the time. We have this special machine that can record the electrical activity without cutting inside the body. It causes no pain. A series of electrodes in a special foamy adhesive tape is placed on various locations on the chest over the heart. The series of spikes and dips, like a rollercoaster, are documented. These waves record normal or abnormal activity of the heart.

Normal EKG

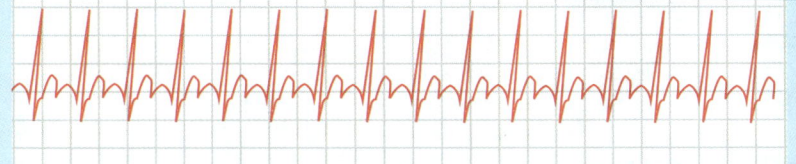

In some people, the heart beats too fast. This is called tachycardia. Tachy means fast.

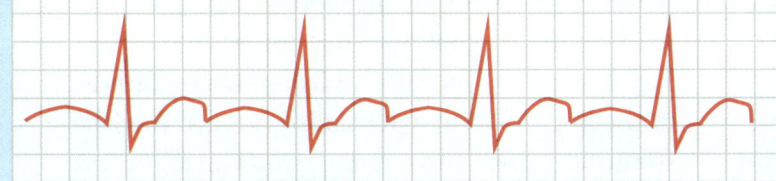

Sometimes the heart beats too slowly. This is called bradycardia. Brady means to slow.

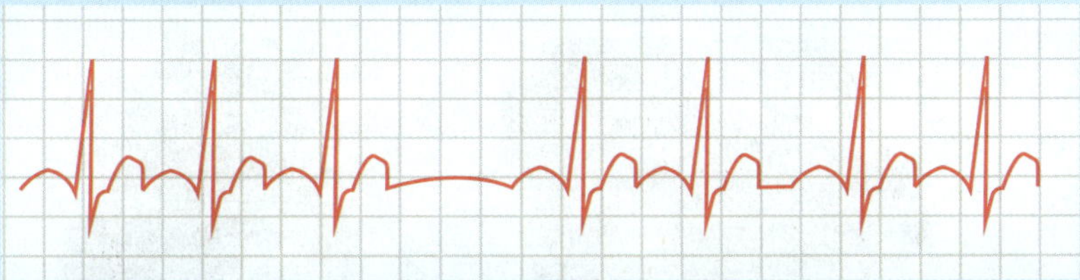

Sometimes the heart's electrical activity is irregular and inconsistent. This is a tracing called fibrillation. The muscle of the heart does not beat in a synchronized fashion. When this happens, the heart is unable to pump blood. This is dangerous.

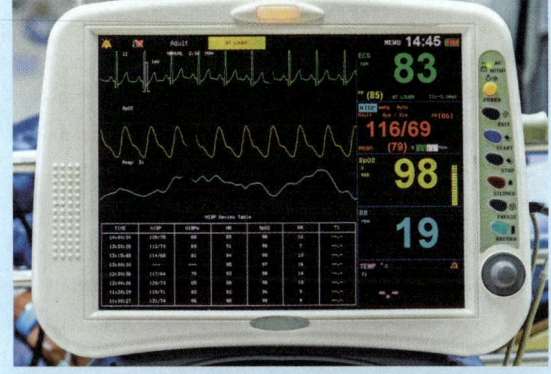

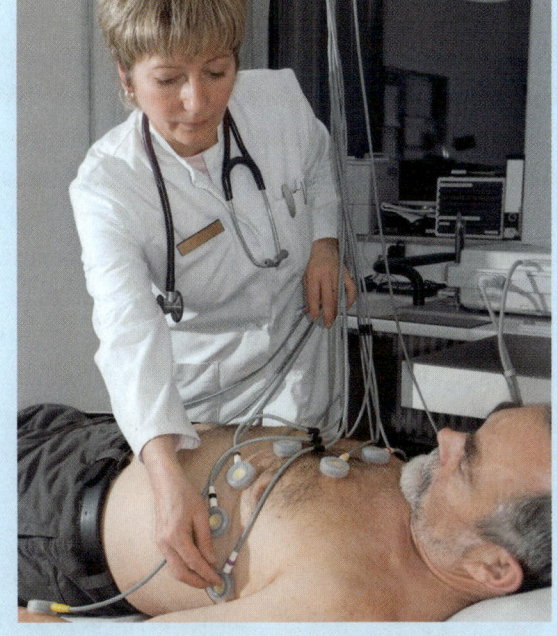

All of these types of rhythms can be unhealthy for a person. These are called arrhythmias (irregular rates). God has given doctors, scientists, and technicians the reasoning ability to find solutions to some of these problems. A pacemaker can be a useful tool in controlling an irregular rhythm. It is a small electrical device surgically placed in someone's chest or abdomen under the skin to assist in controlling abnormal heart rates. It monitors the heart internally. If an irregular rhythm occurs, it sends a very low electrical pulse to prompt the heart to get back on track.

Unit 3: The Complex Circulatory System

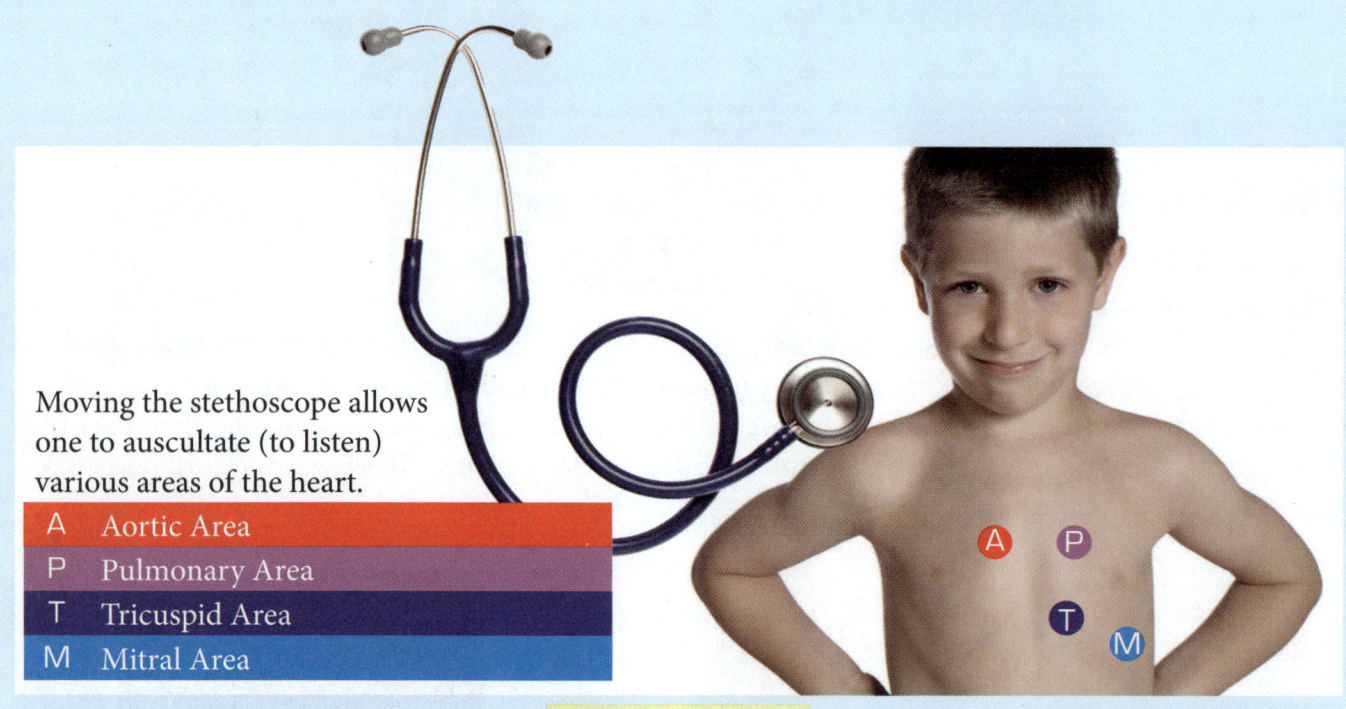

Moving the stethoscope allows one to auscultate (to listen) various areas of the heart.

A	Aortic Area
P	Pulmonary Area
T	Tricuspid Area
M	Mitral Area

Listen to My Heart

It is truly incredible what God will do in our lives when we turn our hearts to Him and listen. Listening is one of the most powerful tools we can develop in learning about our world and growing in our faith. Listening is a skill that doctors must develop in caring for their patients. It is essential to listen to someone as they explain their symptoms. It is also critical to listen to the sounds of the body. As a pediatrician, a children's doctor, I have seen that many of my smallest patients are unable to use words to explain what troubles them. When I listen to the hearts of my patients, I close my eyes and focus intently on the sounds. In the same way, I prefer to close my eyes and bow my head when I pray. It takes all the other distractions away. I am better at concentrating and listening.

During a visit to the doctor, you may have noticed that the doctor listened to your chest with a stethoscope. The stethoscope is a medical device that doctors, nurses, and other health professionals use to listen to the sounds of the body. You may have also noticed that the stethoscope was moved to various locations on your chest. Moving the stethoscope allows one to auscultate (to listen) various areas of the heart.

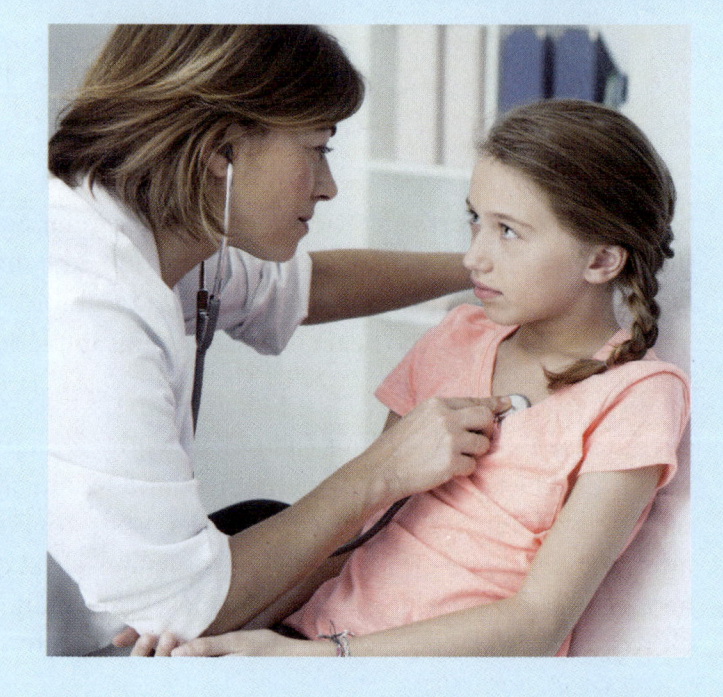

But in your hearts revere Christ as Lord. Always be prepared to give an answer to everyone who asks you to give the reason for the hope that you have. But do this with gentleness and respect (1 Peter 3:15).

I AM wonderfully made

God's Wondrous Machine

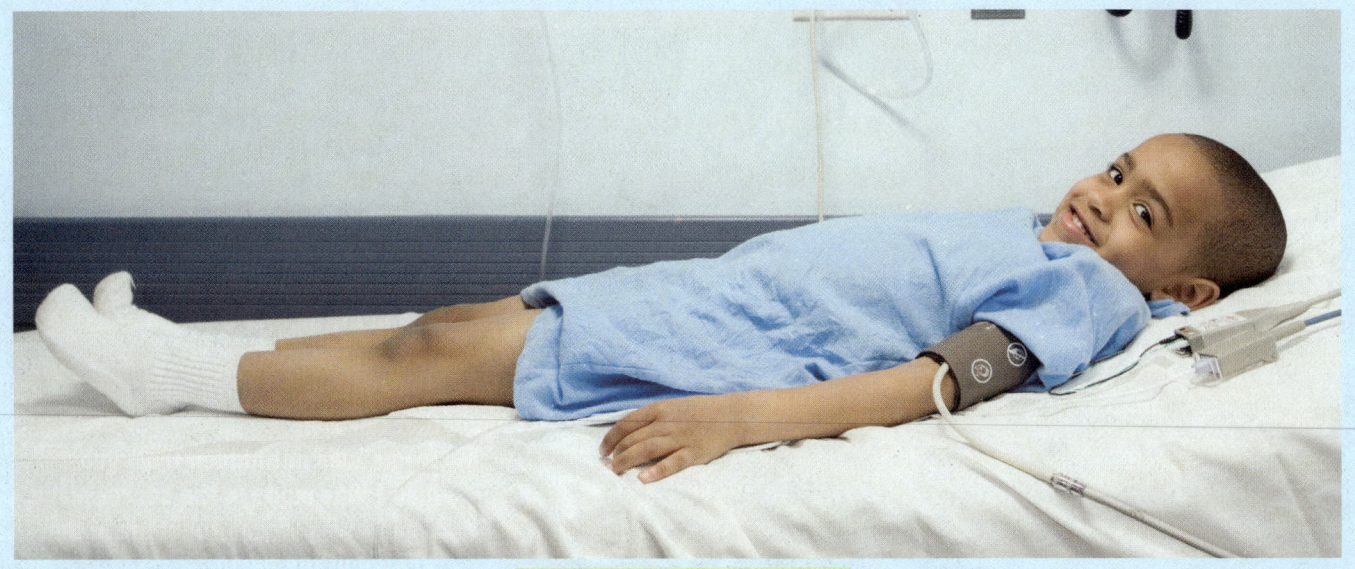

Feeling Under Pressure

As your heart beats, it forces the blood through the blood vessels at a certain pressure. Let's say you took a long balloon and filled it with water. You squeeze the water out the other end with a great force. The water would rush out under the pressure generated by the force of your hand. This is what happens in your blood vessels. The higher the pressure in your vessels, the harder your heart works.

We can measure this pressure with an instrument called a sphygmomanometer. Try saying that ten times fast! The cuff is placed around the arm, just above the bend in the elbow. The blood pressure cuff is inflated snug enough to stop the blood flow in the vessels for just a moment. Slowly the air is let out of the cuff. It slowly deflates. Listening with a stethoscope over the vessels in the fold of your arm, you will begin to hear the pulse and rush of the blood through the vessel. The cuff deflates. You will hear a beginning sound. The sound will persist for several beats until no sound is heard anymore. Watching the gauge, you will note when the first sound and last sound is noted. The first reading is the systolic pressure. This is the highest pressure the heart generated at the peak of its contraction. The second reading is the diastolic pressure. This is the pressure during the relaxation of the ventricles.

A normal blood pressure for an adult is 120/80. The pressure in children varies, depending on the age of the child. Healthy newborn babies will have lower blood pressure. Typically, their blood pressure is about 64/41. Why do you think there would be such a difference in a baby's blood pressure compared to an adult?

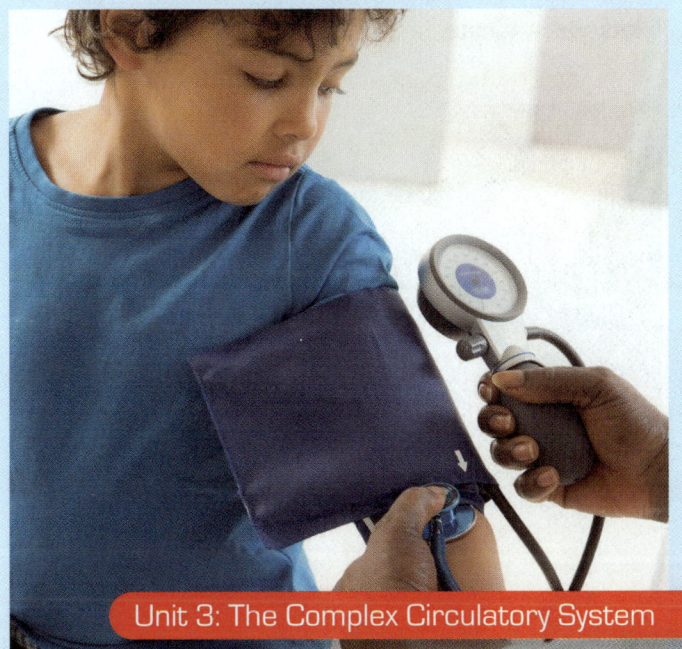

Word Wise!
SPHYGMOMANOMETER is the medical name for a blood pressure cuff device.

Unit 3: The Complex Circulatory System

6 In the Beginning: The Development of the Heart

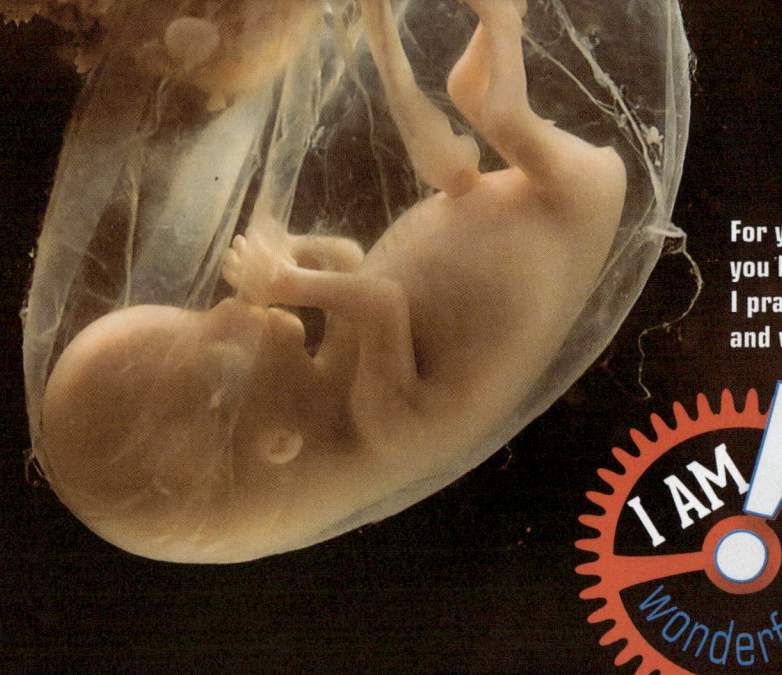

For you created my inmost being;
you knit me together in my mother's womb.
I praise you because I am fearfully
and wonderfully made; your works are wonderful,
I know that full well.
My frame was not hidden from you
when I was made in the secret place,
when I was woven together in the
depths of the earth.
Your eyes saw my unformed body;
all the days ordained for me were
written in your book
before one of them came to be.

— Psalm 139:13–16

I AM wonderfully made

we got the beat

In the mother's womb, after the baby is conceived, by the fifth week, the heart of the baby starts beating and divides into chambers. Six weeks later blood is flowing inside the body. The heart rate is approximately 160 beats every minute.

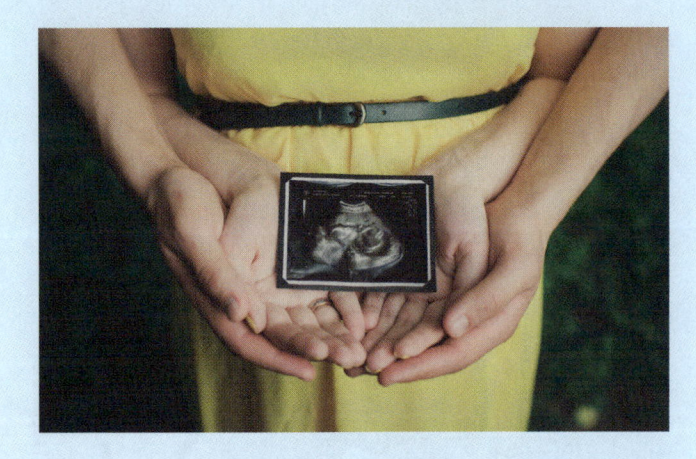

Your heart began development as a simple tube with trunks on each end. It began to beat when you were in your mother's womb, at about 3–4 weeks. The circulatory system is the first major system to function. The heart tube grows longer and then bends back on itself as a loop. The folding of the heart tube only takes 6 days. A four-chambered heart is formed from this convoluted tube. The dividers between the chambers are called septa. They form from the grooves between the folds. The dividers fuse to make walls between the chambers. However, a small hole does remain between the top atrium to allow the blood to be taken directly from the right to the left side of the heart. It is called the foramen ovale. This allows the blood to bypass (go around) the lungs.

God's Wondrous Machine

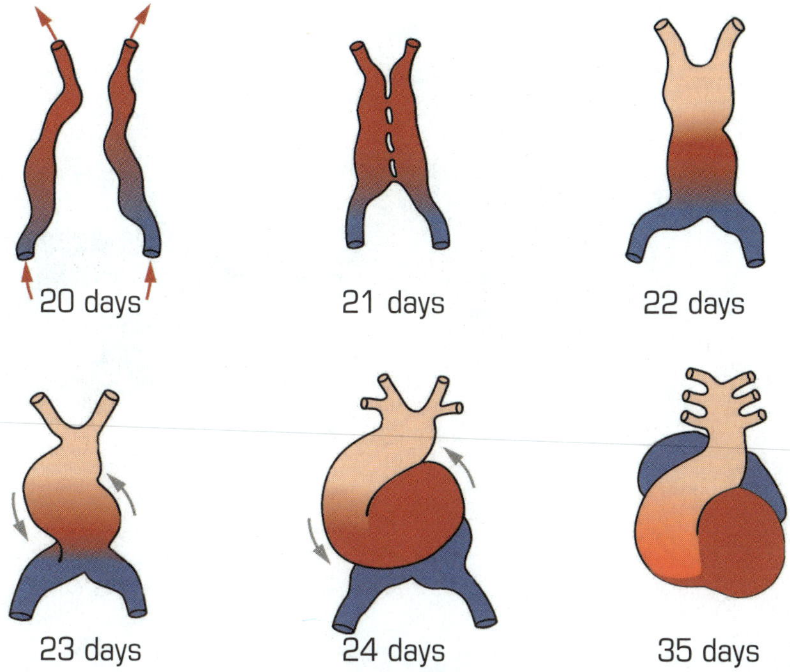

20 days   21 days   22 days
23 days   24 days   35 days

Your heart begins as two tubes that fuse together, and it folds and molds itself into a two-system pump. The right side of the heart pumps blood to your lungs. The left side of the heart pumps the blood to the rest of the entire body.

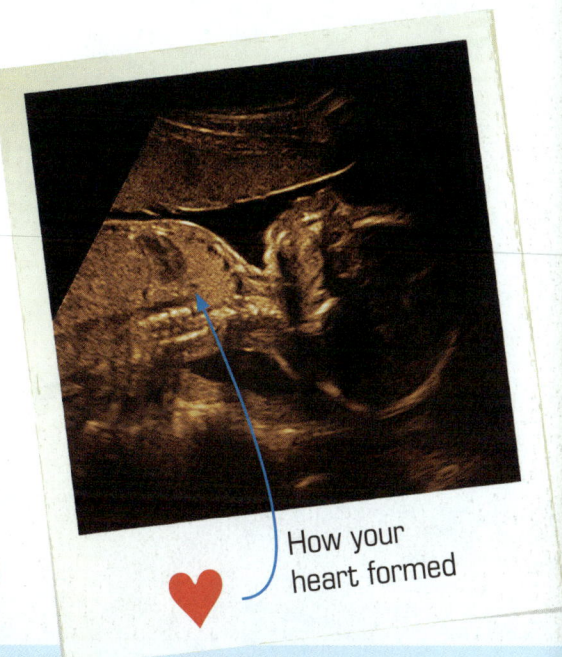

How your heart formed

FETAL HEART RATES

Starting at week 5 the fetal heart rate accelerates by 3.3 beats per minute (bpm) per day for the next month.

The fetal heart begins to beat at the same rate as the mother's, which is typically 80 to 85 beats per minute.

Week 5	starts at 80 and ends at 103 bpm
Week 6	starts at 103 and ends at 126 bpm
Week 8	starts at 126 and ends at 149 bpm
Week 9	the fetal heartbeat tends to beat within a range of 155 to 195 bpm

At this point, the fetal heart rate begins to decrease, and generally falls within the range of 120 to 160 bpm by week 12.

In the womb, the lungs receive blood for nourishment purposes only. The lungs do not provide oxygen for the baby. The blood circulation in a fetus, a baby in the womb, is different than the blood circulation in you and me. There are two major shunts (short cuts). The shunts are small passageways that bypass the lungs and liver. The liver and lungs are not fully developed while the fetus is in the womb. The placenta, the structure that connects the mother to the baby, does the work of these organs. The placenta provides all the oxygen and nourishment the baby needs from the mother. Babies do not "breathe" inside the womb. The environment that the baby lives in is filled with fluid.

Unit 3: The Complex Circulatory System

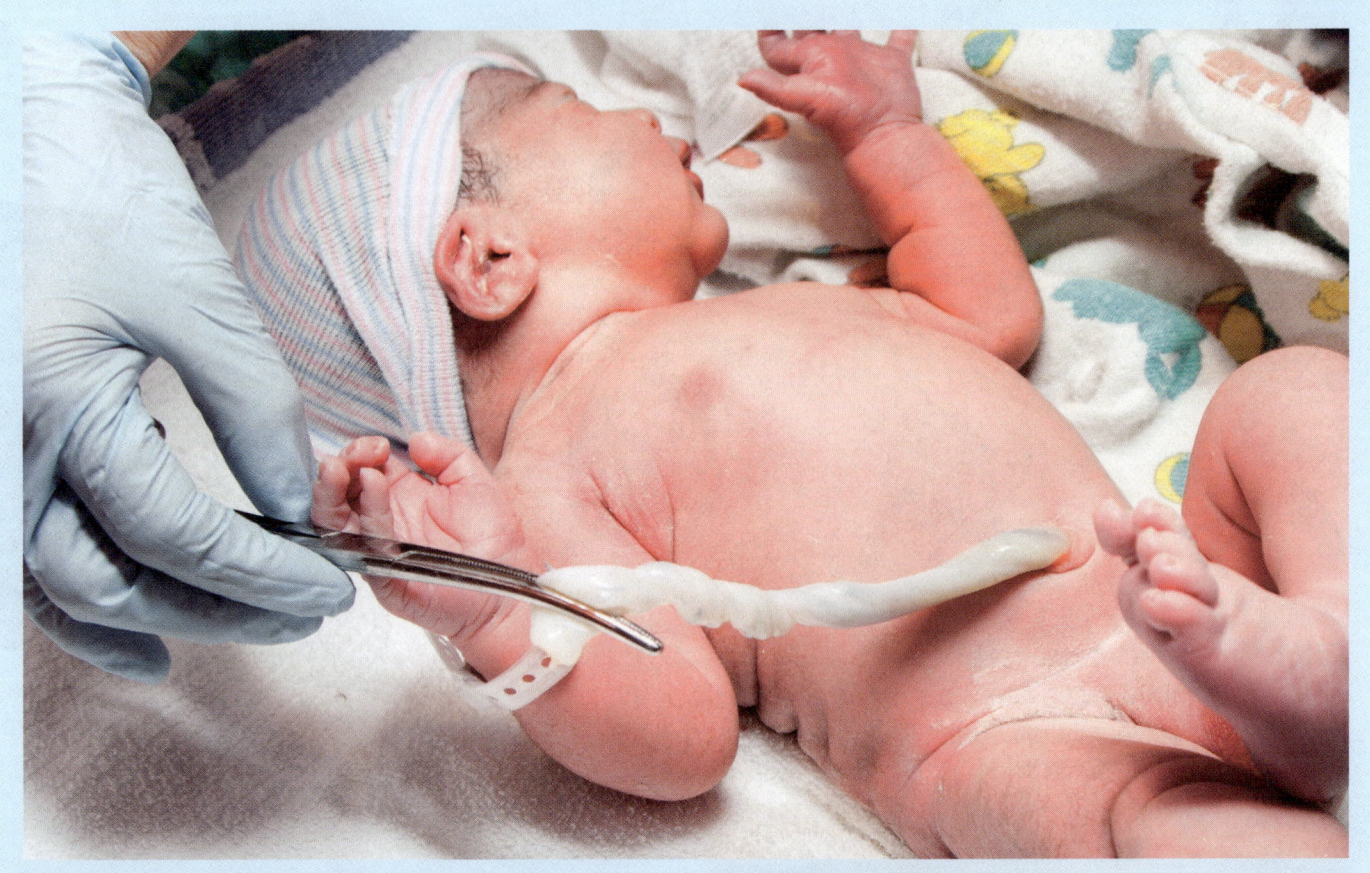

At birth, the baby's first cry starts the miraculous conversion of the fetal circulation to the baby breathing on its own. The umbilical cord, the tube that connects the mother to the baby by way of the placenta, is clamped off at birth.

Now the baby must do things on its own. What is left of your umbilical cord dries up and falls off. You don't need it any more. You are left with your wonderful belly button. Your first cry rushes oxygen into your lungs. This oxygen signals the shunts in your body to close down. They did a great job for you when you were in the womb. They are no longer needed now.

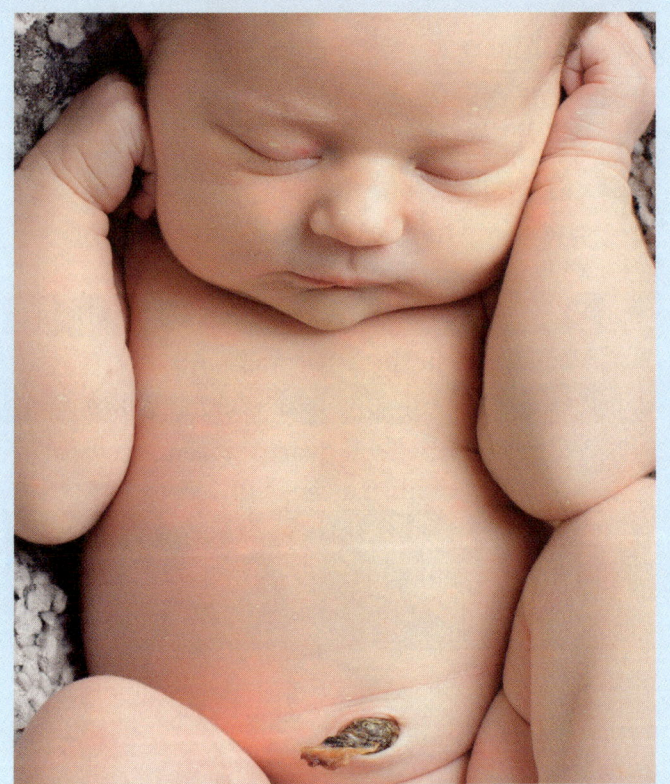

God's Wondrous Machine

The picture below illustrates fetal circulation. The five vessels in the box below (formen ovale, umbilical vein, umbilical artery, ductus arteriosus, and ductus venosus) are vessels that close down at birth. They are no longer necessary after birth.

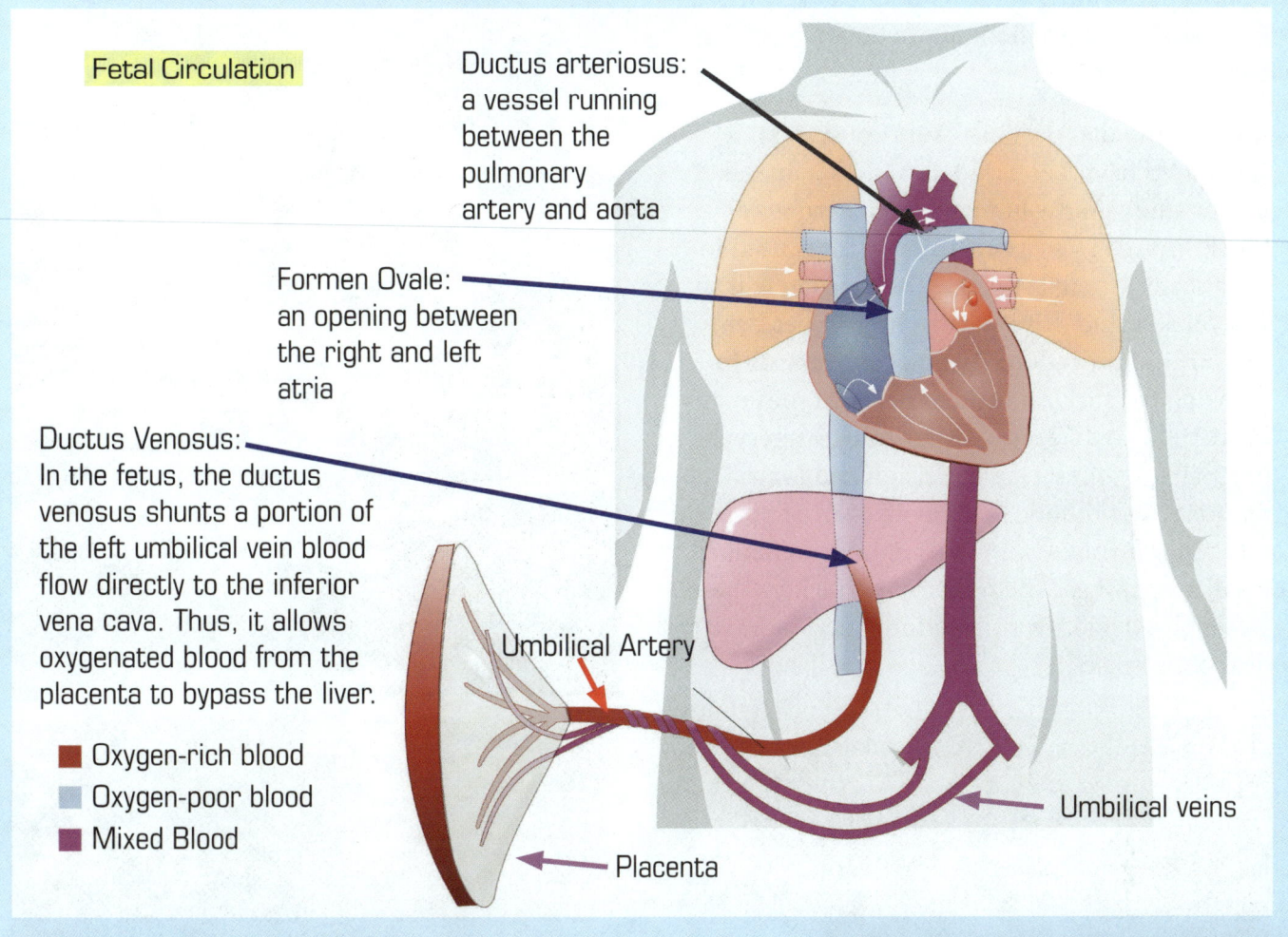

Fetal Circulation

Ductus arteriosus: a vessel running between the pulmonary artery and aorta

Formen Ovale: an opening between the right and left atria

Ductus Venosus: In the fetus, the ductus venosus shunts a portion of the left umbilical vein blood flow directly to the inferior vena cava. Thus, it allows oxygenated blood from the placenta to bypass the liver.

- Oxygen-rich blood
- Oxygen-poor blood
- Mixed Blood

Umbilical Artery

Umbilical veins

Placenta

Some children are born with heart defects. At some point when the heart was developing, it did not form correctly. You may have heard of someone who was born with a "hole" in their heart. This is a defect or hole in the walls between the ventricle or atrium. Some of the blood does not go to the lungs and goes directly from the right side of the heart to the left side. There are many different types of defects. Millions of people have been born with a heart defect, which are among the most common birth defects. Some defects don't need to be treated. For those that do, thanks to medical advances and new types of surgeries, today most are able to have the defect repaired.

Word Wise!

CONGENITAL is a word often used when talking about heart defects. It simply means that the defect has been present in the child since its birth. Sometimes the same defect can appear within multiple people in a family or within different generations of the same family.

Unit 3: The Complex Circulatory System

7 Technology

Heart Surgery Robots

Robots performing surgery? Sounds like the stuff from which science fiction movies are made. It truly is a reality!

Introducing the "da Vinci" surgical system. It is inspired from Leonardo da Vinci's namesake for his study on the human body. It is a new breakthrough in surgery. This system is used for robotically assisted surgery. The surgeon will sit at a console and drive the machine to perform the surgical procedure. The machine assists in allowing the surgical team to perform minimally invasive heart surgeries. Open-heart surgery normally requires a large incision and longer recovery. The robotic system offers an opportunity to perform the same surgery through much smaller openings. The recovery is quicker. There is less blood loss. This procedure offers a great deal of promise.

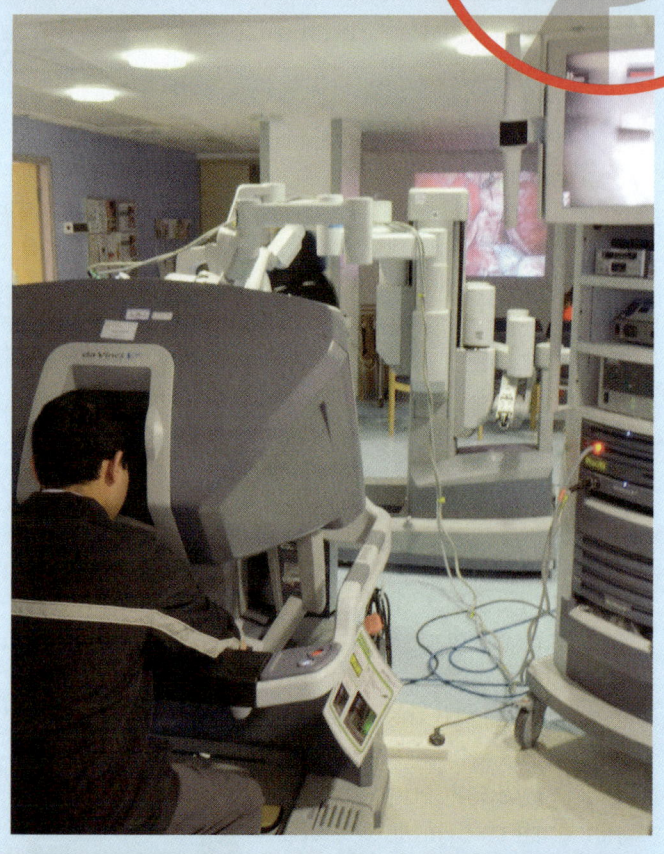

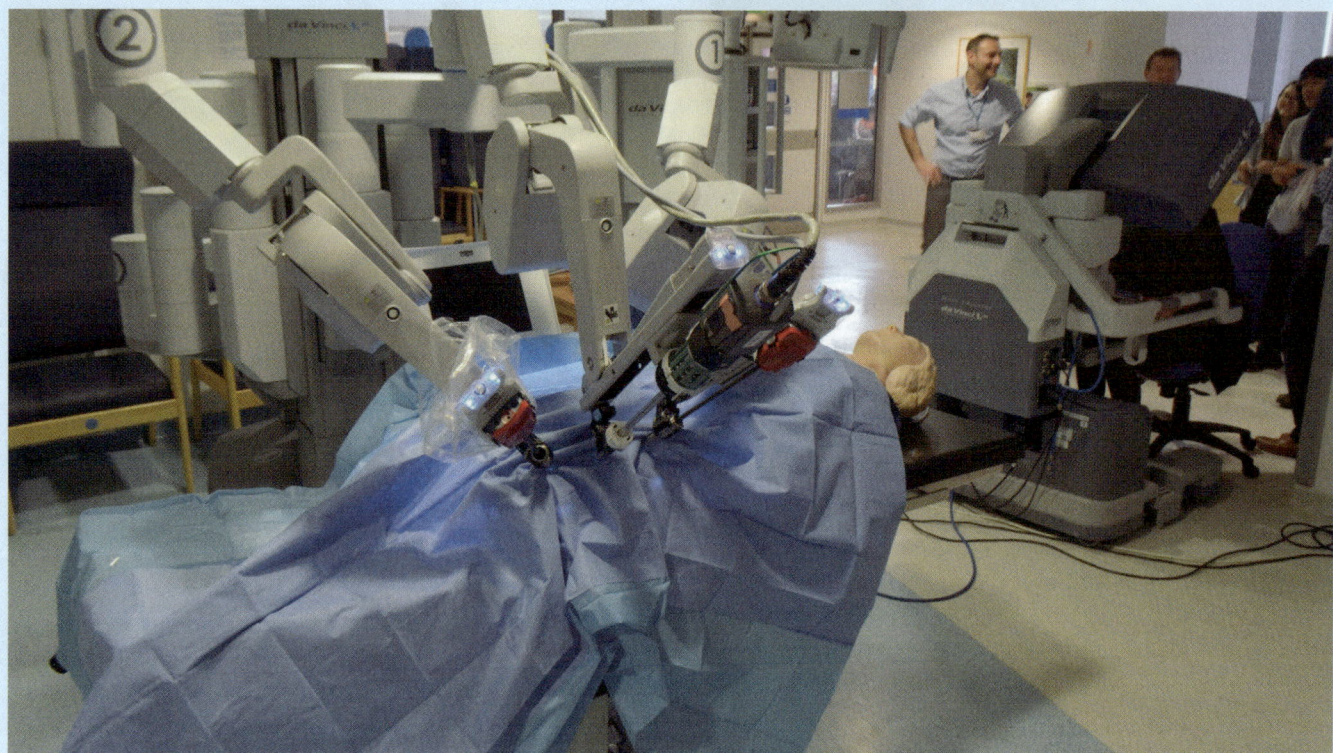

Heart-Lung Machine

The "heart-lung machine," also known as the cardiopulmonary bypass pump, has been a revolutionary invention on the forefront of saving people's lives.

Operating on a moving, beating heart is very challenging. In 1953, Dr. John Gibbon, with his wife Mary, invented the first heart-lung machine after 20 years of development.

Since the Gibbons' invention, the heart-lung machine has improved a great deal. The machine allows blood to bypass (go around) the heart while the surgeons perform delicate surgery. The machine is attached to the patient's large veins that feed into the heart. The blood is re-routed to the heart-lung machine, where oxygen is added. It is pumped back to the body at the large arteries leaving the heart. The heart can be stopped for many hours to perform complicated surgeries.

Sometimes people have problems because one or more of their heart valves do not work properly. Heart valve replacement surgery can be done to correct the problem. Patients are given either a manufactured valve or one that has been donated. A lot of people wait each year for various types of organ donations.

Heart-lung machines are very beneficial during certain heart-related surgeries, as shown below. It temporarily takes the place of the heart and lungs for the patient. Doctors have to be careful not to use it for more than 6 to 10 hours.

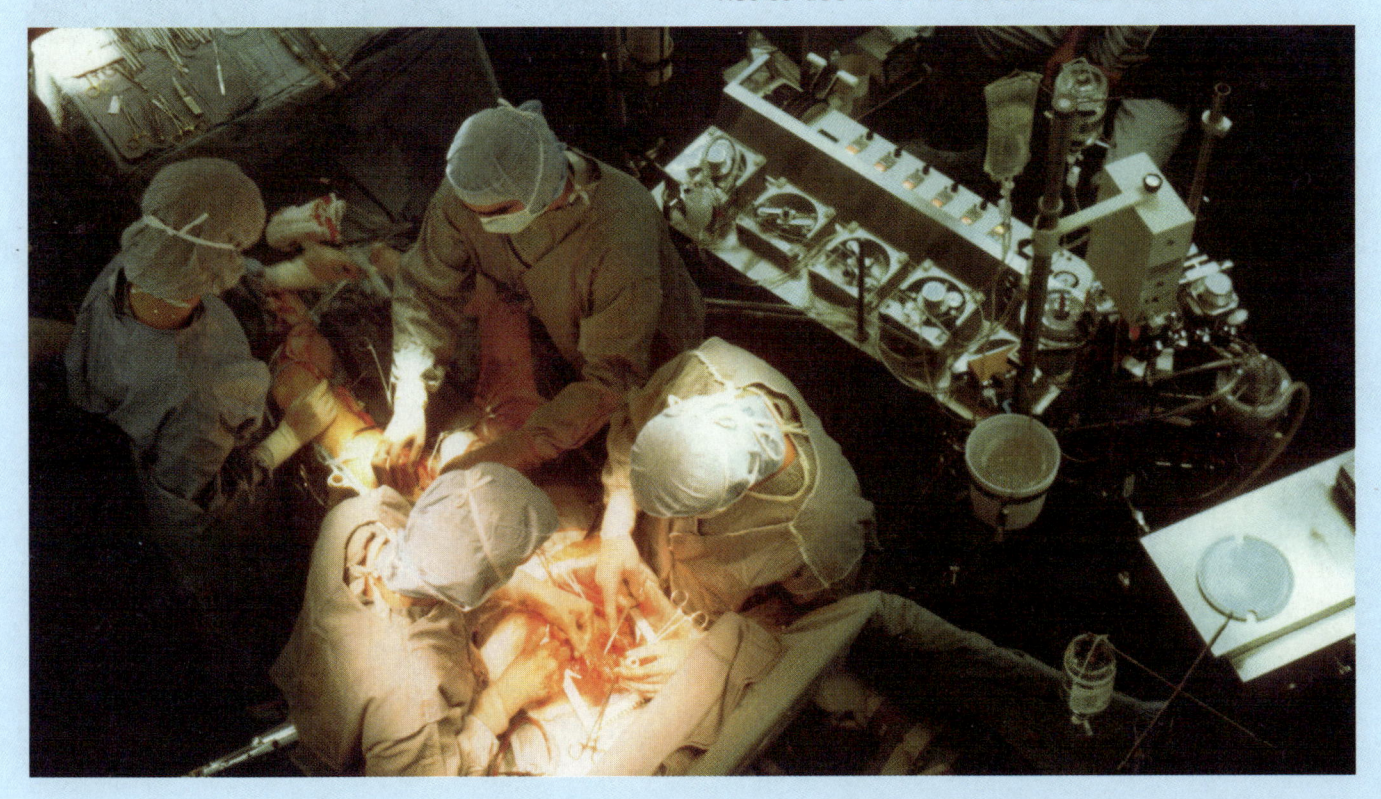

Heart Transplant

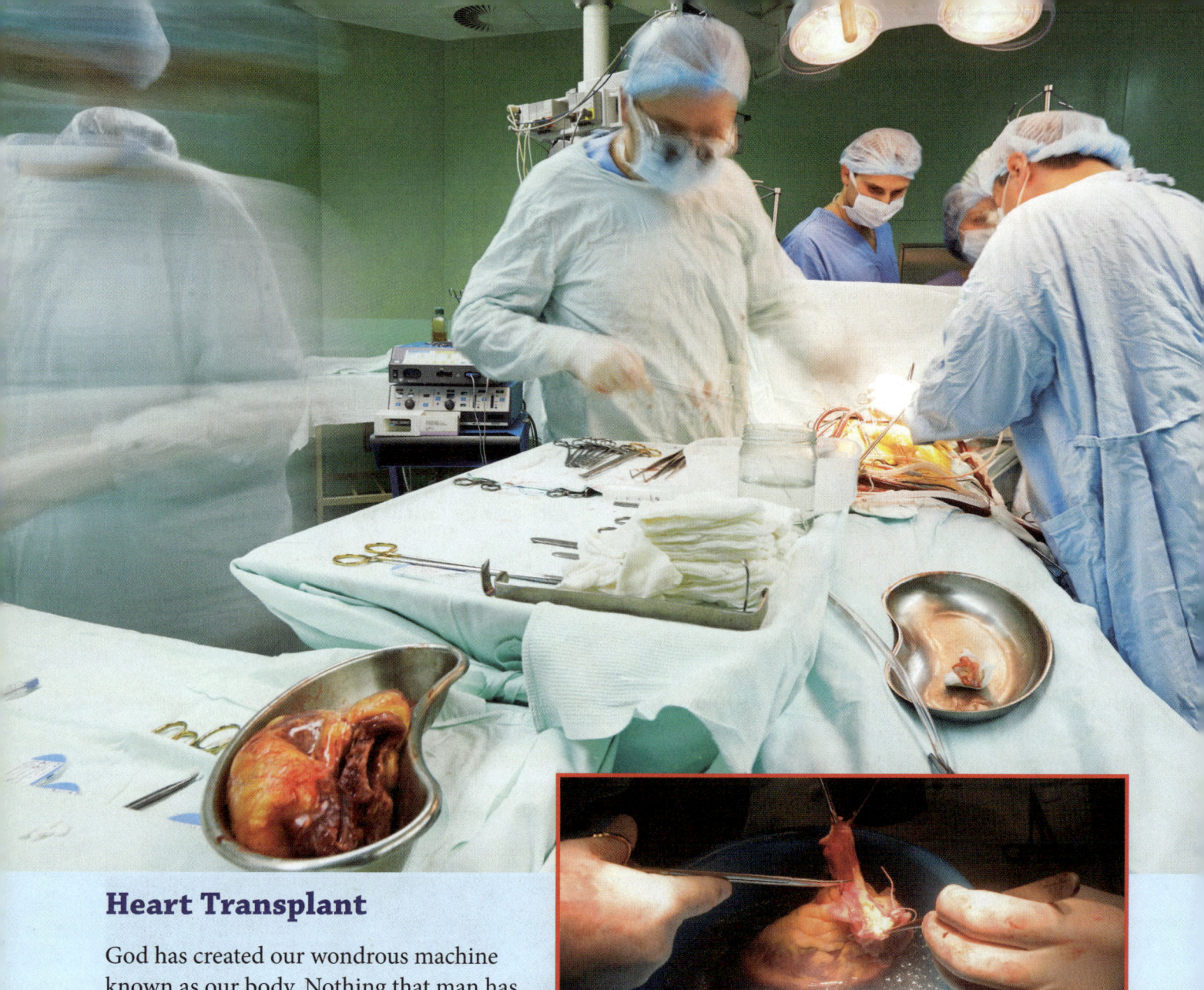

God has created our wondrous machine known as our body. Nothing that man has designed comes close. We continue to design better machines and medical devices. None has been able to perform at the level, the duration, or with the precision of God's machines. Organ transplantation has offered many a new lease on life. Sometimes organs begin to fail before the rest of the body. Failures in organs can be due to birth defects, trauma, and disease. Replacement of the diseased organ with a healthy donor organ has saved and allowed patients to live longer.

The first successful heart transplant was performed by Dr. Christiaan Bernard in 1967. It is estimated that a total of 5,000 heart transplants are performed worldwide each year, and approximately 2,000 are performed in the United States alone. The youngest heart transplant patient in the United States was little Oliver. He was born with a heart problem seven weeks early. It was a problem that would have been fatal. He underwent a heart transplant at six days of age. Dick Cheyney, former vice president of the United States, is one of the oldest recipients of a "new" heart at the age of 71.

God's Wondrous Machine

Coronary Angioplasty

The heart has its own circulatory system. The vessels that travel on the surface of the heart supply it with oxygen. These arteries can become blocked with a buildup of substances called plaque. These plugs can be composed of things like cholesterol and clotted red blood cells. These blocks can happen slowly or suddenly. An artery can become completely blocked, and a heart attack can occur.

Angioplasty can come to the rescue. Angioplasty is a procedure that can open the blocked artery and restore the blood supply. A small, thin tube with a deflated balloon is threaded through an artery in the arm or thigh, and it is floated up to the heart to the location of the blockage.

❶ The small tube is threaded into the blockage.

❷ Once within the blockage, the small balloon is inflated. This pushes the plaque and flattens it to the walls of the artery to allow the blood to flow. In addition to the balloon on the end, a wire stent can be placed over the balloon. When the balloon is inflated, the stent also expands.

❸ The stent is left in place like the scaffolding in a building.

Oliver's surgery was done after his birth, and he is doing well now. But surgeons can also perform heart surgeries on babies still in the womb. There is window of time between 18 and 30 weeks when a variety of surgical procedures can normally be done.

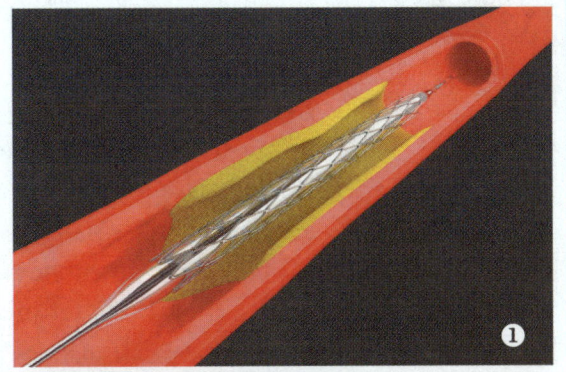

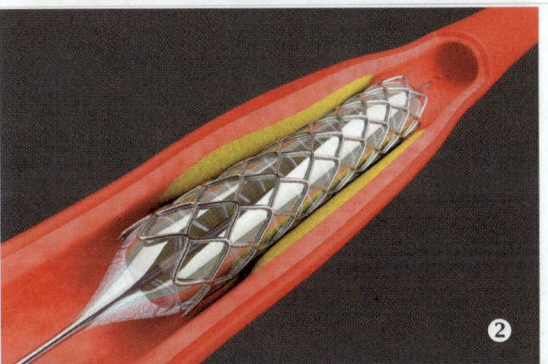

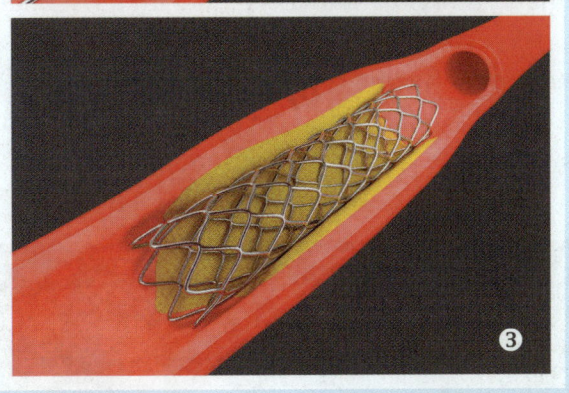

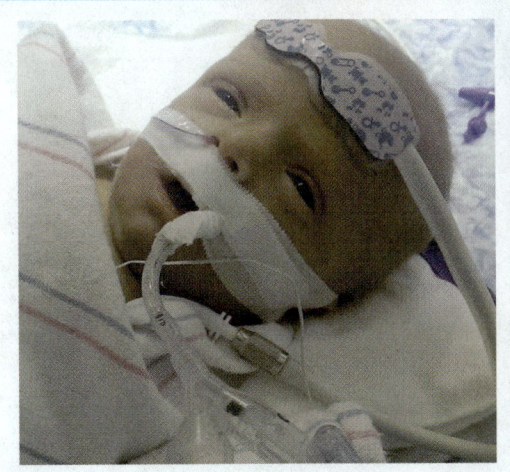

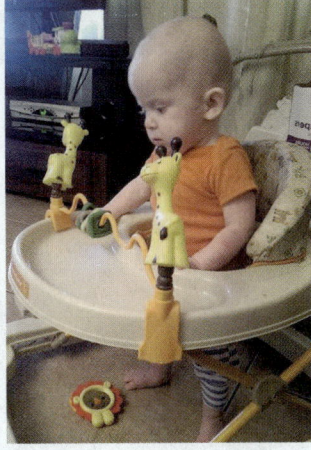

Unit 3: The Complex Circulatory System

8 An Apple a Day Keeps the Doctor Away: Good Heath

Being "heart" healthy seems to be on everyone's minds these days. There are new exercise gadgets and new diets promising good health. It is sometimes hard to discern which of these things will work best for you. There are some foolproof measures that you can do to take good care of your heart.

Get Moving!

Exercise works your heart muscle. When you engage in heart-pumping exercise, your muscles demand more blood to keep up with its demands for oxygen. There is an increased blood return to your heart. The heart muscle strengthens, and the left ventricle adapts and becomes more efficient. It will be able to eject more blood per minute per beat at work and at rest. Exercise helps with

According to National Geographic, the resting rate of Miguel Indurain, a five-time winner of the famous bike race Tour de France, was once recorded at 28 beats per minute!

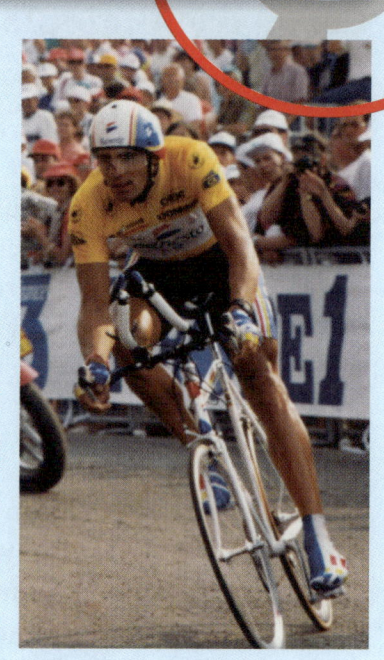

weight loss or maintaining a healthy weight. A normal resting heart rate for most adults is in a range of 60–100 beats per minute. Highly trained athletes can have heart rates as low as 40 beats per minute at rest.

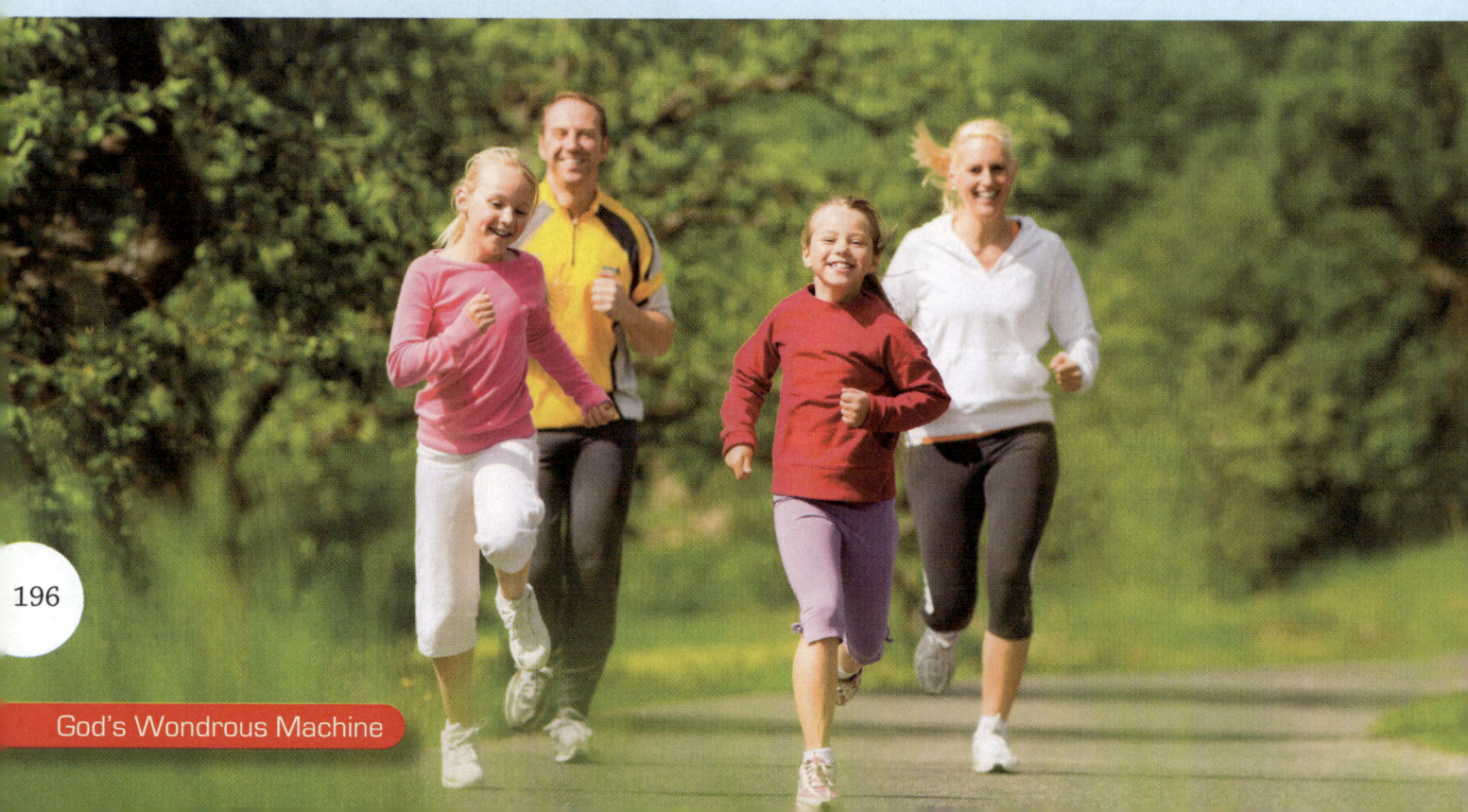

God's Wondrous Machine

Be Colorful!

Have you ever heard the expression "Eat a Rainbow"? What exactly does that mean? The whole rainbow thing is referring to placing a colorful variety of food on your plate when you eat. Eat your fruits and veggies. No, deep-fried French fries do not count. Eating fruits and vegetables is a great way to put money away in your health bank account.

God has infused fruits and vegetables with antioxidants. Antioxidants are helpful in protecting blood vessels and arteries from the damage that high cholesterol, sugar, and high starchy fatty foods can do. Eating a variety of colors gives you a variety of good stuff for your heart and body. Can you think of good healthy foods that are red, orange/yellow, purple/blue, green, white, and brown? Here are some, see if you can think of more.

- Red: tomatoes, raspberries
- Orange/yellow: squash, carrots
- Purple/blue: blueberries, eggplant
- Green: green peas, kiwi
- White: banana, pear
- Brown: lentils, almonds

Expand Your Universe

Many kids only like starchy carbohydrates like sugary cereals, white hot dog buns, and buttery crackers. Grains like whole grain breads, cereals, and pasta are good in a diet. How about expanding your universe by trading out some of that pasta and bread for a starchy vegetable? You can add corn to a tossed salad. Quinoa is a great intact whole grain. Beans and lentils make a wonderful addition to a diet.

God is our Alpha Omega: Let's Add a Bit More Omega

Fish like salmon, tuna, and herring are types of oily fish that are rich in omega-3 fatty acids. These types of omega-3 rich foods have been shown to decrease blood pressure, protect the heart, help joints in your body, and decrease unhealthy fat in your blood. Eating this type of fish once a week has its benefits.

Unit 3: The Complex Circulatory System

9 Ponder This

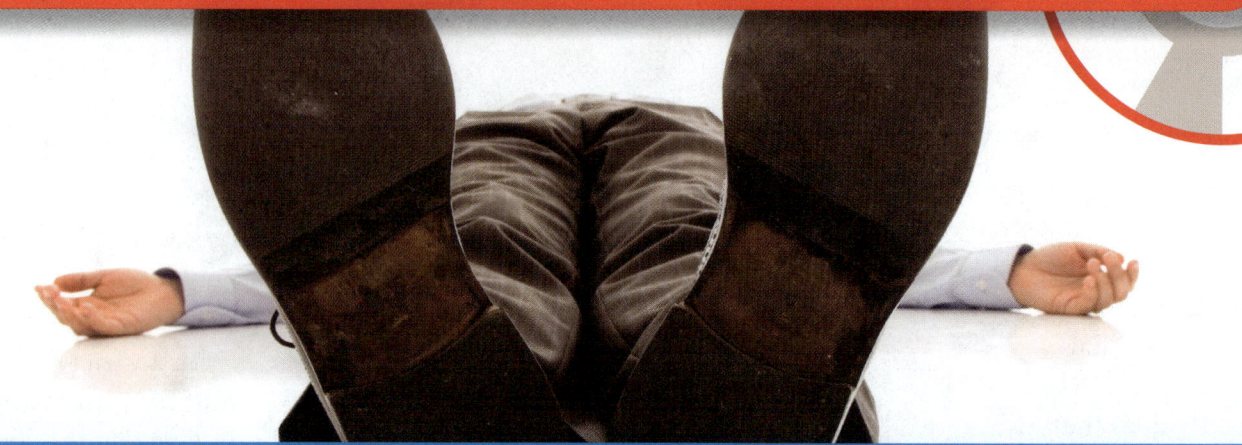

Why do some people pass out at the sight of blood?

Some people feel queasy at the sight of blood. I have even seen people pass out at the sight of a needle. They simply can't control this reaction. Fainting may have its roots in a reflex in our brain. The fancy term we doctors use in describing this phenomenon is called "vasovagal syncope." This name is derived from the vagus nerve that originates in the brain stem. In Latin, vagus means "wandering." This is a perfect name for a nerve that has many branches. One of the branches runs to the heart.

Intense emotion can activate the vagus nerve. Activation of the vagus nerve in a fainting episode causes a drop in the heart rate. It causes blood vessels to dilate, become wider. This causes a drop in blood pressure. This may be a protective reflex. If you lived in ancient times and you encountered something that could rip off your arm, a fainting response might be a good way to slow down the bleeding. You would look dead, and the animal may lose interest and walk away.

Intense emotion does not have to be unpleasant. Some people faint with intense emotional joy. Case in point — back in the 1964 when the Beatles, a rock group from Liverpool, England, came to the United States. Beatlemania was at its peak. Teenage girls would flock just to get a look at them. Young girls were passing out just at the sight of the members of the rock band.

Why do I sometimes become light-headed when I stand up fast? Why do some people pass out after standing for long periods of time?

The veins in your legs have valves, which help to keep blood from flowing backward. The contraction of the muscles in your legs, through movement, helps the blood return to your heart. The muscles squeeze the veins. When you stand for prolonged periods without moving, the blood pools in your legs and the blood return to your heart is decreased. This also means the blood flow to your brain is less. Your body responds by having you take a brief "rest." You pass out. This places you in a horizontal position. This increases the blood return to the heart. Your body is happy, and unconsciousness is of a short duration. This is a protective response.

God's Wondrous Machine

Does living at high altitudes like the mountains of Colorado have an effect on your body?

The Olympic Training Center is located in Colorado Springs, Colorado. This was chosen as the site for training high-level athletes due to its high altitude. This has been thought to improve training performance. The oxygen content of air at high altitudes is less. If you are from areas close to sea level elevation, your body will need to adapt to this high elevation. It takes approximately, on average, 3 to 5 days to adapt to a higher altitude. The bone marrow goes into high gear. It increases red blood cell production to assist with the need for additional oxygen demands of the body. A person whose body has adapted to living at high altitudes may have 30 to 50 percent more red blood cells than those who live at sea level.

What effect do chest compressions have in CPR?

CPR stands for Cardiopulmonary Resuscitation. It is an emergency procedure that a healthcare worker or Good Samaritan can perform in the event that a person's heart or breathing stops. Chest compressions help to keep the blood circulating in an effort to continue the flow of blood and oxygen to the vital organs. The healthcare worker places his or her hands one on top of the other. The hands are placed on the sternum (breastbone). Force on the sternum, pressing it approximately two inches down, compresses the heart between the hard sternum and backbone. This pushes the blood out of the heart. When the person allows the chest to recoil, blood returns to the heart. The cycle is repeated. This can be life-saving in an emergency.

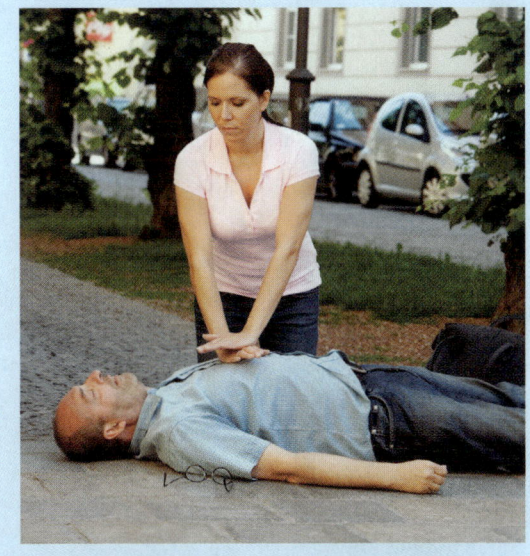

What does it mean when a blood vessel hardens?

Hardening of the arteries is called arteriosclerosis. The arteries become narrowed because fats become loaded on the inside walls. This is called plaque. This plaque grows and hardens. The plaque may even block the artery. This reduces the blood supply to areas of the body like the heart, kidneys, and other organs.

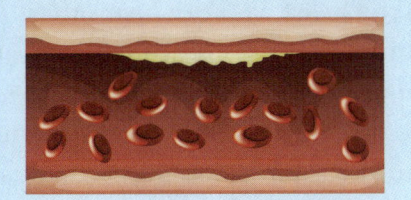

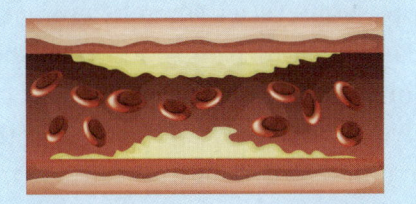

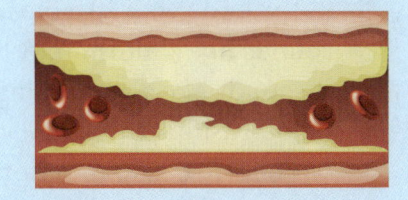

Unit 3: The Complex Circulatory System

What causes a bruise?

A bruise is caused by rupture of small blood vessels under the skin. When you slip and hit your shin on the step, the impact on your skin causes injury to the underlying vessels. Bleeding occurs under the skin, and it becomes painted with a "beautiful" rainbow of colors.

The Bruise Chart

Day 1		Red, swelling
Days 2–5		Swelling decreases, blue, black, and deep purple, RBCs begin to decay
Days 5–9		Bruise turns green to yellow, WBCs clean up the mess and dispose of decaying RBCs
10+ Days		Light brown, gets lighter and lighter

What is a heart murmur?

We describe the sounds of the heart as "lub dub." You can hear many sounds when you listen to the body with a stethoscope. Sometimes when listening to the heart, you can hear other sounds like a murmur. A heart murmur is the additional sound that can be heard with a beating. It sounds like a whooshing or swishing noise. It is a sound caused by the turbulence of the blood rushing through a valve or an abnormal opening in the heart. It can be a normal sound or abnormal sound. A normal murmur is an innocent murmur heard in some children. This murmur disappears in adulthood.

God's Wondrous Machine

Conclusion

So glad you joined up with me in awe of God's handiwork on our journey through *The Complex Circulatory System*. I don't tire talking about this wondrous creation inside you and me. As we learned, the circulatory system is indeed a vast expanse with a network of passages that stretch for 60,000 miles. There are between 20-30 trillion red blood cells in your entire body! Lets look at these numbers from another way. One million seconds is about 11.5 days. One billion seconds is about 32 years and ….wait for it….one trillion seconds is equal to approximately 32,000 years! Mind blowing. I struggle to grasp even how much 20-30 trillion must be.

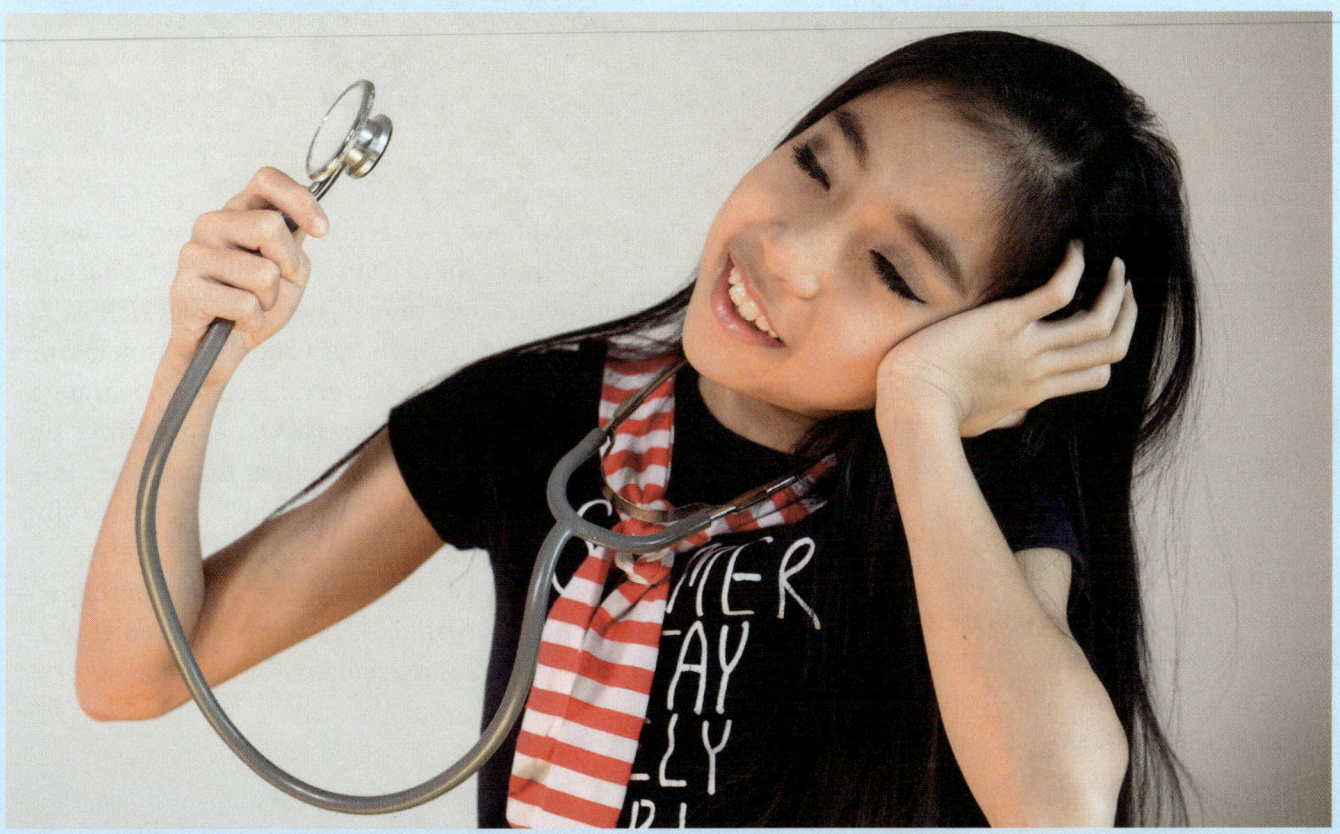

How in the world does God do it? All of this is packed in such small packages. This brings to mind the Psalms in the Bible. The Psalms are wonderful expressions of worship. In Psalm 9:1 it states, "I will praise you, O LORD, with all my heart; I will tell of all your wonders." Learning and talking about science is one of many ways to tell of God's wonders. The only object of praise when we gaze at His wonderment is our heavenly Father. Continue to wonder. Continue to praise Him. Continue to tell of His wonders.

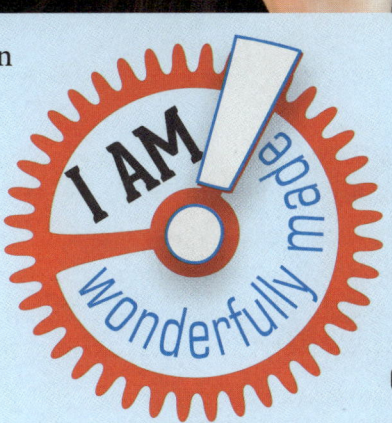

Blessed are the pure in heart, for they shall see God (Matthew 5:8).

Unit 3: The Complex Circulatory System

10 Facts: Bizarre and Gross

Thumbs Up

In ancient times, it was believed that putting blood on the right ear lobe, right thumb, and right big toe symbolically cleansed every part of a person's life. Blood on the thumb was to atone for the bad things one did. Blood on the toe was to atone for the places one went that were not God-honoring. Blood on the ear was to cover for the bad things one heard and thought.

Sleep Tight, Don't Let the Bedbugs Bite

When I was a little girl, my mother would always say to me after kissing me goodnight, "Sleep tight, don't let the bedbugs bite." I always felt warm and would slip off to sleep contently. I had no idea what that old saying meant.

This expression takes its origins back in the 1800s. Mattresses back then were made of items like straw, leaves, pine needles, or other organic type materials. The problem with beds such as these was that they were a haven for rats, mice, and bedbugs! Yikes! Bedbugs are "charming" little pests. They are insects that love to feast on the blood of animals and people. They do not fly. These little critters sure are fast. They hang out on bedding, near beds, and in walls.

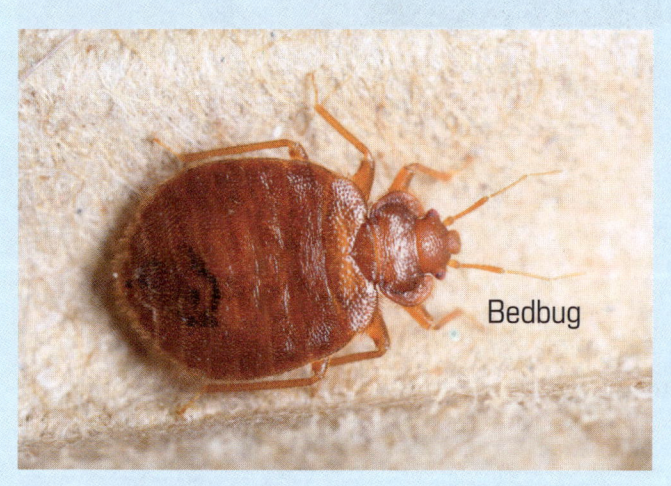

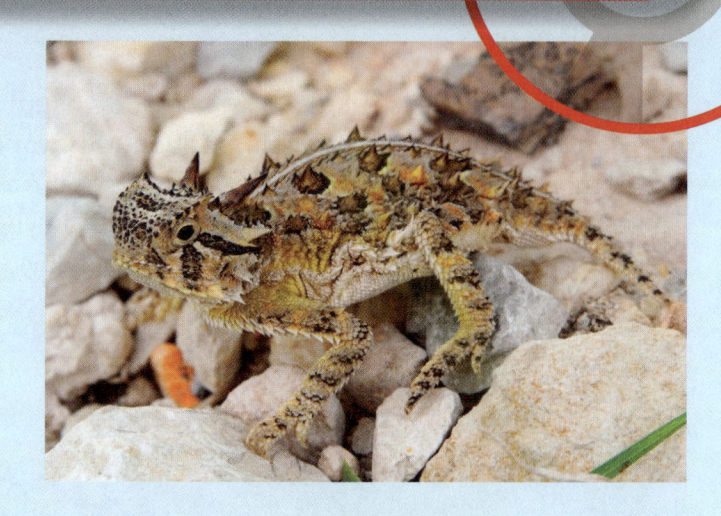

Bedbug

Blood Squirters

"Horned toads" are really horned lizards. Many people think these lizards look like frogs because their bodies are round. They eat a diet rich in harvester ants, which has venom for protection. Horned lizards have a very effective and strange way of defending themselves from predators, like coyotes, foxes, and dogs. When threatened, they actually squirt blood from their eyes. The canines hate this. It is not known why this discourages the predators so much. One theory is that perhaps some of the chemicals from the lizard's diet of harvester ants is excreted with the blood squirt.

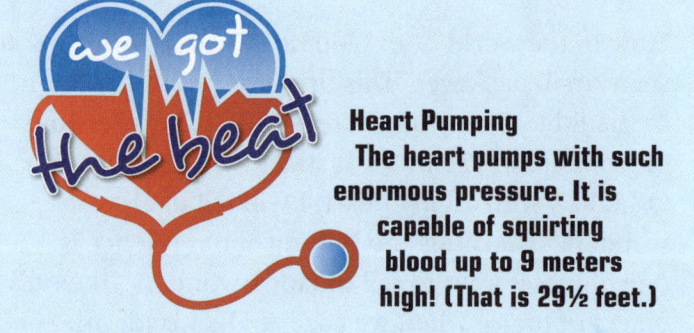

we got the beat

Heart Pumping
The heart pumps with such enormous pressure. It is capable of squirting blood up to 9 meters high! (That is 29½ feet.)

God's Wondrous Machine

Bloodless

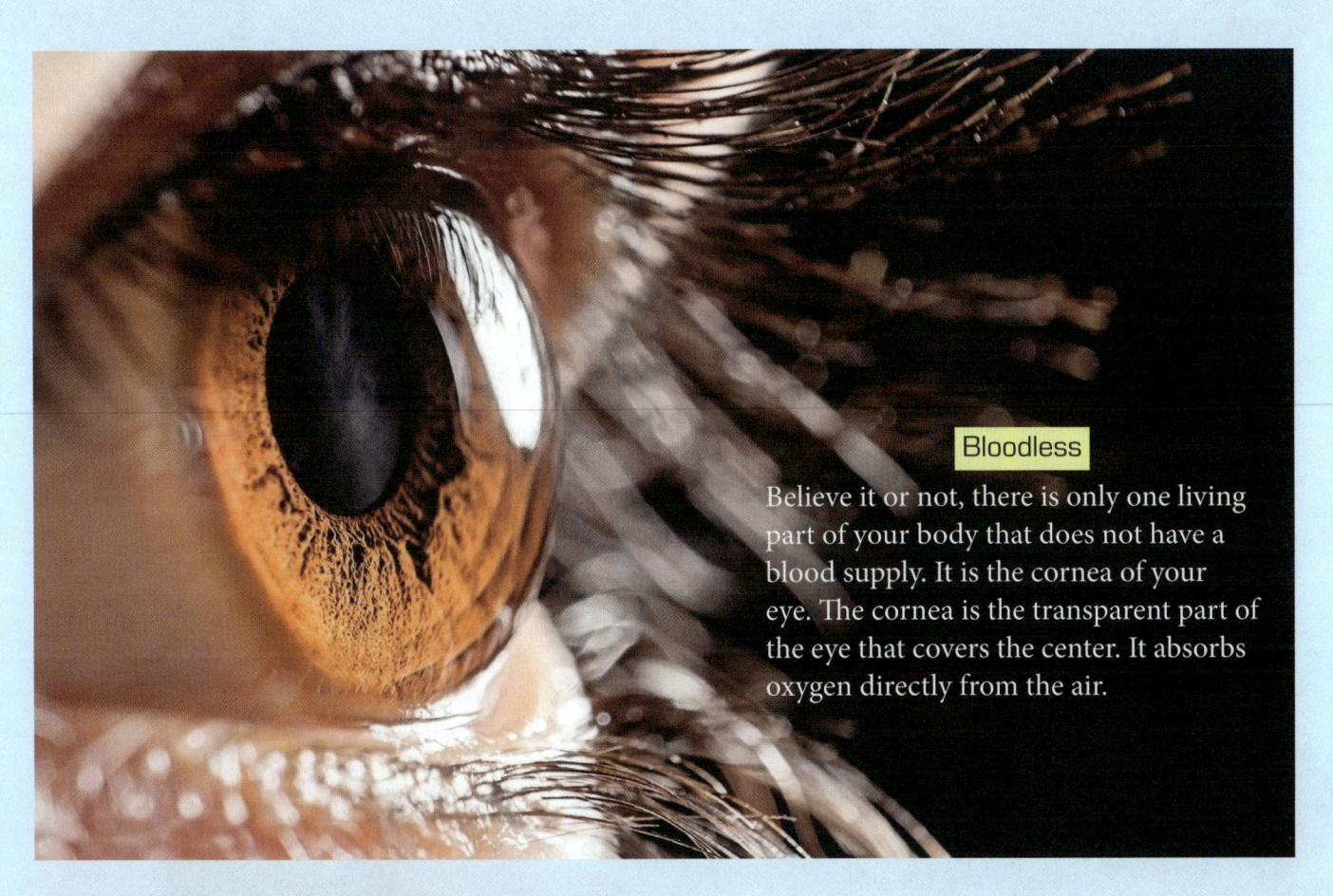

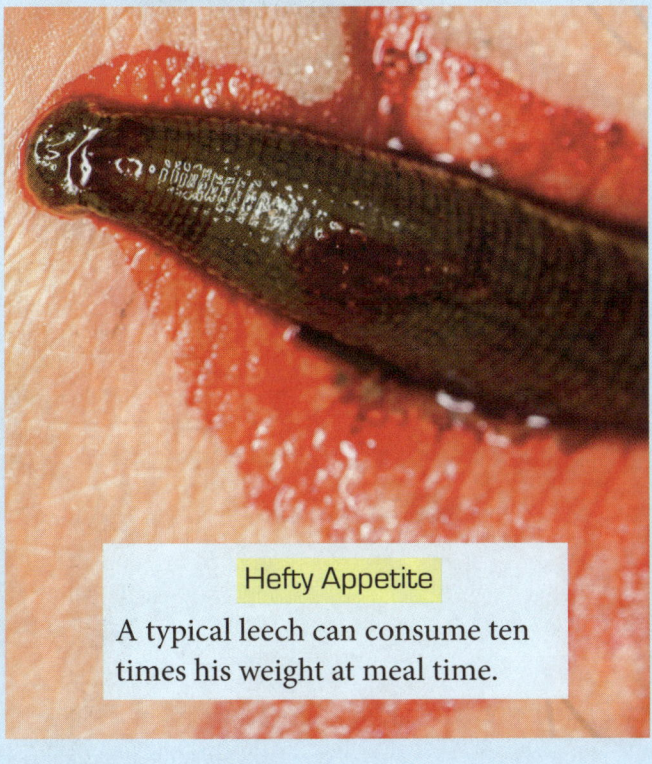

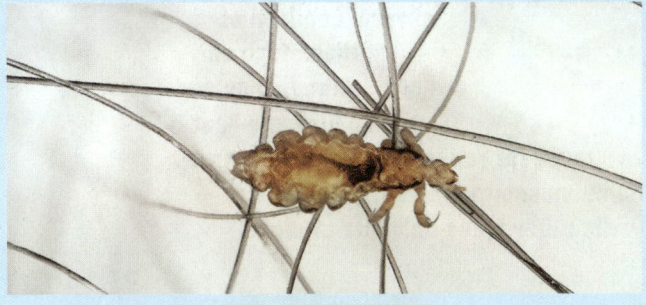

Believe it or not, there is only one living part of your body that does not have a blood supply. It is the cornea of your eye. The cornea is the transparent part of the eye that covers the center. It absorbs oxygen directly from the air.

Hefty Appetite

A typical leech can consume ten times his weight at meal time.

Feeling Lousy?

Another critter that feasts on blood is the head louse. The head louse (one is a louse; more are called lice) brings its terror by infesting and clinging to the hair of its prey. They are tiny, wingless insects that tend to love little kids. Head lice are spread by sharing hats and combs of someone infected with these little guys. They lay their eggs, called nits, close to the scalp and have easy access to a quick meal.

Unit 3: The Complex Circulatory System

11 Fun Stuff

You've Got to Be Kidding

What did Mother bat say to her daughter in the morning:	Hurry up and eat your breakfast before it clots.
Why did the young bat follow his father's profession?	Because it was in his blood.
Why should you never warm up to a snake?	Because they are cold-blooded.
Why did the mosquito go to the dentist?	To improve his bite.
What has antlers and sucks blood?	A moose-quito!
Why are mosquitos religious?	Because they prey on you.

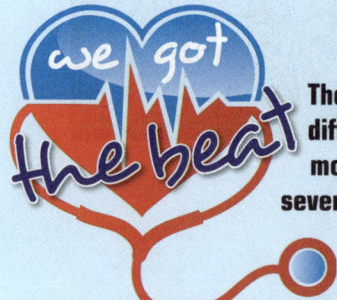

we got the beat

There are over 3000 different types of mosquitoes, but only several hundred of these type eat blood. They use your body heat to locate you when they need a meal. Some mosquitoes bite during the day while other types only bite at night!

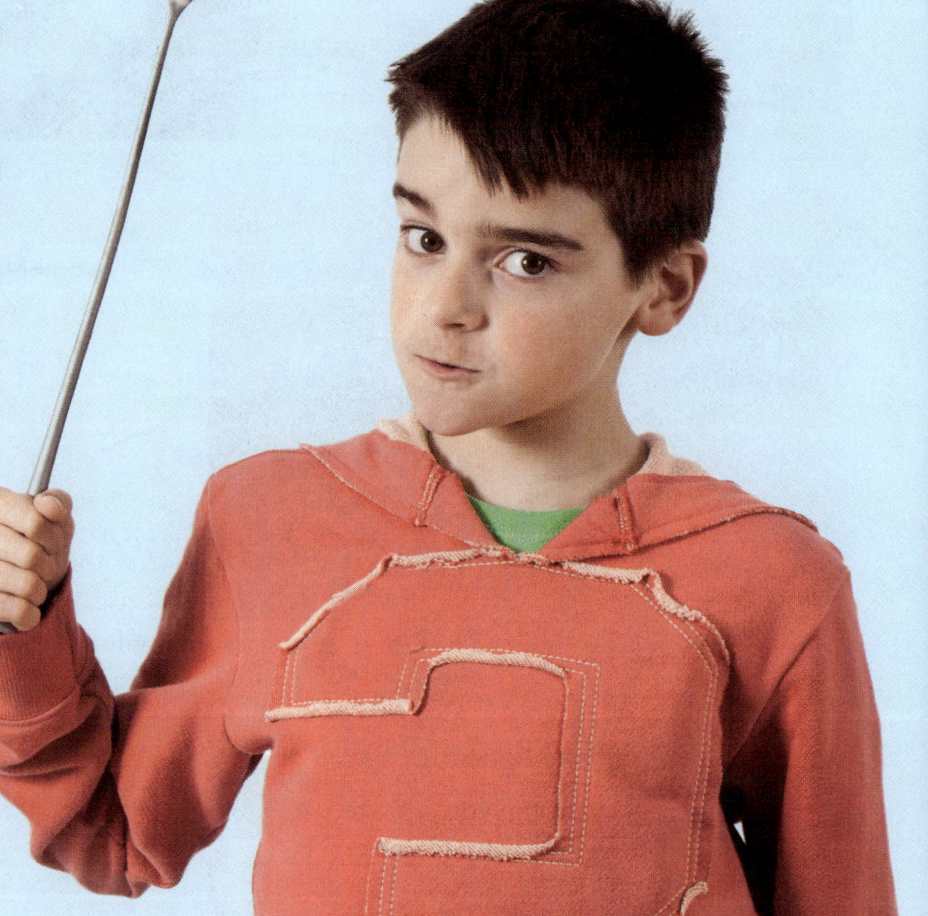

God's Wondrous Machine

Idioms: An idiom is an expression in which the words used mean something different than what they usually mean. Let's play a new game called "Fun with Idioms." You will find heart and blood idioms below. See if you can guess what they mean. See if you can stump your friends and family.

Expression	Meaning
Bleeding heart	A person considered overly emotional about political and other issues
Heart of gold	A very kind and good-natured person
Eat your heart out	Declaring, jokingly or boastfully, that someone is better than someone else
Be all heart	To be kind and generous
Faint of heart	Someone is squeamish, has an upset stomach for something that is unpleasant
Have heart in one's mouth	To feel strongly emotional about someone or something
Warm the cockles of one's heart	To give one a good warm feeling (cockles = chambers of the heart)
Wear one's heart on their sleeve	To display one's emotions openly
Give someone heart failure	To frighten someone
Heart sinks	Feel sad or worried
Half-hearted	Without energy or enthusiasm
Enshrine someone in one's heart	To keep someone's memory alive
Bad blood	Unpleasant feeling, or having a dislike for another person
Be after blood	Actively pursuing someone in order to punish them
Flesh and blood	One of your relatives
Blood in the water	Exposure of a competitive weakness in an opponent that makes the other increasingly aggressive, like sharks on the attack when blood is in the water
Blood is thicker than water	People who are related have stronger feeling to each other than to nonfamily members
Blood is up	Angry
Blood run cold	To be very frightened
Blue blood	A person of royal lineage or wealthy ancestry
Burst a blood vessel	To exert a great deal of effort doing something
Curdle blood	To frighten someone severely
New blood	A new person
Too rich for my blood	Too expensive for one's budget, or too high in fat to eat

Unit 3: The Complex Circulatory System

Heartfelt Quotes!

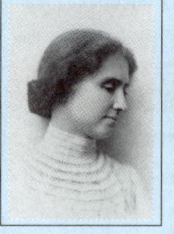

"The best and most beautiful things in the world cannot be seen or even touched — they must be felt with the heart."
—Helen Keller

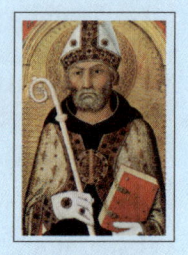

"Sometimes the heart sees what is invisible to the eye."
—H. Jackson Brown, Jr.

"The greatest test of courage on earth is to bear defeat without losing heart."
Robert Green Ingersoll

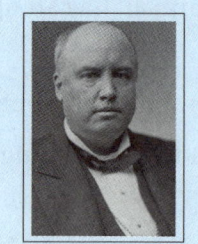

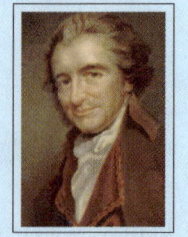

"There is no charm equal to tenderness of heart."
—Jane Austen

"Have a heart that never hardens, and a temper that never tires, and a touch that never hurts."
—Charles Dickens

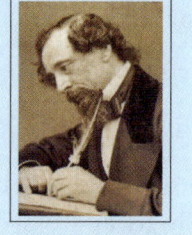

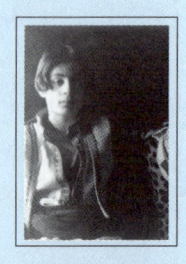

"Only God can perform a spiritual heart transplant."
—Woodrow Kroll

"Because God has made us for Himself, our hearts are restless until they rest in Him."
—Augustine of Hippo

"I love the man that can smile in trouble, that can gather strength from distress, and grow brave by reflection. 'Tis the business of little minds to shrink, but he whose heart is firm, and whose conscience approves his conduct, will pursue his principles unto death."
—Thomas Paine

"Wise leaders should have known that the human heart cannot exist in a vacuum. If Christians are forbidden to enjoy the wine of the Spirit they will turn to the wine of the flesh. . . . Christ died for our hearts and the Holy Spirit wants to come and satisfy them."
—A.W. Tozer

"Faith is knowledge within the heart, beyond the reach of proof."
—Khalil Gibran

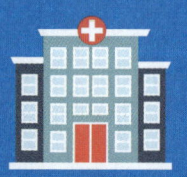

- 5 million patients in the U.S. need blood every year
- Every 2 seconds someone needs a blood transfusion
- 1 pint of blood can save up to 3 lives

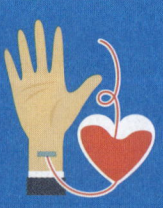

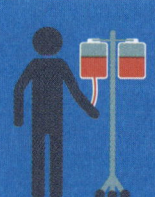

God's Wondrous Machine

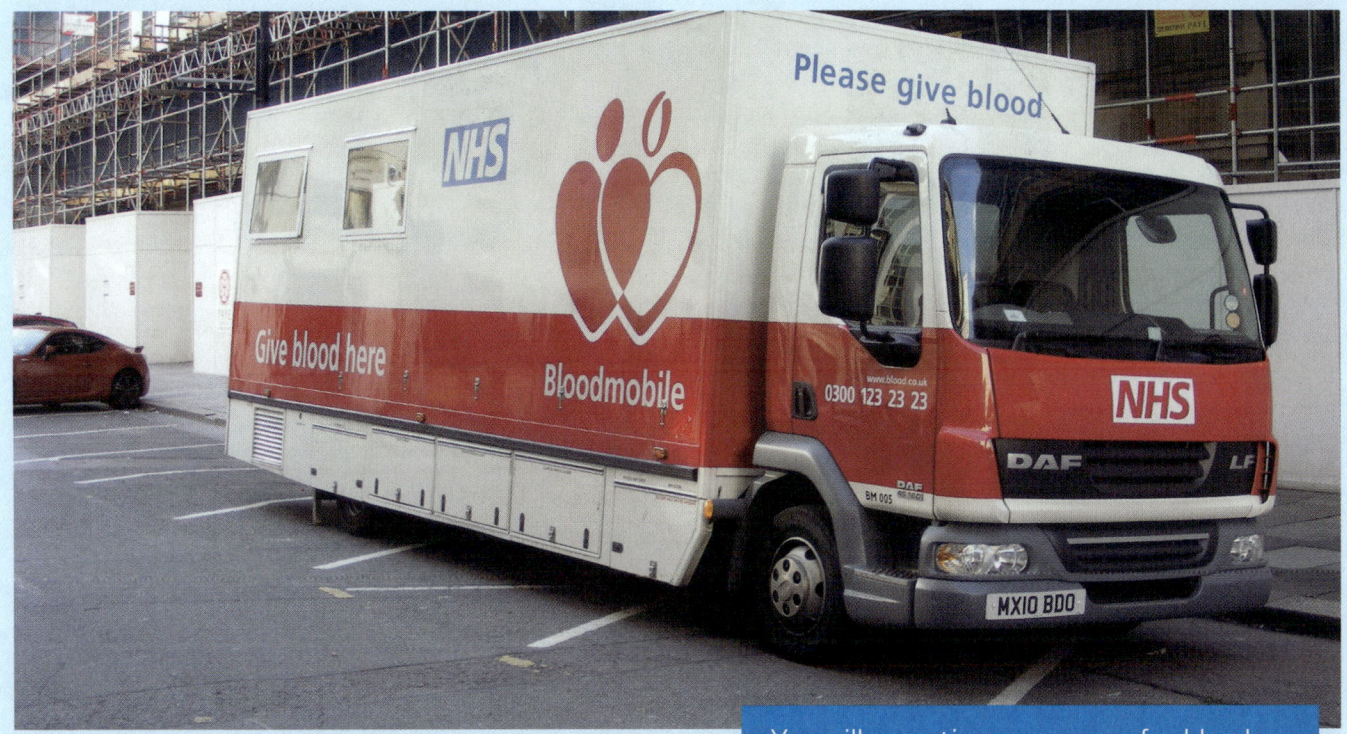

"There is a God-shaped vacuum in the heart of every man which cannot be filled by any created thing, but only by God, the Creator, made known through Jesus."
—Blaise Pascal

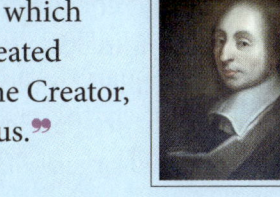

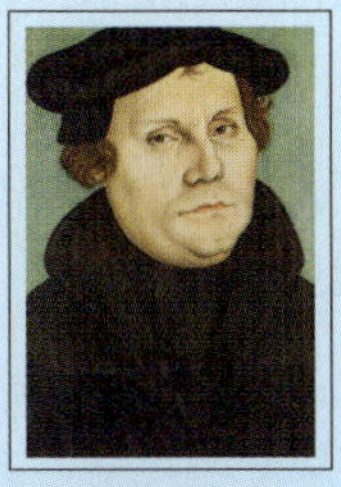

"Grant that I may not pray alone with the mouth; help me that I may pray from the depths of my heart."
—Martin Luther

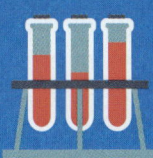

You will sometimes see vans for blood donations in your area. Close to 80% of blood donations that the American Red Cross receives come from these mobile collection sites. You have to meet age and health requirements before you can become a blood donor. According to the American Red Cross, every two seconds someone in the United States will need a blood donation, and around 15.7 million blood donations are collected each year. Donors are vital because blood cannot be created or manufactured.

- Less than 38% of the population is eligible to give blood
- Blood cannot be manufactured; it can only come from donors 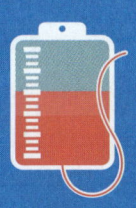
- HONORARY donor
- Donors can give blood every 56 days

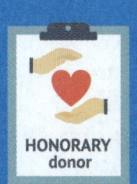

Unit 3: The Complex Circulatory System

MEDI+MOMENT

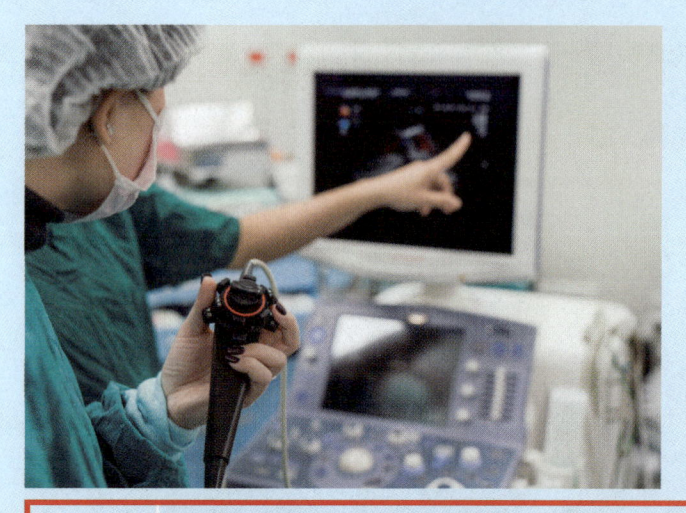

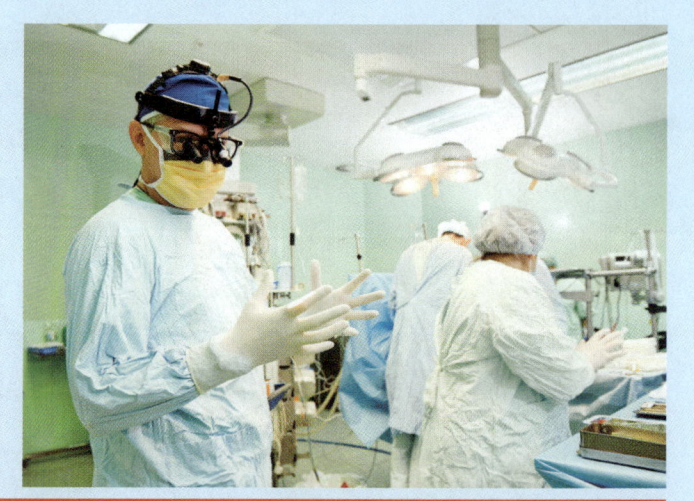

Medical careers can include a lot of different kinds of jobs, including many focused on the heart and circulatory system. Here are just a few:

Biomedical Equipment Technicians	Works in healthcare settings, install, inspect, maintain, repair, modify, and design medical equipment. For example, a perfusionist would operate and manage the heart-lung machine during surgery.
Cardiovascular Technicians	Assist doctors in diagnosing and treating heart and blood vessel problems. They can assist during heart surgery or procedures
Diagnostic Medical Sonographers	Use very specialized equipment that constructs images of the structures in the body that aid doctors in making decisions and diagnosis of problems. They use a machine called an ultrasound. Ultrasound sends sound waves in the body that are painless to the patient. These sound waves bounce off the internal organs. The sound waves are analyzed by a computer and displayed on a screen.
Phlebotomists	People trained to draw blood from a patient for clinical or medical testing, transfusions, donations, or research.
Cardiologist	A doctor that specializes in the care of the heart and blood vessels. There are even pediatric cardiologists. They take care of kids' heart issues.
Cardiovascular Surgeon	Doctors who operate on heart and blood vessels. They repair damage caused by diseases or disorders of the cardiovascular system.
Cardiovascular Rehabilitation Specialist	This specialists work with people who are recovering from heart surgery or people who have heart and lung problems. They educate and design exercise programs to strengthen and improve the health of their patients.

God's Wondrous Machine

Heart Disease Factors

You can make important choices that help keep your heart healthy! Here are a list of things that can play a role in whether you are at risk for heart disease when you become an adult.

Age		Heart disease can occur at any age, but usually affects people as they get older.	Obesity		Being overweight can lead to high blood pressure and diabetes.
Gender		Men have a higher risk of heart disease than women at any age.	Family History		A risk of heart disease can be inherited from your biological parents.
Tobacco		The chemicals in it hurt the heart, blood cells, and lungs.	Blood Pressure		If it is too high, it can damage blood vessels, making them clogged or weak.
Physical Inactivity		Your heart is a muscle. Thirty minutes a day, five days a week make it stronger.	Diabetes		This impacts insulin levels so your body can't create the fuel it needs.
Alcohol		Drinking raises blood pressure and creates unhealthy fat levels in the blood.	Cholesterol		Too much of it can clog or block your arteries.
Unhealthy Diet		Too much salt, fat, or sugar keeps your body from working at its best.	Stress		This can cause your blood pressure to be too high to be healthy.

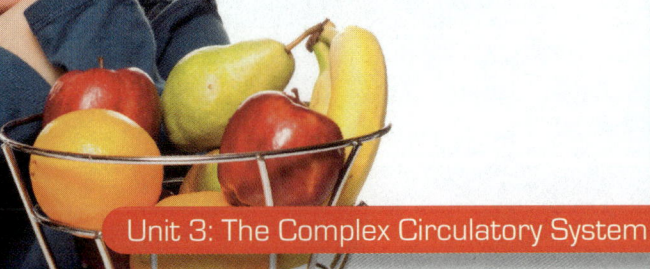

Unit 3: The Complex Circulatory System

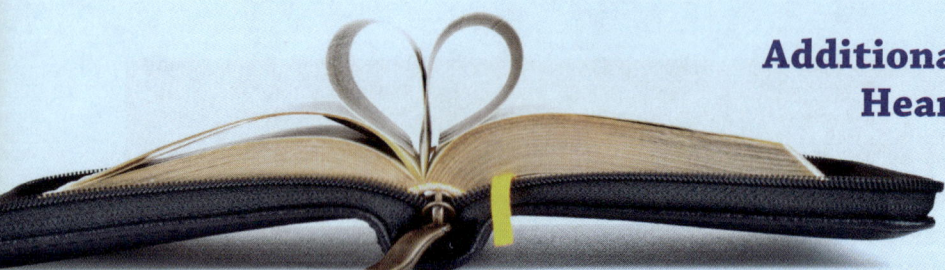

Additional Bible Verses on Heart and Blood

Scripture in this section is from the English Standard Version (ESV)

HEART	Jeremiah 17:10	I the Lord search the heart and test the mind, to give every man according to his ways, according to the fruit of his deeds.
	Matthew 5:8	Blessed are the pure in heart, for they shall see God.
	Hebrews 4:12	For the word of God is living and active, sharper than any two-edged sword, piercing to the division of soul and of spirit, of joints and of marrow, and discerning the thoughts and intentions of the heart.
	Proverbs 3:5–6	Trust in the Lord with all your heart, and do not lean on your own understanding. In all your ways acknowledge him, and he will make straight your paths.
	Psalm 34:18	The Lord is near to the brokenhearted and saves the crushed in spirit.
	James 4:8	Draw near to God, and he will draw near to you. Cleanse your hands, you sinners, and purify your hearts, you double-minded
	1 Samuel 16:7	But the Lord said to Samuel, "Do not look on his appearance or on the height of his stature, because I have rejected him. For the Lord sees not as man sees: man looks on the outward appearance, but the Lord looks on the heart"
	1 Timothy 1:5	The aim of our charge is love that issues from a pure heart and a good conscience and a sincere faith
	Psalm 26:2	Prove me, O Lord, and try me; test my heart and my mind
	2 Timothy 2:22.	So flee youthful passions and pursue righteousness, faith, love, and peace, along with those who call on the Lord from a pure heart
	Hebrews 10:22	Let us draw near with a true heart in full assurance of faith, with our hearts sprinkled clean from an evil conscience and our bodies washed with pure water
	1 Thessalonians 2:4	But just as we have been approved by God to be entrusted with the gospel, so we speak, not to please man, but to please God who tests our hearts
	Psalm 119:10	With my whole heart I seek you; let me not wander from your commandments!
	Proverbs 16:1	The plans of the heart belong to man, but the answer of the tongue is from the Lord
	Matthew 11:29	Take my yoke upon you, and learn from me, for I am gentle and lowly in heart, and you will find rest for your souls

God's Wondrous Machine

HEART	Luke 16:15	And he said to them, "You are those who justify yourselves before men, but God knows your hearts. For what is exalted among men is an abomination in the sight of God
	Proverbs 22:11	He who loves purity of heart, and whose speech is gracious, will have the king as his friend
	Proverbs 6:18	. . . a heart that devises wicked plans, feet that make haste to run to evil
	Ezekiel 11:19–21	And I will give them one heart, and a new spirit I will put within them. I will remove the heart of stone from their flesh and give them a heart of flesh, that they may walk in my statutes and keep my rules and obey them. And they shall be my people, and I will be their God. But as for those whose heart goes after their detestable things and their abominations, I will bring their deeds upon their own heads, declares the Lord God
	Proverbs 17:3	The crucible is for silver, and the furnace is for gold, and the Lord tests hearts
	Proverbs 14:30	A tranquil heart gives life to the flesh, but envy makes the bones rot
	Psalm 84:2	My soul longs, yes, faints for the courts of the Lord; my heart and flesh sing for joy to the living God
	Ephesians 3:14–20	For this reason I bow my knees before the Father, from whom every family in heaven and on earth is named, that according to the riches of his glory he may grant you to be strengthened with power through his Spirit in your inner being, so that Christ may dwell in your hearts through faith — that you, being rooted and grounded in love, may have strength to comprehend with all the saints what is the breadth and length and height and depth
	Psalm 119:11	I have stored up your word in my heart, that I might not sin against you
BLOOD	1 John 5:6	This is the one who came by water and blood — Jesus Christ; not by the water only but by the water and the blood. And the Spirit is the one who testifies, because the Spirit is the truth
	1 John 1:7	But if we walk in the light, as he is in the light, we have fellowship with one another, and the blood of Jesus his Son cleanses us from all sin
	Romans 5:9	Since, therefore, we have now been justified by his blood, much more shall we be saved by him from wrath of God
	1 Peter 1:1–2	To those…according to the foreknowledge of God the Father, in the sanctification of the Spirit, for obedience to Jesus Christ and for sprinkling with his blood: may grace and peace be multiplied to you
	Matthew 26:28	… for this is my blood of the covenant, which is poured out for many for the forgiveness of sins

Unit 3: The Complex Circulatory System

Bibliography

Adler, Robert E. *Medical Firsts: From Hippocrates to the Human Genome.* Hoboken, NJ: John Wiley and Sons, 2004.

Aliki. *My Five Senses.* New York: Crowell, 1989.

Allison, Linda. *Blood and Guts.* New York: Yolla Bolly Press, 1992.

Alton, Steve. *Blood and Goo and Boogers Too! A Heart-Pounding Pop-up Guide to the Circulatory and Respiratory Systems.* New York: Dial Books, 2008.

Artell, Mike. *Backyard Bloodsuckers: Questions, Facts and Tongue Twisters About Creepy, Crawly Creatures.* Parsippany, NJ: Good Year Books, 2000.

Barnhill, Kelly Regan. *The Bloody Book of Blood.* Mankato, MN: Edge Books/Capstone, 2010.

Barnhill, Kelly R. *Sick, Nasty Medical Practices.* Makato, MN: Capstone Press, 2009.

Beccia, Carlyn. *I Feel Better with a Frog in My Throat.* New York: Harcourt Publishing Company, 2010.

Becker, Christine. *Gross Anatomy.* Toronto, Canada: RGA Publishing Group, Inc., 1996.

"blood"— *McGraw-Hill's Dictionary of American Slang and Colloquial Expressions.* 2006. McGraw-Hill Companies, Inc. 27 Aug. 2015, http://idioms.thefreedictionary.com/blood.

Bragg, Georgia. *How They Croaked: The Awful Ends of the Awfully Famous.* New York, NY: Bloomsbury Publishing, 2011.

Branzei, Sylvia. *Grossology and You: Really Gross Things About Your Body.* New York: Penguin Putnam Inc., 2002.

Branzei, Sylvia. *Really Gross Things About Your Body.* New York, NY: Penguin Putnam, 2002.

Brynie, Faith Hickman. *101 Questions About Blood and Circulation with Answers Straight From the Heart.* Brookfield, CT: Millbrook Press, 2001.

Brynie, Faith Hickman. *101 Questions About Sleep and Dreams That Kept You Awake Nights . . . Until Now.* Minneapolis, MN: Twenty-First Century Books, 2006.

Carter, Rita, Susan Aldridge, Martyn Page, Steve Parker. *Human Brain Book.* New York: Dorling-Kindersley Publishing, 2009.

Childress, Kim. *Wacky Bible Gross Outs.* Grand Rapids, MI: Zonderkidz, 2014.

Claybourne, Anna. *100 Most Disgusting Things on the Planet.* New York, NY: Scholastic, 2010.

Conley, Kate A. *Joseph Priestley and the Discovery of Oxygen,* Hockessin, DE: Mitchell Lane Publishers, 2006.

Cunningham, Kevin. *Disease in History: Flu.* Greensboro, NC: Morgan Reynolds Publishing, Inc., 2009.

Cunningham, Kevin. *Pandemics.* New York, NY: Scholastic Inc., 2012.

Dawson, Ian. *The History of Medicine, Prehistoric and Egyptian Medicine,* New York, NY: Enchanted Lion Books, 2005.

De La Bedoyere, Camilla. *Ripley's Human Body: Believe it or Not!* Bromall, PA: Mason Crest, 2011.

Dendy, Leslie, and Mel Boring. *Guinea Pig Scientists: Bold Self-Experimenters in Science and Medicine.* New York, NY: Henry Holt and Company, 2005.

Despopoulos, Agamemnon, and Stefan Sibernagl. *Color Atlas of Physiology.* New York: Thieme Medical Publishing, 1991.

Diamond, Marian C., Arnold B. Scheibel, and Lawrence M. Elson. *The Human Brain Coloring Book.* New York: Barnes and Noble Books, 1985.

DiConsiglio, John. *Blood Suckers! Deadly Mosquito Bites.* New York, NY: Franklin Watts, 2008.

Ditkoff, Beth Ann, Andrea Ditkoff, and Julia Ditkoff. *Why Don't Your Eyelashes Grow? Curious Questions Kids Ask About the Human Body.* New York, NY: Penguin Group, 2008.

Dorland's Illustrated Medical Dictionary. Philadelphia, PA: W.B. Saunders Company, 1994.

Dowswell, Paul. *Medicine.* Chicago, IL: Reed Educational and Professional Publishing, 2002.

Eldon, Dorry. *Lyrical Life Science: Volume 3 — The Human Body,* Corvallis, OR: Lyrical Learning, 1998.

Emery, Joanna. *Gross and Disgusting Things About the Human Body.* Canada: Blue Bike Books, 2007.

Evans, Michael, and David Wichman. *The Adventures of Medical Man: Kids' Illnesses and Injuries Explained.* Buffalo, NY: Annick Press, 2010.

Fardon, John. *1000 Things You Should Know About: Human Body.* Essex, UK: Miles Kelly Publishing, 2000.

Ferguson Books. *Careers in Focus: Medical Technicians and Technologists.* New York, NY: Infobase Publishing, 2009.

Fleischman, John. *Phineas Gage: A Gruesome, but True Story About Brain Science.* New York: Scholastic, 2003.

Fleming, Deena. *More Gross Jokes.* New York, NY: Tangerine Press, 2005.

Foster, Michael, and Patricia Twohey. *The Human Body.* Greensboro, NC: The Education Center Inc., 2000.

Fradin, Dennis. *Medicine: Yesterday, Today and Tomorrow.* Chicago, IL: Children's Press, 1989.

Getz, David. *Purple Death: The Mysterious Flu of 1918.* New York, NY: Henry Holt and Company, 2000.

Gleason, Carrie. *Feasting Bedbugs, Mice, and Ticks.* New York, NY: Crabtree Publishing, 2011.

Guyton, Arthur. Basic *Neuroscience*. Philadelphia, Pennsylvania: W.B. Saunders Co., 1992.

Haslam, Andrew. *Make it Work! Body*. Chicago, IL: World Book Inc., 1998.

Helleman, A., and Bryan H. Bunch. *The Timetables of Science: A Chronology of the Most Important People and Events in the History of Science*. New York: Simon and Schuster, 1991.

Herlihy, Barbara L., and Nancy K. Maebius. *The Human Body in Health and Illness*. Philadelphia, PA: W.B. Saunders, 2000.

Hollar, Sherman. *Pioneers in Medicine: From the Classical World to Today*. New York, NY: Encyclopedia Britannica, 2013.

Johnson, Jinny. *Under the Microscope. Breathing — How We Use Air*. Danbury, CT: Grolier, Inc. 1988.

Kalman, Bobbie. *Early Health and Medicine*. New York, NY: Crabtree Publishing, 1991.

Kapit, Wynn, and Lawrence M. Elson. *The Anatomy Coloring Book*. New York: Harper Collins, 1993.

Kyi, Tanya Lloyd. *50 Body Questions: A Book That Spills Its Guts*. Buffalo, NY: Annick Press, 2014.

Kyi, Tanya Lloyd. *Seeing Red: The True Story of Blood*. Buffalo, NY: Annick Press, 2012.

Kruszelnicki, Karl. *Munching Maggots, Noah's Flood and TV Heart Attacks and Other Cataclysmic Science Moments*. New York, NY: John Wiley and Sons, 2000.

Lambert, Mark. *How Our Bodies Work: The Lungs and Breathing*. Englewood, NJ: Schoolhouse Press, Inc., 1988.

Lambert, Mark. *The Brain and Nervous System*. Englewood Cliffs, NJ: Schoolhouse Press, Inc, 1988.

Larsen, C.S. *Crust and Spray: Gross Stuff in Your Eyes, Ears, Nose, and Throat. Gross Body Science*. Minneapolis, MN: Millbrook Press, 2010.

Law, Kristi. *Clot and Scab: Gross Stuff About Your Scrapes, Bumps and Bruises*. Minneapolis, MN: Millbrook Press, 2010.

Lawry, James V., and H. Craig Heller. *Nervous System: Human Biology*. Chicago, IL: Everyday Learning Corporation, 1999.

Lew, Kristi. *Bat Spit, Maggots, and Other Amazing Medical Wonders*. Mankato, MN: Capstone, 2011.

Llamas, Andreu. *Respiration and Circulation*. Milwaukee, WI: Gareth Stevens Publishing, 1988.

Markle, Sandra. *Faulty Hearts: True Survival Stories*. Minneapolis, MN: Lerner Publishing, 2011.

Masoff, Joy. *Oh Yikes! History's Grossest Wackiest Moments*. New York, NY: Workman Publishing, 2006.

Masoff, Joy. *Oh Yuck! The Encyclopedia of Everything Nasty*. New York, NY: Workman Publishing, 2000.

Martini, Federic, H., and Kathleen Welch. *Clinical Issues in Anatomy*. San Francisco, CA: Pearson Education, 2006.

Mason, Estate of Martha. *Breath: A Lifetime in the Rhythm of an Iron Lung: A Memoir*. New York: First Bloomsbury USA, 2010.

Miller, Connie Colwell. *The Snotty Book of Snot*. Mankato, MN: Capstone Press, 2010.

Moore, K. and A. Dalley. *Clinically Oriented Anatomy*. Baltimore, Maryland: Lippincott Williams and Wilkins, 1999.

Moore, Keith, and T.V.N. Persaud. *The Developing Human: Clinically Oriented Embryology*. Philadelphia, PA: W.B. Saunders, 2003.

Murphy, Glenn. *Why Is Snot Green? And Other Extremely Important Questions (and Answers)*. New York: Scholastic, 2007.

Netter, Frank. *Atlas of Human Anatomy*. East Hanover, New Jersey: Novartis, 1997.

Orr, Tamra. *Avian Flu*. New York, NY: The Rosen Publishing Group, Inc., 2007.

Parker, Steve. *Brain Surgery for Beginners and Other Major Operations for Minors: A Scalpel-Free Guide to Your Insides*. Brookfield, CT: Millbrook Press, 1995.

Patton, Kevin T. *Survival Guide for Anatomy and Physiology*. St. Louis, MO: Mosby Inc., 2014.

Perl, Lila. *Don't Sing Before Breakfast, Don't Sleep in the Moonlight: Everyday Superstitions and How They Began*. New York, NY: Clarion Books, 1988.

Petechuk, David. *The Respiratory System*. Westport, CT: Greenwood Press, 2004.

Peters, Stephanie True. *The Battle Against Polio*. Tarrytown, NY: Benchmark Books, 2005.

Peters, Stephanie True. *The 1918 Influenza Pandemic*. Tarrytown, NY: Benchmark Books, 2005.

Pinnock, Dale. *Healing Foods: Prevent or Treat Common Illnesses with Fruits, Vegetables, Herbs, and More*. New York, NY. Skyhorse, 2011.

Platt, Richard. *Plagues, Pox and Pestilence*. New York, NY: Kingfisher, 2011.

Porter, Cheryl. *Gross Grub*. New York: RGA Publishing Group, 1995.

Reilly, Kathleen. *The Human Body: 25 Fantastic Projects: Illuminate How the Body Works*. White River Junction, VT: Nomad Press, 2008.

Rhatigan, Joe. *Gross Me Out! 50 Nasty Projects to Disgust Your Friends and Repulse Your Family*. New York: Lark Books, 2004.

Rhatigan, Joe. *Ouch!* Watertown, MA: Charlesbridge Publications, 2013.

Rodgers, Kara. *Blood: Physiology and Circulation*. New York, NY: Britannica Educational Publishing, 2011.

Rodgers, Kara. *The Cardiovascular System*. New York, NY: Britannica Educational Publishing, 2011.

Rodgers, Kara. *Medicine and Healers Through History.* New York, NY: Britannica Educational Publishing, 2011.

Romanek, Trudee. *ZZZ . . . The Most Interesting Book You'll Ever Read About Sleep.* Tonawanda, NY: Kids Can Press, 2002.

Rooney, Anne. *The Story of Medicine.* London: Arcturus Publishing Limited, 2009.

Rosaler, Maxine. *Cystic Fibrosis.* New York, NY: The Rosen Publishing Group, Inc., 2007.

Sadler, Thomas W. *Langman's Medical Embrology,* Philadelphia, PA: Lippincott Williams and Wilkins, 2011.

Sadler, T.W. *Langman's Medical Embryology.* Philadelphia, PA: Williams and Wilkins, 2006.

Sadler, T.W. *Langman's Medical Embryology.* Baltimore, Maryland: Williams and Wilkins, 1995.

Silver, Donald M., and Patricia J. Wynne. *The Body Book: Easy-to-Make Hands-on Models That Teach.* New York: Scholastic, 1993.

Silverstein, A., V. Silverstein and Nunn Silverstein. *Sleep.* Danbury, Connecticut, 1992.

Silverstein, Dr. Alvin, Virginia Silverstein, and Laura Silverstein Nunn. *Sleep.* New York: Grolier Publishing, 2000.

Simon, Seymour. *The Brain: Our Nervous System.* New York: Morrow Junior Books, 1997.

Singleton, Glen. *Gross Jokes. Kingley,* Australia: Hinkler Books, 2004.

Stein, Sarah. *The Body Book.* New York: Workman Publishing Company, 1992.

Stewart, Melissa. *Up Your Nose! The Secrets of Schnozes and Snouts. The Gross and Goofy Body.* New York: Marshall Cavendish, 2009.

Stille, Darlene R. *Extraordinary Women of Medicine.* Danbury, CT: Children's Press, Grolier Publishing, 1997.

Stimola, Aubrey. *Ebola.* New York, NY: The Rosen Publishing Group, Inc., 2011.

Strom, Laura Layton. *Dr. Medieval: Medicine in the Middle Ages.* New York, NY: Children's Press, 2008.

Sutherland, Stuart. *Discovering the Human Mind.* London: Stonehedge Press, Inc., 1982.

Szpirglas, Jeff. *Gross Universe: Your Guide to All Disgusting Things Under the Sun.* Toronto, Canada: Maple Tree Press, Inc., 2004.

Tangerine Press. *More Jokes.* New York, NY: Scholastic, 2005.

Thompson, Richard. *The Brain: An Introduction to Neuroscience Primer.* New York: W.H. Freeman and Company, 1993.

Time. *Your Brain: A User's Guide.* Des Moines, IA: Time Home Entertainment, 2011.

Tiner, John Hudson. *Exploring the History of Medicine: From the Ancient Physicians of Pharaoh to Genetic Engineering.* Green Forest, AR: Master Books, 1999.

Treays, Rebecca. *Understanding Your Brain: Internet-Linked, Lifting the Lid on What's Inside Your Head.* New York: Scholastic Inc., 2005.

Van Cleave, Janice. *The Human Body for Every Kid: Easy Activities That Make Learning Science Fun.* Chichester, England: John Wiley and Sons Inc., 1995.

Veglahn, Nancy. *American Profiles- Women Scientists.* New York, New York: Facts on File, Inc., 1991.

Walker, Richard. *Under the Microscope: Heart- How the Blood Goes Around the Body.* Danbury, Connecticut: Franklin Watts, 1998

Ward, Brian. *The Brain and Nervous System.* New York: Franklin Watts Limited, 1981.

Weitzman, I., Eva Blank, Alison Benjamin, and Rosanne Green. *Jokelopedia: The Biggest, Best, Silliest, Dumbest Joke Book Ever.* New York, NY: Workman Publishing Company, Inc., 2000.

West, David. *Brain Surgery for Beginners and Other Major Operations for Minors.* New York, New York: Scholastic, 1993.

Winner, Cherie. *Circulating Life: Blood Transfusion from Ancient Superstition to Modern Medicine.* Minneapolis, MN: 21st Century Books, 2007. Woods, Michael, and Mary Woods. *Ancient Medicine: From Sorcery to Surgery.* Minneapolis, MN: Runestone Press, 2000.

Bibliography for Activities in *The Complex Circulatory System*

Aims Education. *From Head to Toe: Respiratory, Circulatory and Skeletal Systems, Book 3.* Fresno, CA: Aims Education Foundation, 1986.

Branzei, Sylvia. *Grossology.* New York, NY: Price Stern Sloan, 2002.

Conway, Lorraine. *Superific Science Series: Book IX. Body Systems.* New York, NY:Good Apple, 1984.

Foster, Michael and Patricia Twohey. *The Human Body.* The Education Center, 2000.

Hixson, B.K. *Cow Eyes, Beef, Hearts and Worms.* Salt Lake City, UT: Wild Goose Company, 1992.

Kalumuck, Karen. *Exploratorium Human Body Explorations: Hands On Investigations of What Makes Us Tick.* San Francisco, CA: Exploratorium, 2003.

Reilly, Kathleen. *The Human Body: Illuminate How the Body Works.* White River Junction, VT: Nomad Press, 2008.

Rhatigan, Joe, Rain Newcomb, and Clay Meyer. *Gross Me Out! 50 Nasty Projects to Disgust Your Friends and Repulse Your Family.* New York, NY: Lark Books, 2004.

Romanek, Trudee. *Mysterious You: Squirt! The Most Interesting Book You'll Read Ever About Blood.* Toronto, ON: Kids Can Press, 2005.

VanCleave, Jance. *Play and Find Out about the Human Body: Easy Experiments for Young Children.* New York, NY: Scholastic, 1998.

Haslam, Andrew, and Liz Wyse. *Body — Make it Work! The Hands-on Approach to Science.* New York, NY: Scholastic, 1997.

Endnotes

1. http://en.wikipedia.org/wiki/Counting_sheep
2. Adapted from "What Makes Us Yawn?" by Melanie Radzicki McManus, http://science.howstuffworks.com/life/inside-the-mind/human-brain/question5721.htm
3. Adapted from "20 Amazing Facts About Dreams that You Might Not Know About" by Simon Andras, http: www.lifehack.org

INDEX

Abb ad al-mu'tadid 67
abdominal 34, 100, 174
ability 11, 17, 31, 35, 51, 88, 93, 98, 108,
.... 116, 118, 124, 130, 168, 172, 185
abnormal 14, 19, 22, 33, 53, 112, 169, 185
absorb 75
aches 122
acid 128, 171
activities 6–7, 14, 45, 65, 98, 214-215
Adam's apple 96
adapt 107
adrenalines 50
aerosol 91, 125
afflicted 130
ailment 69, 142
air 31, 52, 55, 60, 80-85, 88-101, 103-104, 106-107,
.... 110-112, 114, 118, 120, 123, 125-129, 133,
.... 142-143, 152-154, 160, 167, 172, 187, 203, 213
airway 99, 124, 127
allergen 126
allergic 126-127
allergies 94, 127
allergy 76, 126
aluminum 99, 160
alveolar 98, 101, 103, 109, 120
alveoli 76, 83, 98-99, 101, 103-104, 106, 109-110, 120, 127
alveolus 98, 101
Alzheimer's 62
ammonia 88
amniotic 108
anatomy 6, 9, 14, 18, 28, 30, 46, 62, 83,
.... 95-96, 155-157, 180, 212-213
Anaximenes 84
anemia 146, 168-169, 171, 174
anesthesia 85
Anesthetic 85, 178
anesthetizing 85
Angioplasty 195
anosmia 76, 93
anterior 12-13, 32, 38, 52, 92
anterior nerve 52
antibiotics 111
antibodies 130, 146, 165, 172-173
antigens 146, 172-173
antioxidants 62, 197
antiseptic 76, 91
anti-viral 111
aorta 146, 174, 180, 182-183, 191
Aphasia 18
apneustic center 76, 107
apparatus 133
appetite 88, 203
approval 21
arbor vitae 10-11, 36
areas 10, 12, 22-23, 29, 31, 34-35, 41, 46, 58, 70, 102-103,
.... 113, 117, 122, 124, 153, 167, 169-170, 177, 179, 184, 186
Aristotle 17, 84, 152
arm 27, 34, 53, 113, 125, 132-133, 156, 159, 161, 187, 195
arteries 146, 152-154, 157, 159, 161,
.... 174-175, 180, 183, 193, 195, 197

arteriole 98
arterioles 146, 174-175
artery 114, 153, 174-175, 181-183, 191, 195
artificial 115, 160-161
artificial heart 160-161
aspiration 97
asthma 76, 112, 118-119, 127-128, 140
astrocytes 46
Astroglia 10-11, 25
atrium 146, 150, 182-184, 188, 191
auditory 12-13, 32, 38
aura 33
auscultate 146, 186
autonomic 10-11, 37, 39, 50
autonomic nervous system 10-11, 37
autonomic system 50
awake 33, 56-58, 212
axon 10-11, 25
Babies 42, 53, 56, 86, 110, 124, 187, 189, 195
Babinski reflex 19, 53
back 13, 31-32, 47-48, 50, 53-54, 56-57, 83-84, 91, 95, 97,
.... 99-101, 116, 123, 152, 169, 174-175, 178, 185, 188, 193, 202
backbone 47-48
bacteria 54, 76, 91, 121-123, 129, 158
bacterial 54, 129
bacterium 86, 123
Barnard, Christiaan N. 159
base 13, 37, 41, 47, 65, 84
BBB 46
beating 14, 112, 180, 188, 193
behaviors 42, 58
Bible 9, 16, 21, 65, 83, 88, 108, 150-151, 154, 162, 201, 210, 212
bile 124, 153
billions 14, 21, 24, 40, 82
BioLung 115
biomass 121
birth 17, 40-42, 86, 88, 95, 99, 108, 190-191, 194-195
bladder 48, 50-51, 118
blood 17, 25-26, 35, 37, 39, 45-46, 50, 54-55, 70,
.... 81-82, 84-85, 89, 92-93, 101, 103-104, 106-107, 114-115,
.... 121, 123-124, 127, 146, 150, 152-162, 164-185, 187-189,
.... 191-193, 195-197, 201-204, 206-207, 210, 212-215
blood-brain 10, 46, 89
blood-brain barrier 10-11, 46, 89
bloodhound 93
bloodstream 46, 89, 101, 103, 106, 114
blood type 172-173
blood vessels 11, 25, 45-46, 50, 54-55, 84, 92, 101,
.... 157, 159-161, 167-169, 174-175, 180, 187, 197
Blundell, James 157, 202
bodies 14, 16, 20, 52, 54, 82, 89, 91, 101, 103, 108,
.... 116, 119, 121, 133, 157, 171, 176, 178, 180, 202, 213
body 11-14, 16, 18-25, 29, 34-35, 37, 39-41, 44, 46-48,
.... 50, 54, 56-60, 62, 64-66, 70, 72, 83-85, 89, 91, 94,
.... 97, 99, 101-104, 106-107, 110, 112-113, 115-116, 118,
.... 121-124, 126, 129-130, 132-133, 140, 150-154, 156, 158,
.... 160-161, 163, 165-170, 172, 174, 180, 182-186,
.... 188-190, 192-194, 197, 201, 203-204, 212-215
body temperature 12, 37, 54, 57
bone marrow 146, 166-167

216

God's Wondrous Machine

booger	92
Bordet, Jules	158
born	17, 37, 40, 42, 53, 60-61, 84, 88-89, 108, 110, 119, 135, 152, 159, 167, 169, 172, 191, 194
braces	132, 135
Brachial Plexus	27, 48
Bradycardia	146, 185
brain	10, 14-26, 28-31, 33-47, 51-55, 58, 61-62, 65-67, 70-73, 89, 93, 103, 107, 123, 153, 168, 184, 212-214
brain freeze	55
brain stem	28, 184
branch	36, 50, 99
break	114, 117-118, 129
breath	60, 80, 82-84, 88, 100, 105-107, 110, 112-113, 116, 123, 127-128, 139, 157, 168, 180, 213
breathe	39, 50, 82-83, 87, 90, 93, 97-99, 101, 103, 106-108, 114, 118, 128, 133-134, 140, 152, 175, 189
breathing	14, 48, 50, 55, 76, 84, 88-89, 98, 100, 104, 107-108, 110, 119, 125, 128, 130, 133-134, 142, 190, 213
breathtaking	90, 103, 142
bridge	38, 126
Broca's area	18, 35
bronchi	76, 98-99
bronchioles	76, 90, 98-99, 101-102, 127
bronchus	98-99
buffy coat	146, 165
C1-C5	48
C5- T1	48
canary	89
cancer	20, 62, 117-119, 159
capillaries	46, 82, 84, 101, 104, 109, 157, 174-175
capillary	101, 146, 174-175
carbon	76, 82, 89, 99, 101, 103-104, 107, 115, 120, 165, 175, 177
carbonated	103
carcinogen	118
cardiology	159, 161
Cardiopulmonary Resuscitation	229
care	10, 17, 42, 54, 70, 111, 116-117, 119, 157, 196
cartilage	96-97, 99
Cataplexy	57
cause	17, 45, 48-50, 91, 93, 96, 101, 107, 118, 121, 123-125, 129, 159, 168-169, 178, 182
cavities	25, 95, 126, 180
cavity	90, 93-95, 100, 107, 120, 180-181
cells	10, 14, 25, 41, 49, 72, 76, 82, 90-91, 93, 100-103, 106, 108, 118, 121, 124, 146, 158, 165-175, 184, 195, 201
center	14, 18, 28-29, 76, 107, 115, 152, 154, 203, 212, 215
central nervous system	10, 24-25, 41
centrifuge	146, 164-165
centuries	16, 152, 154, 156
cerebellum	10, 18, 28, 36, 38
cerebral cortex	18, 28
cerebral hemispheres	10, 29, 36
Cerebral Palsy	10
cerebral spinal fluid	10, 25
cerebrospinal fluid	44
cerebrum	10, 18, 26, 28-30, 32-33, 37
Cervical Area	48
CFTR	125
chambers	89, 182, 188
cheekbone	31
chemical	44, 101, 103, 107, 125, 177
chemistry	107
Chemoreceptors	76, 107
cherry bark	128
chicken pox	49
childhood	37, 49, 143
chloride	125
Chloroform	86
chocolate	62
choking	97
Chordae tendineae	146, 182
Christ	16, 116, 186, 206
Chromosome	125
chronic	66, 118, 127
Cigarette	100, 117-118
cilia	76, 93, 100, 102, 118
circulation	84-85, 103-104, 156, 179, 189-191, 212-213
Clark, Barney	190
closed circulatory system	146, 154, 180
clot	114, 165, 169-170, 178, 213
clotting	169-170, 177-179
coils	12
cold	49, 54-55, 94, 128, 150, 157, 168
Cold sores	49
combustion	85
common mullein	140
communications	13
complex	19, 39, 65, 84, 121, 150, 201, 215
composition	91
compound	111
comprehension	13, 32
compressor	128
Computed Tomography Angiography	161
Computerized Tomography	22
concha	93
conducting	13
congenital	221
connects	37, 47, 84, 189-190
conscious	29, 37, 39, 50
contagious	60, 123, 170
control	14, 17-18, 24, 28, 34, 36-37, 50, 54-55, 59, 66, 107, 130, 184
convolution	12
COPD	118
Coronary	146, 180, 182, 195
corpus callosum	10, 28-29, 37
cortex	18, 28, 34-35, 59
cough	86, 99, 112-113, 118, 121-122, 129, 140
cranial meninges	44-45
cranial nerves	41
cribriform plate	76, 92-93
crippling	130
croup	129
crying	14, 82
crystallography	111
CSF	25, 44
CT Scans	22, 113
cure	55, 67, 87, 128, 140, 170
cycle	18, 56
cystic fibrosis	76, 86-87, 124-125, 214
damage	20, 30, 35, 42, 45-46, 55, 83, 93, 116-117, 119-121, 168, 197
dander	126

Index

data	38, 70
Da Vinci, Leonardo	186, 222
death	16-17, 19, 37, 66, 70, 72, 96, 123, 125, 130, 133, 206, 212
DeBakey, Michael	189, 191
decision-making	31
decompression	103
defecate	50
defect	99, 124-125, 191
deformities	130
dementia	228
dendrites	10, 25
depth	179
dermatomes	10, 49
design	10, 25, 52, 65, 76, 88, 108, 194
detectors	103
developed	17, 19, 21, 41, 67, 70, 86-87, 89, 95, 111-112, 125, 130, 161, 165, 173, 189
diagnose	23, 104-105, 161
diagnosed	19
diagnosis	70, 85, 113, 125
diaphragm	48, 81, 98, 100, 107, 130, 133
diarrhea	121, 125
Diastole	146, 184
dieffenbachia	96
diencephalon	10, 37-38, 54
differences	18, 121, 133, 172
diffuse	101, 103
digestion	51, 121, 124
dioxide	76, 82, 88-89, 99, 101, 103-104, 107, 115, 165, 175, 177
disability	132
disease	14, 20, 66, 86, 105-106, 118, 121-125, 127, 130, 132, 153, 161, 165, 168-171, 177, 194, 212
disorder	37, 57, 125, 171
dissenter	88
dizziness	103, 168
doctor	17, 21, 23, 31, 42, 52, 70, 85-86, 105, 112, 124, 135, 155, 158, 172, 186, 196
dormant	49
dorsal	38, 49, 52
dorsal root	49, 52
dreaming	58, 61
Drew, Charles Richard	159, 161, 173
duct	101, 109
ears	177, 213
eating	37, 66, 97, 197
ECMO	115
EEG	22
egg	45, 113, 177
Einthoven, Willem	158
electrical	22, 25, 33, 42, 47, 72, 107, 125, 128, 133, 158, 184-185
Electrocardiogram	146, 158, 185
electrode	125
Electroencephalogram	22
element	85
embolism	114
embolus	114
Emission	23, 113
Empedocles	84
emphysema	118, 120
Endocardium	146, 181
enterovirus	111
Ependymal Cells	10, 25
Epicardium	146, 181
epidemic	66, 76, 122, 130, 132-133
epiglottis	76, 90, 97
epilepsy	17, 33
epithelium	76, 102
Erasistratus	85, 152
Erythrocytes	146, 166
esophagus	97, 99
ether	85
EV-D68	111
evolution	171
exhalation	100, 110
exhale	76, 82, 101, 104, 118, 133, 175, 177
experiments	46, 88-89, 215
expiration	107
Expiratory	107, 110
exquisite	93
external	16, 34, 160
eye	31, 34, 203, 206
eyes	38, 40, 50, 56, 58-59, 126, 142, 157, 161, 186, 188, 202, 213, 215
fat	197
feet	14, 30-31, 37, 48, 52, 91, 133, 202
female	37, 178
fetus	108, 146, 189, 191
fever	54, 121-122, 126, 177
fibers	47, 115, 169
fibrinogen	165
fibrosis	76, 86-87, 124-125, 214
fibrous	44-45
Fight or Flight	50-51
flavonoids	62
fluid	10, 25, 44, 108, 112, 124, 150, 158, 165, 169, 180, 189
fold	159, 187
formula	21, 103
Forssmann, Werner	159
fracture	93
fragment	92
fragrance	93
frontal	10, 18-19, 31-33, 42, 94-95
fumes	30, 103
function	20, 25, 28, 48, 72, 90, 92, 94, 100, 104, 106, 108, 110, 114-115, 118, 153, 168, 188
gadgets	128, 196
Gaffney, Drew	160
Galen	18, 85, 152, 154-155
gap	13
gene	87, 125
genetic	86, 124-125, 168, 170-171, 173, 214
germ	86, 94
germy	91, 94, 121
gestation	76, 108, 110
Gibbon, John	193
gland	10, 18, 37, 51, 59
glands	50, 124
glia	25
glucose	62
gluteal region	48
God	10, 16, 25, 35, 39, 41, 45, 50-52, 56, 65, 72-73, 76, 82-84, 88, 91, 93, 97, 99, 101, 103, 106-108, 116-117, 119, 121, 124, 128, 135, 139, 150-151, 154, 161-162, 170-171, 185-186, 194, 197, 201, 206-207

grasp reflex	53
gray matter	10, 29, 43
groove	12
growth	14, 37, 41, 59
gyrus	10, 34
Harvey, William	154, 156
hazards	89
head	18, 26, 31, 34, 38-39, 41-42, 46, 48, 53, 55-56, 67-68, 110, 112, 133, 177, 180, 186, 203, 214-215
headache	39, 67, 103
headaches	17, 89, 122
heal	94, 115, 129
health	14, 21, 41, 54, 58, 70, 116-118, 123, 133, 186, 196-197, 207, 213
hearing	26, 28, 51
heart	14, 17, 39, 50-51, 72-73, 81, 84-85, 98-99, 112, 115, 118, 127, 142, 150-154, 156, 158-161, 168, 174-175, 180-189, 191-197, 201-202, 206-207, 210, 212-213
heart-lung machine	193
heart rate	39, 50-51, 183-184, 188, 196
Hematophagic	146, 176
Hematopoiesis	146, 167
hemisphere	18, 34
hemoglobin	146, 166-169, 171
Hemophilia	146, 170-171
hemostasis	146, 165, 169-170
herbal	140
herbs	68, 140, 213
Herophilus	155
HGH	59
highway	14, 25, 99
Hippocrates	17, 155, 212
Hippocratic Oath	17
histology	14
History	15, 70, 72, 84, 135, 152, 154, 171, 178, 212-214
homunculus	10, 19, 33-34
hormones	37, 50
human growth hormone	37, 59
humors	91, 153, 155, 178
hundreds	14, 121, 154, 184
hydrocyanic	128
hygienic	117
hypothalamus	10, 28, 37, 41, 51, 54, 59
illness	17, 49, 58, 99, 116, 121-122, 129, 132, 134, 153-154, 165, 171, 177, 213
imaging	20, 23, 95, 113
immune	49, 54, 126, 130, 158, 172
immunity	165, 171
impulses	14, 24-25, 33, 35, 50, 107
Infantile	87, 132
infect	123
infection	37, 49, 94
Inferior	38, 92, 182-183, 191
inflamed	94, 127, 181
inflammation	94, 126-127, 129
Inflammatory	120
Influenza	76, 122, 213
information	24, 36-38, 42, 47, 49, 52, 73
inhalation	100, 128
inhale	76, 82, 93-94, 101
innovation	84
innovative	72

insatiable	89
insect	101
insight	16, 42-43
inspiration	107
Inspiratory	107
insulates	12
integral	14
intelligence	17, 121
interactions	31
intercostal	100, 107
internal	16, 54, 59, 184
interprets	35
intestinal	117
intestines	91, 124
investigation	14, 134
involuntary	60, 107
IPPB	125
iron	30-31, 76, 87, 130, 133-134, 166-167, 213
irritants	126
itching	14
Jivaros	68
joints	103, 197
kidney	123
King James II	117
knowledge	15-17, 43, 65, 84, 89, 112, 117, 140, 150-152, 154, 159, 161, 206
kuru	66
L1-5	48
laboratory	89
Landsteiner, Karl	158, 172
language	18, 35, 65, 167
Laryngitis	76, 129
laryngopharynx	95-96
laryngotracheobronchitis	129
larynx	76, 81, 90, 96-97, 129
lateral	13, 32
lead	17, 41, 48, 66, 96-97, 123, 130
learning	42, 65, 88, 157, 186, 201, 212-214
leeches	155, 178-179
left	18, 20, 29, 31, 34-35, 90, 93, 99, 130, 140, 152-153, 158, 174, 182-184, 188-191, 195-196
leg	34, 48, 52, 114, 125, 135
life	16, 33, 36, 41-43, 53, 56, 72, 82-85, 88, 108, 116, 119, 123, 133-135, 158, 162, 171, 177, 184, 194, 202, 212, 214-215
life-threatening	33, 48, 103, 128, 171
lining	25, 91-93, 102, 127, 167
lipid	—
lobe	10, 18, 31-33, 42, 98, 202
logic	29, 65
loss	17, 33, 48, 51, 85, 93, 132, 192, 196
lower	48, 52, 76, 90, 96, 98, 156, 167, 182-184, 187
Lower, Richard	156
lung	22, 76, 80, 83, 86-87, 98-99, 102, 104, 106, 108-110, 114-115, 117-120, 123-124, 127, 130, 133-134, 140, 157, 159, 183, 213
lycopene	62
machine	14, 20, 44, 48, 72, 83-84, 106, 115, 119, 133-134, 161, 164-165, 185, 192-194
magnetic resonance imaging (MRI)	20
malaria	146, 169, 171, 177
male	37, 178

219

Index

malfunctions	124
malnutrition	124
Malpighi, Marcello	157
Mankind	16
maxillary	94
medical	17-19, 22-23, 26, 31, 67, 70, 84, 87, 89, 115, 119, 123-124, 134, 140, 156-157, 159-160, 178, 186, 191, 194, 212-214
medicine	16-17, 21, 39, 70, 81, 87, 110, 114, 154-155, 158-161, 172, 178, 212-214
medulla	10, 28, 39, 107, 184
medulla oblongata	10, 28, 39, 107
Membrane	101, 115
membranes	180
memory	10, 29, 43, 51, 58, 65, 72
meninges	10, 44-45
mercury poisoning	69
Mesencephalon	10, 38
microbiologist	87
Microglia	10, 25
microscope	84, 157, 166, 213-214
microscopic	14, 99, 169, 171
midbrain	28, 38
middle	31, 37, 67, 80, 91-92, 98, 140, 151-152, 155, 166, 168, 178, 181, 184, 214
miles	24-25, 73, 82, 91, 93, 135, 169, 174-175, 201, 212
mind	16-18, 26, 65, 73, 88-89, 201, 214
mites	126
molds	126, 189
molecule	103
monoxide	89, 103
Moro reflex	53
mosquitoes	171, 177, 204
motor homunculus	34
motor root	52
motor speech	11
mouth	49, 51, 53, 55, 87, 95-97, 102, 104, 121-122, 130, 177, 207
mouthpiece	85, 104, 128
movement	29, 34, 41, 45, 59, 101, 104, 108, 125
mucus	76, 91-92, 94, 100, 102, 118, 124, 126-127
muscle	17, 26, 28, 34, 48, 50, 66, 100, 110, 127, 158, 180-181, 184-185, 196
myelin sheath	10, 25
myelin sheaths	25
Myocardial infarction	146, 180
Myocardium	146, 181
Narcolepsy	57
Nares	76
nasal	55, 76, 90, 93-95, 126, 129
nasal turbinate	76, 93
nasopharynx	95
nebulizer	128
neck	26, 34, 39, 48, 53, 96, 133, 177
nerve	18, 25, 29, 41, 47-49, 52, 93, 184
nerve column	47
nerve plexus	48
nerves	24, 27, 39, 41-42, 47, 49, 55, 92-93
neural plate	41
neural tube	41
Neuroglia	10
neuroglial cell	25
Neurologists	70
neurons	10, 22, 24-25, 29, 40, 42
neuroscience	16, 19, 30-31, 33, 213-214
nicotine	117
nitrogen	85, 88
nitrous	84-85, 88
Non-Rapid Eye Movement sleep (NREM)	56
nose	34, 53, 90-95, 104, 121-122, 126, 129, 140, 143, 213-214
nosebleed	93
nose-picking	129
Nostril	90
nutrients	25, 44, 165, 174, 181
oblongata	10, 28, 39, 107, 184
Occipital Lobe	10, 32
olfactory	92-93
Oligodendroglia	10, 25
omega-3 fatty acids	197
Open circulatory system	146, 180
oral	87, 95, 130
order	24, 29, 42, 55, 72, 89, 95, 97, 99, 103, 105-107, 110, 113, 116-117, 124, 151, 178
organ	14, 19, 72, 83, 108, 124, 130, 151, 193-194
organisms	12
organogenesis	76, 108
organs	21, 48-49, 99, 103, 106, 108, 115, 121, 124, 156, 166, 168, 174-175, 180, 189, 194
originate	14, 29, 41, 168
oropharynx	95
ossuaries	69
outbreak	66, 111, 122
oxide	84-85, 88, 167
oximeter	106
oxygen	25, 76, 82, 84-85, 88-89, 99, 101, 103-104, 106, 110, 114-115, 165-168, 174-175, 181-182, 184, 189-190, 193, 195-196, 203, 212
oxygenated	115, 161, 174, 182-183, 191
pain	33, 39, 55, 81, 85-86, 94, 113, 129, 168, 178, 185
palate	55, 92
pancreas	124
Pandemic	76, 122, 213
paralysis	17, 57, 61, 87, 130, 132-133
paralytic	133
parasympathetic branch	50
Parietal Lobe	10, 32
part	24-26, 28, 31, 35, 37, 50, 56, 59, 65, 70, 84-85, 89, 91, 93, 96-97, 114-115, 139, 159, 181-182, 202-203
passage	30, 97
passageway	90, 92, 98, 127
pathologist	86, 124
pathology	14
pediatrician	186
perceive	14
perception	13, 29, 32
perfluorocarbon	103
pericardial sac	146, 180-181
peripheral nervous system	24, 52
pertussis	86
PET scan	23, 113
pharynx	34, 76, 90-91, 95-96
phlegm	91, 153
photic	111

phrenology	18, 67
physical	51, 60, 65, 72, 98, 113
physician	17-18, 73, 85, 112, 152, 156-160, 172
physics	91
physiologist	76, 89, 158
Physiology	14, 28, 83, 87, 158-159, 212-213
Piccolomini	18
pituitary gland	10, 37, 51, 59
plasma	165, 173
platelets	146, 165-166, 168-170
pleura	76, 99
plumbism	17
pneuma	84-85, 152
pneumocyte	109
pneumonia	112
pneumotaxic	76, 107
poisoning	17, 69, 103
polio	76, 87, 111, 130, 132-135, 213
Poliomyelitis	130
pollens	126
Pons	10, 28, 38, 107
Positron Emission Tomography	23
posterior	38, 52
posterior nerve	52
pound	40, 42, 55, 180
power	16, 26, 65, 121, 134, 139, 160
Praxagoras	152
pregnancy	41, 110, 150
prescription	21
pressure	39, 45-46, 49-50, 110, 118, 125-126, 133, 165, 187, 197, 202
Primary	109
procedure	14, 19, 67, 99, 115, 155, 159, 172, 192, 195
processing	29
protect	25, 46, 50, 89, 119, 130, 162, 172, 197
protector	13
Prothrombin	146, 169
pseudostratified	102
puberty	37, 96
pulmonary	98, 104, 114, 118, 182-184, 191
pulse	106, 185, 187
pumped	17, 115, 158, 174, 180, 193
pupils	50-51
puzzles	65
pyrogens	10, 54
quadriplegia	48
quadriplegic	48
quality	16, 89, 94
Queen Elizabeth	140
Queen Victoria	86, 171
quest	16
Quotes	72, 142, 206
radiation	46
railroad	30
Rapid Eye Movement sleep (REM)	192
rash	149
rashes	121
reaction	38, 126, 130, 158, 172-173
reasoning	42, 152, 185
receptor	90
receptors	52, 93, 107
red blood cells	82, 101, 103, 106, 146, 158, 166, 168-169, 172-173, 175, 195, 201
reflex	19, 52-53, 99
region	18, 29, 33-35, 44, 48-49, 61, 70, 93, 101, 122, 167
relay station	149
remedy	112
Remote Monitoring	70
Respiration	89, 104, 134, 213
respirator	48, 133
respiratory	39, 76, 82-84, 87, 89-90, 96-99, 101-102, 105, 107, 110-111, 115, 119, 122, 140, 142, 212-213, 215
response	38, 50-51, 54, 120, 126-127, 130, 169
rhinitis	126-127
rhinorrhea	126
Rhinotillexomania	129
ribs	85, 99-100, 110, 167
right	29, 33-34, 84, 93, 96, 99, 102, 112, 117, 119, 135, 143, 150, 159, 162, 167, 170, 175, 177, 182-184, 188-189, 191, 202
rocket	91
rooting reflex	53
running	14, 169, 184, 191
runny	122, 126
ruptures	121
S1-S5	48
sacculi	109
sacs	83, 98-99, 101, 118
saturation	106
scan	23, 31, 113-114
scanners	23
scent	93
seasonal	126
secretes	37, 51, 184
seizure	22, 33
sensation	48
sensations	17, 49
sense	18, 35, 39, 51, 72, 82, 90, 93
sensors	22, 107
sensory	19, 34, 36-38, 47, 49, 52
sensory homunculus	34
sensory root	52
septum	93, 109, 120, 184
Servetus, Michael	156
shakiness	17
shingles	10, 49
sick	56, 110-111, 122, 124, 134, 212
sickle cell anemia	146, 168-169, 171, 174
side	16, 42, 53, 89, 93, 153, 159, 174-175, 182-183, 188-189, 191
signals	14, 25-26, 39, 43, 51, 59, 172, 190
singing	14, 96
Sinoatrial node	146
sinus	94-95, 126
sinuses	76, 90, 94-95, 124
sinusitis	94
Skeeter	135
skeletal	29, 108, 215
skin	44, 48-50, 52, 54, 68, 102, 122-126, 140, 157, 164, 167-169, 175, 177-179, 185
skipping	14
skull	14, 37, 44-45, 67, 93-94, 108, 167
sleep	17-18, 56-59, 61, 72, 202, 212-214
sleepwalking	58

221

Index

slime	112
slimy	91
smell	33, 51, 90, 93, 177
smiling	14
smoke	116, 119
smoking	100, 117-118, 159
sneeze	91-92, 111, 116, 122
sneezing	14, 91, 111, 123, 126
Sniff	93, 126
snot	91, 213
social	31
Somnambulism	58
speech	18, 35, 58, 66, 94, 96
sphenoid	94-95
Sphenopalatine ganglioneuralgia	55
sphygmomanometer	187
spina bifida	41
spinal	10, 23-28, 41, 46-49, 52, 130
spinal cord	23-24, 26-28, 41, 46-47, 49, 52, 130
spinal fluid	10, 25
Spinal ganglion	49
spinal nerve root	49
spine	41, 47-49, 100, 108, 123, 167
spirometer	104-106
spit	117, 123, 213
spongy	83, 90, 99, 166
sputum	123
stages	56-57, 95, 170
Starling, Ernest Henry	158
stem	28, 38, 101, 146, 168, 170, 184
stem cell	146, 168, 170
sternum	100, 167, 180
steroids	110
stethoscope	76, 86, 112, 146, 186-187
stimulus	52-53
Store-and-Forward	70
Stress hormones	50
stroke	35, 70, 158
structures	18, 25, 28, 30, 37-38, 44, 72, 98, 100, 102, 107
subconscious	29
subdural	45
substance	25, 91, 101, 110, 118, 163, 165, 167, 178
support	25, 33, 48, 132, 134-135, 160
surface	22, 29, 76, 83, 93, 101-104, 110, 121, 180, 195
surfactant	76, 101, 108
swallowed	91, 99-100
swallowing	34, 37, 66
sweat	54, 86, 124-125, 140, 177
swell	55, 96
sympathetic	50
symptoms	58, 66, 69, 111, 121, 126, 128, 186
synapse	10, 42-43
Syncope	146
systems	21, 24, 28, 39, 50, 65, 89, 103, 124, 130, 212, 215
Systole	146, 184
T2-T12	48
Tachycardia	146, 185
taste	90, 93, 124, 177
Taussig, Helen Brooke	159
technology	20, 22, 70, 112, 115, 133-134, 192
teen	42, 58
Telemedicine	70
Temporal Lobe	10, 32
tension	101, 110
terminal	25

testing	21, 41, 70, 104, 154, 164
thalamus	10, 28, 37-38, 59
thinking	14, 28, 43, 52, 65, 69, 107, 180
thorax	100
throat	95-97, 100, 122, 129, 157, 212-213
Ticks	177, 212
time	15-18, 40-42, 49-50, 56, 58, 61, 66, 70, 83-84, 89, 92, 97, 103, 107, 115, 121, 126, 132-135, 140, 150-152, 154-155, 158, 166-167, 169, 177-178, 183-185, 195, 203, 214
tobacco	117
Tomography	22-23, 113, 161
tongue	34, 41, 55, 96-97, 212
tonic neck reflex	53
touch	49, 112, 206
trachea	76, 90, 97-99
tracheostomy	76, 99
tract	76, 90-91, 96-99, 102
tracts	29, 124
traffic jams	14
transfusion	157-158, 161, 172, 206, 214
transmembrane	125
transplant	115, 159, 161, 194, 206
treated	19, 117, 128, 191
Tricuspid valve	146, 182
tube	41, 85, 97, 99, 112, 133, 159-160, 164, 188, 190, 195
tubercular	123
tuberculosis	86, 123, 140
tubing	99
tumors	23
tunnel	47, 51, 90, 97
ultrasound	41
understanding	16, 18, 33, 65, 72, 83, 89, 140, 150-152, 155, 160, 214
Universal donor	146, 172
Universal receiver	146
upper	76, 90, 96-98, 117, 182-183
urinate	50
vaccine	87, 111, 130
valve	85, 146, 175, 182-184, 193
valves	146, 156, 182, 184, 193
vapor	101
vein	113-114, 153, 159, 164, 170, 174-175, 183, 191
veins	146, 152-153, 155, 157, 167, 175, 179-180, 182-183, 191, 193
ventilation	76, 104, 114
ventilator	134
ventral	38, 52
ventral root	52
ventricles	10, 44, 146, 182, 184, 187
venule	98
venules	146, 174-175
Vertebra	47, 167
vertebrae	41, 167
vertebral canal	47
Vesalius, Andreas	156
vessels	25, 45-46, 50, 54-55, 84, 92-93, 101, 151, 157, 159-161, 165, 167-169, 174-175, 179-180, 182, 187, 191, 195, 197
vestibule	92
vibration	13, 32
viral	54, 129
virus	49, 76, 87, 111, 121-122, 130, 132
vision	26, 51, 58
visual	19, 34, 38, 59, 165
Visual cortex	59

vital	25, 37, 46, 108, 153, 165, 207
vitamin E	62
vitamin K	62
vomiting	89, 103, 121
Wakley, Thomas	157
Washington, George	157
waste	25, 44, 101, 107, 174
water	22, 83-84, 91-92, 101, 103, 112, 121-122, 124, 165, 187
waves	22-23, 41, 94, 167, 185
weight	26, 35, 40-41, 85, 123, 132, 196, 203
Wernicke's area	18, 35
wheezing	127
white blood cells	121, 146, 165-166, 168-169, 172
white matter	10, 18, 29, 36
whooping	86, 140
Williams, Daniel Hale	158
windpipe	97-98
womb	40-41, 82, 108, 150, 167, 180, 188-190, 195
work	18, 26, 30, 33, 56, 65, 67, 82, 89, 93, 106, 108, 111, 115, 122, 124, 133, 151, 168-170, 175, 180, 189, 193, 196, 213, 215
workings	15-16, 18, 140
wounds	121
x-ray	22, 95, 111, 123, 161
yawn	56, 60, 215
zinc	62
zones	12

Photo credits:

Photo Credits: T-top, B-bottom, L-left, R-right, C-Center, BK-Background

Photos from Thinkstock.com and shutterstock.com unless specified.

Centers for Disease Control and Prevention: p 86 TL; p 87 BR; p 111 BL; p 123 B

Dr. Damadian/Fonar Inc: p 20 (3)

Dreamstime.com: p 23 CR; p 39 BL; p 47 (2); p 49 CL; p 53 CR; p 60; p 63 TR; p 64 BC; p 131 R

Flickr Creative Commons: p 38 TL (Keith Allison); p 138 B; p 152; p 155 C; p 161 TL; p 207 T

Flickr: p 53 TL & p 53 TR (dianabog, baby Emmalyn); p 89 (Philip Dunn)

istock.com: pg. 26 R; p 54; p 58 BL; p 61 TL; p 113 (2); p 163;

Lee Hardwin: p 58 T

Library of Congress: p.14; p 19 TL; p 87 TR (2); p 123 T, C

NLPG: p 109 (7); p 154

Parents of Oliver, Carolyn Otto and Chris Crawford: p 195 (2)

Science Photo Library: p 27 (Springer Medizin); p 30 (BSIP); p 33 (James King-Holmes); p 34 (Natural History Museum, London); p 37 (New York Public Library); p 41 TL (Gschmeissner); p 46 (John Bavosi); p 53 CL (bsip Asteir); p 96 B (2); p 99 TR; p 102; p 104 B; p 108; p 125 B; p 156 BL; p 160 TR; p 160 B; p 161 C; p 173 TR; p 176 (Candiru)

Superstock.com: p 130 BR; p 131 BL; p 155 B;

Wikimedia Commons: Images from Wikimedia Commons are used under the CC-BY-SA-3.0 license (or previous creative commons licenses) or the GNU Free Documentation License, Version 1.3. U.S.

p 16 BL & CL; p 17 (4); p 18 (2); p 19 BL; p 231 TL; p 31; p 66 BR; p 67 (2); p 68)2); p 69 (2); p 70 T; p 72 (5); p 73 (2); p 84; p 85 (3); pg 85 TR; BL; C; p 87 BL; C; p 88 C; p 96 TR; p 97 BR; p 104 C; p 106 T; B; p 114 T; p 115; p 130 T; BL (2); p 132; p 133; p 135; p 138 T; p 142 (5); p 143 T (4); p 155 C (2); p 156 T (5); p 157 T (5); p 158 T (5); p 159 T (5); p 160 T L (2); p 167 BR; p 171 TL; p 176 (Botfly Larvae; Tsetse Fly; Lamprey); p 179 C; p 181 (2); p 189 T; p 192 (2); p 193 B; p 196 TR; p 206 (7); p 207 C (2);

CREATION BASED
MasterBooks® CURRICULUM

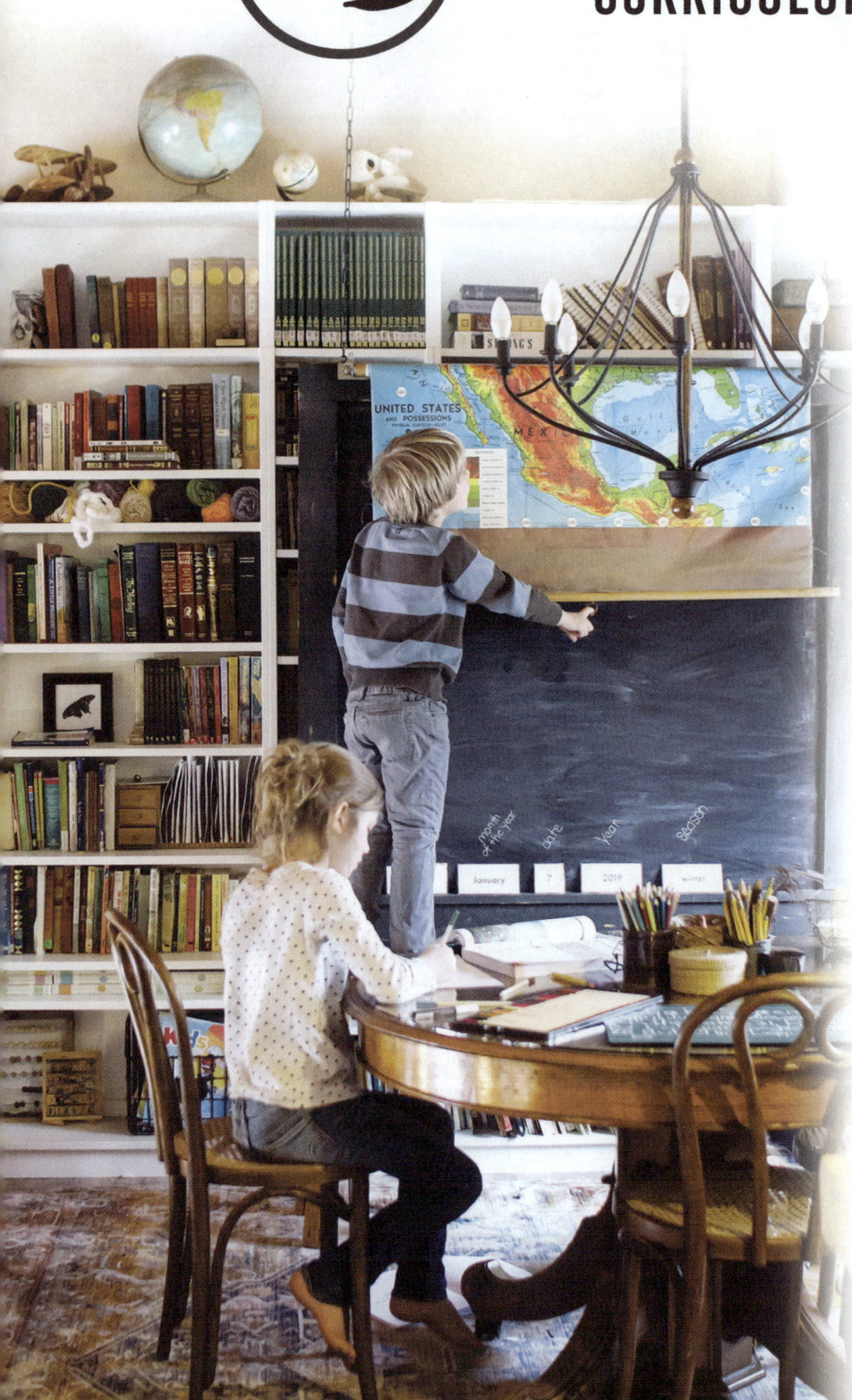

Designed for "Real World" Homeschooling

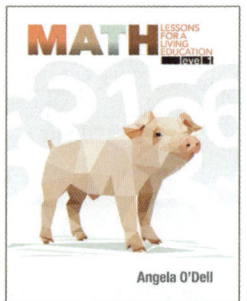

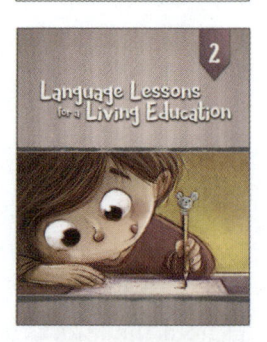

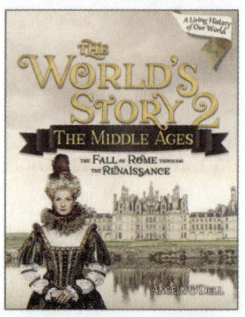

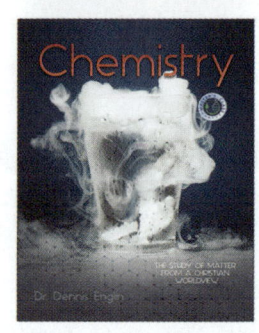

TO SEE OUR FULL LINE OF FAITH-BUILDING CURRICULUM

MasterBooks.com
Where Faith Grows!